Paul T. Bartone

Prediction of Life Span

Prediction of Life Span

Recent Findings

edited by
Erdman Palmore and
Frances C. Jeffers
Duke University

Heath Lexington Books
D.C. Heath and Company
Lexington, Massachusetts
Toronto   London

To the thousands of persons
whose cooperation
in longevity studies
made these findings possible.

Table of Contents

viii

List of Tables

List of Figures

Foreword

I am pleased to be able to provide a brief introduction for this volume, *Prediction of Life Span*. The Duke University Center for the Study of Aging and Human Development has had a longstanding interest in human longevity and its predictors. Even prior to the founding of the Center many investigators at Duke had been involved in studies of the aging process, including those physical, behavioral, and social factors related to decline in function and eventual death, as well as those variables related to the maintenance of optimal functioning and longevity. The Duke Geriatric Project, one of the first interdisciplinary longitudinal studies of noninstitutionalized aged in the country, was initiated with a panel of 260 aged participants and is now in its seventeenth year. For every member of the longitudinal panel, over 700 pieces of information were coded during each person's periodic two days of evaluation at Duke. Nine separate professional disciplines were involved in a coordinated study of the aging process. This history of multidisciplinary collaboration placed us in the fortunate position of being able to obtain a mass of information which can now be related to the longevity of panel members. At this time almost half of the initial group of participants are still alive, and we are able to identify those variables which appear to be related to increased longevity in those participants still part of the panel.

The work of the Center has been described primarily through reports in the scientific literature. During the thifteen years of its existence, hundreds of articles and several books have appeared in the professional literature authored by Center investigators. A recent book, *Normal Aging*, edited by Erdman Palmore and published by the Duke University Press in 1970, is a compilation of findings related to the longitudinal study. A survey of the theoretical and practical implications of the Center findings, coupled with those of others in gerontology, has been organized by Busse and Pfeiffer in their volume, *Behavior and Adaptation in Late Life*, published by Little, Brown and Company in 1969.

In an effort to test a number of hypotheses stemming from the first longitudinal study and to project backwards the aging processes which are believed to originate in the middle years of life (45-69), a second longitudinal study of 500 middle-aged persons was organized at the Center and initiated in 1968. This second study, which focuses primarily on adaptation to stress, also included many variables directly related to longevity in the middle and later years of life.

At this time, both longitudinal studies are part of a comprehensive program of research and training involving some eighteen laboratories and two training programs at Duke University. One of these programs is in collaboration with the Department of Psychiatry and is a two year gero-psychiatric program for fellows who have completed two or three years of psychiatric residency and who wish specialized training in working with the elderly. The second is a pre- or post-doctoral (Ph.D. or M.D.) research training program focusing upon some aspects of the behavioral sciences or behavioral physiology related to aging and human development. Another recent development at the Center was the organization of an information and counseling service for older persons (ICSOP), which offers a comprehensive evaluation, referral, and counseling program for older persons in the Durham area; as well as for agencies and younger individuals who are having difficulty with an aged relative.

In this volume two senior associates at the Center, Erdman Palmore and Frances Jeffers, make an important contribution to our understanding of longevity. They summarize much of the relevant recent findings from the Center and, by bringing together the contributions of others who are beginning to focus on this crucial question, they cover the area in a most comprehensive way. This is a focus not just on predictors of longevity but on two central questions of profound theoretical and practical significance to man: how can we live longer and how can we sustain the highest quality of life throughout our years?

Carl Eisdorfer
Director, Duke Center for the Study of
Aging and Human Development
Durham, North Carolina

**Part I
Introduction**

1

The Promise and Problems of Longevity Studies

ERDMAN PALMORE

The Promise

The search for longer life seems to be almost universal throughout history and in most societies. It is related to the basic drive for self-preservation, without which no individual or group will survive very long. Many of the most ancient writings show the high value placed on long life by early societies. For example, the Old Testament promises long life as a reward for obeying the Commandments. Ponce de Leon is only the most famous of a long line of men who spent their life seeking a longer life. Most of medical science is dedicated to preserving longer life through combating disease and death. One of the ways of increasing life span is to find out what factors contribute to longer life and then to attempt manipulation of these factors in order to increase longevity.

In addition to this practical interest in longevity, there is the theoretical scientific probability that longevity research may be a key to unlock the mysteries of human aging processes and the finite life span. By identifying factors related to early death or to longevity, better theories and understanding of the basic aging processes may be developed. There is the methodological advantage that the number of years lived can usually be measured easily and precisely. Longevity research has few of the validity and reliability problems which plague research dealing with more abstract and vague dependent variables such as adaptation, functioning, and life satisfaction. Actually, the sheer fact of survival can be viewed as a minimum test of adequate functioning. Furthermore, it appears probable that those factors associated with longevity may also be associated with life satisfaction, productivity, and other generally desirable characteristics. Thus, longevity studies should contribute to improving the quality of later years and as well as increasing the quantity of those years. Such are the promises.

Problems of Heredity Studies

But there are many methodological and theoretical problems involved in longevity research. Perhaps the chief problem is the general one of untangling

Erdman Palmore is Associate Professor of Medical Sociology, Center for the Study of Aging and Human Development, Duke University, Durham, North Carolina.

3

the relative influence of the many factors involved: hereditary, health, psychological, and social. Looking first at the studies which have attempted to show the influence of hereditary factors on longevity, there are so many problems involved as to render quite doubtful the semi-humorous assertions that "the best way to assure oneself of long life is to choose long-lived parents" (Lansing 1959).

It should be understood that hereditary factors usually include both genetic (transmitted by genes) and nongentic factors in heredity (cyto-plasmic inheritance, maternal age influences, etc.). The main weakness of these studies is that they do not in fact separate hereditary factors from environmental factors. As Rose points out, the genealogical studies and the studies showing association between longevity of parents and offspring cannot demonstrate that such association is due to hereditary factors (Chapter 2). It is at least theoretically possible that the entire association between longevity of parents and children could be accounted for by the similar environments of parents and children. We know that parents from upper-class homes with better income, better standards of living, better health care, better education, etc., tend to rear their own children in homes with better standards of living, better health care, more education, etc.

The same criticism applies to twin studies which show that identical twins have more similar life spans than do their siblings, for it is quite probable that twins have more similar environments than do their siblings. The same criticism also applies to the ingenious comparison of identical and fraternal twins by Kallmann and Jarvik (1959), who found that identical twins had more similar life spans than fraternal twins. Here again it is quite probable that identical twins experience greater similarity in their environment than do fraternal twins, for fraternal twins are more likely to be treated differently than are identical twins. Furthermore, Kallman and Jarvik found no overall statistically significant difference in their latest analysis, but rather a trend toward declining differences in life span comparisons of their identical and fraternal twins (p. 248).

Much of the belief in the human inheritance of longevity is based on an extrapolation from animal studies, which have demonstrated conclusively that longevity among animals is strongly influenced by parental longevity (Lansing 1959). In animal studies the environment can be controlled fairly well. But such extrapolations to humans from animal research is extremely dubious because humans are obviously more influenced by psychological and social factors. In addition to the general problem of not controlling for differences and similarities in environment, most human studies of longevity inheritance have serious methodological problems such as nonrepresentative samples, incomplete and inaccurate data (see Chapter 2). It is significant that at least two recent studies have found little or no relationship between longevity of parents and their offspring (Chapter 17).

The fact that women in industrialized companies generally live longer than men is often interpreted as support for the importance of hereditary factors in longevity. But there are obviously profound differences in the psychological and social environments of men, as compared to women, which could account for most, if not all, of the sex differences in longevity. Women generally have a more protected environment, less dangerous occupations, fewer violent deaths, accidents, suicides, and less smoking and lung cancer, etc. A recent study concluded that the greater mortality of men could be entirely accounted for by their more extensive smoking (Grannis 1970). The one study which attempted to equate environmental influences compared the longevity of male and female Catholic teaching orders (Madigan and Vance 1957). However, even in this study there were no controls for environmental differences in childhood between the sexes prior to admission into the teaching order. Differences in sex role are inculcated early in life, and could well continue to play an important part in the differing reactions of the Brothers and Sisters to fairly similar environments during adulthood. Furthermore, it is possible that there were important differences between the brothers and sisters in initial selection (the orders may have attracted less physically fit men), in the amount of smoking, overweight, and stress produced by the vows of chastity and obedience, etc. A later article by Madigan reports that priests in another teaching order tended to smoke more than average, to be more overweight than average, and to experience great stress from their vows of chastity and obedience and the other demands of their order (Madigan 1962).

Problems in Studying Physical, Psychological, and Social Predictors

Despite the commonsense assumption of a relation between good health and longevity, surprisingly little seems to be known about the influence of general health or even of specific diseases on longevity. There are massive statistics about causes of death in the vital statistics literature and several isolated studies on select populations of the chances of recovery or death from very specific types of illness (such as have appeared in the *Metropolitan Statistical Bulletin*), but there appear to be few studies comparing the longevity of persons with generally good health to those with generally poor health, or long-term follow-up studies of the longevity of persons having contracted various kinds of disease or illness. The present book contains studies of the relationship of brain impairment with longevity (Chapter 8), studies of physical factors related to longevity among institutionalized persons (Chapters 4, 7 and 12), a report on the Framingham study of factors related to death from heart disease (Chapter 5), and reports from the Duke Longitudinal Study of Aging relating health to longevity (Chapters 17 and 18). But in general, most of the studies relating health to longevity fail to have controls for psychological and social factors that may affect longevity. Many also fail to control adequately for age of the persons (see "Control for Age" below).

As for the relationship of psychological factors to longevity, such as reaction time, cognitive functioning, and attitudes, substantial research has begun to appear only recently. Several chapters in this book report recent findings of such studies (Part 3). Problems that remain with this type of research are adequate controls for age, hereditary factors, and social stress.

As for social factors related to longevity, it is well known that upper-class persons, whites, and females tend to live longer than their counterparts. Much or most of these differences have been attributed to differences in the social environment which lead to less role stress, adequate nutrition and medical care, less exposure to contagious diseases and violent death, and so forth. A recent book attempts to relate a measure of social stress to mortality (Dodge and Martin 1970). However, these linkages are largely assumptions at this point, and the careful studies which would show the direct relationships and mechanisms linking social factors to longevity remain to be done. Chapter 18 shows that in the Duke Longitudinal Study, psychosocial factors such as work satisfaction and adjustment show a greater relationship to longevity than do measures of health and other factors when the age factor is controlled.

One particular social factor, retirement from work, deserves special comment. There seems to be a widespread belief that retirement from work tends to lead to an early death. This is probably based on the common observation that many persons who retire die shortly thereafter. But apparently this is a spurious relationship due chiefly to the tendency of those in poor health to retire. Myers did find that the death rates of retired workers tend, during the first year or two of retirement, to be considerably higher than the general level. However, he concludes that these rates could be explained by the tendency of those in poor health to retire voluntarily, and he finds that this increase in death rate does not occur among those under compulsory retirement plans (1954). Similarily, studies of retirees from a Canadian communications company showed no upward fluctuation in rates immediately following retirement but rather a tendency of retirees to fulfill the life expectancy for the general population of the same age (Tyhurst 1957). Furthermore, the general health status of older persons appears to be largely unaffected or possibly even benefited by retirement (Tyhurst 1957, Thompson and Streib 1958, Schneider 1964). It may well be that retirement from stressful or unpleasant occupations contributes to longevity among those who were forced to engage in such occupations prior to becoming eligible for retirement pensions. On the other hand, if retirement is accompanied by withdrawal from all socially meaningful roles, this decline in involvement and activity may contribute to a shorter longevity (Chapter 18).

Measuring Longevity

There are three general and related problems faced by predictions of longevity studies which may affect the validity and accuracy of their findings. These are the problems of developing an accurate and reliable measure of longevity, of controlling for age effects, and of controlling for secular changes in the society. In prospective studies, when one takes a given group of people and gives them a series of tests in order to measure possible factors related to their longevity, he has three alternative ways of measuring their longevity. First, the most accurate way would be to wait until all members of the cohort had died so that he could be sure exactly how long they lived after the examination. The difficulty with this method is that the required time period could be twenty to fifty or more years, depending on the age of the persons examined. While this method may be feasible in the future for those longitudinal studies of aging which have already been in existence for ten or more years, this method is not possible at present because many of the members of the current longitudinal panels are still living. A more practical method for the present is using mortality rates, or constructing life tables based on mortality rates, for different subgroups in the studies. The difficulty here is that in order to secure stable rates, the number of persons in each subgroup must be relatively large. Longitudinal studies to date have included only relatively small numbers because of the expense of complete examinations and continuing follow-up studies.

A similar method is to use the dichotomous variable, living or dead, and attempt discriminant function analysis to see which combination of predictor factors best discriminate between those who are still living and those dead at a later point of time (see Chapters 10, 12, 13, 14, and 15). A similar difficulty applies to this method: a relatively large number of cases is required for stable results. Furthermore, there are no measures made of how long those still living will continue to live, nor of how long those who died survived after the beginning of the study. In other words, this measure of longevity is simply a dichotomous one rather than a continuous individual variable which would take into account individual life spans, and would allow the more high-powered correlation and multivariate techniques to be used in predicting longevity.

A third alternative was developed for use in the Duke Longitudinal Study (Chapter 18). In this method, the measure of longevity is the number of years of actual survival of those persons who had died by the time of the follow-up study, and for those who are still living an estimate is made of how long they are likely to survive after their initial examination. This estimate is made by adding the number of years survived at the present time since examination to the number of additional years they are expected to survive based on actuarial tables of their present life expectancy differentiated by age, sex, and race. The difficulty with this estimate, of course, is that it will often turn out to be inaccurate by a few years one way or the other. We believe that when the subjects are relatively old (most of the Duke subjects are now in their 80's or over) these inaccuracies will be relatively small since there is very little life expectancy left. Furthermore, when the majority of the subjects have already died (at present about two-thirds of the Duke subjects have died) the influence on the total group findings of inaccuracies from the estimates on the living minority will be relatively small. Other longitudinal studies are now trying out this method to estimate the longevity of their subjects, such as the study at the Philadelphia Geriatrics Center and the Baltimore NIMH longitudinal study. We hope this method will be more widely used so that its accuracy and validity can be subsequently tested on various population groups.

Retrospective studies have less difficulty measuring longevity because they usually take a known group all of whom have already died, such as members of a given family or residents in a given institution at an earlier point in time. The difficulties here are that retrospective data are quite limited and subject to inaccuracy and distortion through recall, and that there are problems of secular changes.

Secular Changes

A retrospective study was conducted by Rose and Bell which illustrates the problem of secular changes (Chapter 2). They took a sample of all men dying over age 50 in the Boston area in a given year and did multivariate analysis of various factors related to age at death, drawn from information supplied by next of kin. In addition to the limitations of inaccuracies of such retrospective data, the study had great difficulty in handling the problems of secular changes in the society and behavior patterns of the persons studied. For example, the strongest single factor associated with age at death was smoking behavior: the more smoking, the earlier the age at death. The fallacy of an interpretation which would attribute this earlier death to the greater smoking is that since smoking has increased rapidly over the past few generations, it was the younger men who naturally had smoked more. Thus the relationship of smoking to earlier deaths could be an entirely spurious one due to the secular increase in smoking among younger men.

Similarly, education showed a negative relationship to age at death, but this is probably due to the secular increase in education among the younger men. Rose is now planning a secular free retrospective study design in which persons dying at a given age will be matched with persons of the same age who are still living. This would allow discriminant function analysis to see which factors are associated with those living compared to those who are dead.

Control for Age

Finally, there is the problem of controlling for age of persons at the beginning of the study. We know that in general the risk of dying increases with age at a logarithmic rate, approximating the well known Gompertz Plot (Strehler 1960). Thus, if we want to know what factors *other* than the simple effects of older age contribute to more or less remaining longevity, this general effect of age must somehow be controlled. One solution is to compare the mortality rates for the longevity of similar age groups. Thus, mortality or longevity may be examined separately for ten year age groups, or even five year groups. But this is at best only a partial control on age because *within* each ten year group the older persons will have a greater mortality than the younger ones. In other words, any age-related variable, such as mortality, will still be age-related within the ten year age group.

Another method of partially controlling for age is to compare those who died earlier than their life expectancy with those who die later than their life expectancy (Clement 1969). The difficulty here is that once again a dichotomous dependent variable must be used and there is no discrimination between those who die much earlier than expected and those who die only a little before expected, nor between those who live a little more than expected and those who live much longer than expected.

A more refined control on age is to match individual persons by age. The difficulty with such matching processes is that it cuts down the number of cases available for study rather drastically.

A quite different approach is to study only very old persons and to compare them with younger persons (Chebatorev 1969, Beard 1962). There are several difficulties with this method: the measure becomes a dichotomous comparison; the assumption is made that the younger persons will not live to be as old as the older persons being studied; and there is no way to compare the dead members of the same age cohort, which introduces the problem of secular changes again.

The solution to this problem developed for the Duke Longitudinal Study was to divide the number of years survived after the initial testing by the actuarial life expectancy at that initial testing (Chapter 18). This results in a Longevity Quotient, which is the ratio of actual to expected number of years survived. Thus, it standardizes for age and shows whether a person survives more or less than average for his age group. It is analogous to an intelligence quotient which standardizes actual test scores by dividing through with the average test scores for a given age group. For longevity studies of institutionalized populations, this method can be improved by building a unique life expectancy table based on the mortality rates in that institution. These unique life expectancy tables are more accurate for persons in that institution than life expectancy tables based on the general population. Studies of longevity in Cleveland and Philadelphia are experimenting with this method.

Progress

Despite these many problems, progress is being made on most fronts in the campaign to establish accurate and reliable predictors of longevity. In the past few years there has been a surge of interest and research on longevity. For example, early in 1970 there was a five day interdisciplinary conference on Extension of the Human Life Span, sponsored by the Center for the Study of Democratic Institutions, Santa Barbara, California. At the 1970 annual meeting of the Gerontological Society in Toronto, an entire afternoon session was devoted to research on "Predictors of Survival," along with another session on "Alteration of the Life Span," and several other papers dealing with longevity and mortality. At the 1969 International Congress of Gerontology in Washington, D.C., there were at least thirteen papers reporting on longevity studies. This is a substantial increase over previous meetings of the International Congress and of the Gerontological Society, in which only a few papers on longevity were presented.

This book presents a review and summary of the major recent findings which have emerged from this surge of research on longevity. Some of these findings have been reported in papers at various professional meetings, but most have not been previously published. After the next chapter, in which Rose presents a methodological critique of longevity studies, the findings are organized into three sectons, corresponding to the three types of predictors. The physiological predictors include findings on genetic and cellular factors, brain impairment, physical impairment, health practices, cigarette smoking, exercise, excess weight, and diet. The section on psychological predictors includes findings on intelligence, attitudes, cognitive functioning, behavior, and psychological stress. The section on social predictors includes the relationship to longevity of social behavior of heart patients, of financial status, marital status, work satisfaction, over-all happiness and adjustment. This section concludes with a chapter on the social issues and consequences of increasing longevity. Other psychosocial factors are reported on in earlier sections. The book concludes with a summary and discussion of the future of longevity research.

References

Beard, B. Longevity and the never married. 1962. In *Social and Psychological Aspects of Aging*, ed. C. Tibbitts, and W. Donahue. N.Y.: Columbia University Press.

Chebotarev, D. Longevity and the role of its investigation in the elucidation of the aging processes. 1969. Proceedings of the 8th International Congress of Gerontology, Washington, D.C., vol. 1.

Clement, F. Du pronostic de mort à partir de diverses measures. 1969. Proceedings of the 8th International Congress of Gerontology, Washington, D.C., vol. 2.

Dodge, D., and Martin, W. 1970. *Social Stress and Chronic Illness*. Notre Dame: University of Notre Dame Press.

Grannis, G.F. 1970. Demographic perturbations secondary to cigarette smoking. *Journal of Gerontology*, 25:55-63.

Kallmann, F., and Jarvik, L. 1959. Individual differences in constitution and genetic background. In *Handbook of Aging and the Individual*, ed. J. Birren. Chicago: The University of Chicago Press.

Lansing, A. 1959. General biology of senescence. *Handbook of Aging and the Individual*, ed. J. Birren. Chicago: The University of Chicago Press.

Madigan, F. and Vance, R. 1957. Differential sex mortality: a research design. *American Journal of Sociology* 35:193-199.

Myers, R. 1954. Factors in interpreting mortality after retirement. *Journal of American Statistical Association* 49:499-509.

Schneider, C. 1964. *Adjustment of Employed Women to Retirement*. Ph.D. dissertation. Cornell University, 1964.

Strehler, B. 1960. In *Aging: Some Social and Biological Aspects*, N. Shock, ed. Washington: American Association for the Advancement of Science, 1960.

Thompson, W., and Streib, G. 1958. Situational determinant: health and economic deprivation in retirement. *Journal of Social Issues* 14:18034.

Tyhurst, J. et al. 1957. Mortality, morbidity and retirement. *American Journal of Public Health*, 47:1434-1444.

2 Critique of Longevity Studies

CHARLES L. ROSE

The remarkable increase in life span in this country since the turn of the century has significantly increased the numbers and proportion of older people in the population. This in turn has increased interest in aging research in general and prediction of longevity in particular. This chapter presents a critique of the literature on prediction of life span from the standpoint of problems of methodology. The rationale of this paper is that methodological problems exist which must be identified and solved for the optimal ongoing and future development of the field.

These special problems stem from the long span of human life, the interdiction against experimentation with humans, and the complexity of determining the human life span. The long life span of the human subject discourages the human investigator since he cannot count on outliving his subjects. Also, long human life span coupled with rapidity of social change generate the secular effect as a data contaminant. Length of life and interdiction against human experimentation have been mostly responsible for animal studies. Findings from subhuman organisms, however, present hazards in extrapolating to human cases. The complexity of determining life span raises problems of model and theory building which can be approached in part by an inductive data analysis involving data reduction and multivariate prediction. Methodological problems in data anlysis, however, arise due to the fact that characteristics of the data do not always fit the assumptions of the statistical procedures, and the state of the art of machine-assisted statistical analysis still provides severe limitations.

Another aspect of the complexity of determination is its cross-domain nature. Predictors of life span include four types of variables: genetic, physical, psychological, social, and these interact with each other in complex ways. It therefore becomes necessary not merely to include all of these types in the variable set, but also to investigate their interactions, particularly how one variable sums up, taps, or indexes other variables from other domains, or even from the same domain. Thus, specific variables must be examined as to what other variables they may be indexing. This is a problem, of course, that is not

Charles L. Rose is Research Sociologist, Normative Aging Study, V.A. Outpatient Clinic, Boston, Mass. Material in this chapter was adapted from C.L. Rose and B. Bell, *Predicting Longevity: Methology and Critique*. Lexington, Mass.: Heath Lexington Books, D.C. Heath and Company, 1971.

restricted to life span prediction, but applies to any dependent variable which has a complex determinancy.

A further general problem is the time- and space-bound nature of longevity predictors. Longevity predictors will vary over time because of environmental change and will also vary from country to country because of regional and cultural differences. The first will require replicated studies for periodic updating of the predictor set, and the second requires comparative cross-national studies. Perhaps a simpler way of saying all this is that accurate prediction can only be applied to the population from which it is derived. In addition to environmental differences across time and space, one should also leave open the possibility of genetic differences as a further determinant of life span such that a generic pool may change over time or that genetic pools are different in different places.

With these general considerations out of the way, let us now proceed to a critical examination of the literature. Actually, the literature on longevity goes back many thousands of years, and has been summarized by Gruman (1966). This early voluminous literature, however, is based on mythology, folklore, religious prescriptions, and naïve medical notions of the times. This literature, although prescientific, and not covered in the present review, contains many intriguing ideas which are well worth congitating on as sources of hypotheses for serious systematic study. The earliest published sources that can lay claim to systematic adequacy in that they are based on some quantitative analysis of data are the genealogical studies starting with Beeton and Pearson (1899). Therefore we will start with this group of studies.

Genealogical Studies

The genealogical studies, as might be expected, focused on intergenerational transmission of longevity and so dealt with a tiny slice of the problem. Intergenerational concordance in life span cannot be assumed to be purely due to genetic transmission. For example, long life of parents may well produce a more favorable environment for the offspring as well as a more favorable genetic endowment, so that nongenetic mechanisms may be operating as well. Another problem is that genealogical data are secondary and present pitfalls of highly nonrepresentative populations, selective incompleteness of data, inaccuracy of records, and biasing effect of secular trends. These problems are illustrated in a review of the following studies: (1) Beeton and Pearson's studies of old English genealogical records, Foster's Peerage of Great Britain and Ireland, Burke's Landed Gentry of the British Empire, and the Society of Friends' records; (2) Bell's (the inventor of the telephone) study of a single genealogy (1918), the descendants of William Hyde of Norwich, Conn., who died in 1681; (3) Wilson and Doering's (1926) study of a single genealogy, "The Elder Pierces," descendants of John Pers Weaver of Watertown, Mass.; (4) Yuan's (1931) study of a Chinese family over five centuries; and (5) Jalavisto's (1951) study of Finnish and Swedish genealogies of the middle class and nobility over five centuries. Following the genealogical material, there will be presented data on the intergenerational transmission of longevity based on broader population groups.

Beeton and Pearson's study showed a clear relationship between parental and offspring longevity but there were serious omissions of data. The bulk of the genealogies was confined to males due to the preference of tracing pedigrees through the male line, and the reticence of revealing the age (and therefore age-at-death) of females. Also there was a tendency to omit deaths under 21 years of age (which accounted for 30 percent of deaths in the nineteenth century) and deaths during late adulthood.

Bell included only one-third of the individuals in the genealogy he analyzed and also overrepresented early adult deaths, due to his use of a cutoff point (1864) which tended to eliminate longer lived individuals.

The Wilson and Doering study corrected for this sampling problem by a cutoff data which allowed the population studied to reach an age up to 95. At the same time, however, they introduced a new sampling problem by restricting the data to fathers and to sons who were fathers, which cut out pre-adult death and death of infertile offspring.

The Chinese study was the first to use life table techniques, which give more detailed information than do correlation coefficients as used in previous genealogical studies. Yuan prepared three life tables, one on sons of parents who died at ages 20-29, another on sons of parents who died at ages 50-69, and a third table on sons of parents who died at 70 and over. The results showed progressively better life expectancy, although differences were small especially after age 45, and there was some overlapping between the first and second table. Secular trends of decreasing mortality over five centuries, however, certainly contaminated the findings.

Jalavisto, the most recent student of genealogies, did not use the life table and was subject to the usual genealogical errors of inaccuracy and incompleteness of data and the secular effect.

Special Population Studies

Genealogical studies were popular because they tapped available records. In order to characterize broader and more representative groups, Pearl (1931) collected primary data on age-at-death of parents and offspring in working class families in Baltimore. Pearl took this step, interestingly enough, after he failed to find significant intergenerational relationships through genealogical material. Applying life table analysis, Pearl indeed found that parents of longer-living sons had greater life expectancy at all ages then parents of shorter-living sons; and conversely, that sons of longer-living parents had corresponding higher life expectancies at all ages.

Pearl and Pearl (1934) also developed as an age-at-death predictor an index called "Total immediate ancestral longevity," arrived at by summing age-at-death of parents and four grandparents. This index was then applied to a group of nonagenarians and earlier dying individuals from the Baltimore data, and indeed the index was higher for the more longevous group. It was found, however, that about one-half of the nonagenarians did not have two long-lived parents. This could only be explained on the basis of nongenetic factors neutalizing the effect of genetic influences, or at least of nongenetic determinants also being present (Korenchevsky 1961:16).

The index, however, had certain defects. The requirement that all six ancestors be dead tended to overrepresent those with earlier-dying ancestors. Also, the requirement that age-at-death be known tended to overrepresent those nonagenarians whose ancestors died at later ages because informants would find it easier to recall a more recent death. Another problem in the use of the index was that complete data were only available on a small fraction of the cases, so that analyses were made on a small and selected part of the total sample.

As part of a morbidity study in a rural county of upstate New York, Preas (1945) analyzed the population data for intergenerational concordance in longevity. In this case, the writer was aware that she was not merely studying a genetic effect but more probably the combined effect of the genetic transmission and related favorable environmental conditions. However, the study contained two sampling problems: an overrepresentation of the more fertile parents since they had a better chance to have offspring within the required period; and a large attrition of cases due to missing data.

In another study, van Zonneveld and Polman (1957) took a living population sample 65 years of age and over, and found that more of the octogenarians had parents who had attained that age than did the younger subjects. The finding regarding intergenerational transmission of longevity is based on the assumption that the younger subjects will have a shorter life span than the older subjects. However, this is only actuarially true for large populations and cannot be counted upon for smaller samples. In addition, there was the usual problem of sampling bias due to the fact that about one-fourth of the cases had to be deleted because of lack of information. For example, if the deleted cases had more shorter-living parents among the octogenarians than the younger groups, the true relationship between the generations would be considerably less than that found.

The life insurance industry provides a vast source of data on familial transmission of longevity from records of deceased insurees (Dublin, Lotka and Spiegelman 1949). Insurance records, however, are prone to error. One such is pointed up in the Dublin and Marks (1951) finding that the living or dead status of parents at the time of the offspring's insurance application is a better predictor of offspring's age-at-death than is parents' age-at-death. The explanation offered by Cohen (1964:162) is that insurance companies require applicants with poor family survivorship to have a higher level of health than applicants with a more favorable family history. This would in fact weaken the true relationship between survivorship of insuree and his parents by selection. Another possibility of error is the tendency of the applicant not to reveal a poor family health history, as he knows that this would result in higher premiums.

Maternal versus Paternal Influence

A special question in the field of intergenerational transmission is which parent is the more important influence. The literature is conflicting on this point. In a study of a German religious sect (Korenchevsky 1961:17) the effect of mother or aunt appeared to be more pronounced than that of father or uncle. Jalavisto's genealogical study concurred with this finding and in addition found that the maternal influence was stronger for sons than for daughters. Bell's genealogical data, however, showed an opposite finding: a higher percentage of offspring lived until age 80 when father attained that age than when mother did. Cohen (1964:174) also found a lower probability of survivorship in fathers of shorter-lived offspring than in mothers of shorter-lived offspring. Kallman (1957) on the other hand found there was no difference in the maternal and paternal effect in his identical twin studies. Though there was a definite relationship between parental and offspring age-at-death, there was no difference whether it was the father or mother who lived longer. One wonders whether this particular finding was influenced by the special independent variable of twinning.

In general, the discrepancies in the findings can be understood in terms of the different times and associated different life expectancies represented in the various studies, as well as differences in sampling and methods of recording. With respect to whether a genetic or social effect is involved, one might say the following: greater maternal influence could be explained by a genetic hypothesis, but also by a social one, i.e., a greater factor of nurturance may be operating when the mother lives longer than when the father does. (Nurturance is here defined as operating not only during the early years of offspring, but over a longer period which terminates with the mother's death). The "no difference" finding could also be accounted for under a social hypothesis, even if genetically father's influence was more important. One simply does not know whether these parental influences are primarily genetic or social.

Parental Age

A further specification of parental influence on offspring longevity is age of parent at time of birth of offspring. The general findings, spanning both human and subhuman sources, are that parental age is a predictor of offspring longevity, and maternal age is more important than paternal age. The effect was found in microscopic water organisms (Lansing 1954) as well as in humans (Jalavisto 1951). For an explanation, again one can appeal to a variety of theories. One is that germ cells are deleteriously affected by the cumulative over-time effect of radiation or other physical factors. Since spermatogonia divide continually and ovocytes do not, the deleterious over-time effects tend to be thrown off in the male case while in the female case the effects are retained and passed on to the offspring (Curtis 1963). Thus maternal parental age is the more important factor. On the other hand, one can speculate that social effects are operating.

The older mother may not be in as good position for child rearing both physically and sociologically, as the younger mother is. The father is usually less involved in child rearing and on this basis the paternal age factor may be less important.

The widespread findings that older siblings tend to live longer could be related to parental age, since children born later in birth order are also born when parents are older. Thus, later siblings with their older parents would tend to die earlier (Beeton and Pearson 1901-2; Yerushalmy 1938; Dublin et al. 1949).

Race

Black-white differentials in mortality are well known but they are decreasing. In 1900, the life expectancy of the white was 14.6 years more than that of the black and by 1963 it had dropped to 7.1 years (Chase 1965). If we assume the differential is due purely to socioeconomic factors, the closing gap in mortality may be interpreted as due to reduction of socioeconomic differentials and it could be predicted that the gap would be completely closed when socio-economic parity is achieved. In fact, it is the prevailing theory among demographers that racial differences are socioeconomic in nature (Linder and Grove 1947:12). However, since there are genetically determined biological differences between white and black, it is possible that these differences include genetically determined longevity differences. The question can be settled only by investigating longevity differences with socioeconomic status controlled, in which case the disappearance of the longevity differential would favor a pure socioeconomic hypothesis.

There is, however, a basic problem in relating race to longevity. This is the unreliability of assessing race from skin color and self report, in view of the widespread racial admixture between white and black in this country. This unreliability in the independent variable would weaken the validity of a genetically determined racial differential, and would tend to give more weight to socio-economic factors in explaining so-called racial differences in mortality.

Sex

Just as whites are longer lived than blacks, women are longer lived than men. The trends, however, have been very different in the two cases. Whereas the favorable white differential has been steadily decreasing, the sex differential once favored the male but now favors the female, with females showing a lower death rate at all ages in the United States, as well as in all other industrialized countries (Spiegelman 1966). When social status and health treatment of women was low, including greater exposure to risks of more pregnancies, females had a higher mortality than males. One is reminded of the findings in Bell's genealogical study of the higher mortality in women. Also, those countries which still have lower female longevity (Upper Volta, Cambodia, India, Jordan, Pakistan and Ceylon) are all undeveloped, have generally low life expectancy and low status for females. In India, for example, the male expectancy is 41.9 years and the female expectancy is 40.5 years (Population Index 1968:516).

However, as general mortality decreased and women's status increased, her longevity rose above that of males (Thomlinson 1965:131). By 1964, for example, female life expectancy was higher by 6.9 years (Spiegelman 1966:23). This differential was due to decline in tuberculosis and maternal mortality at younger ages in the female, and decline in disease related to high blood pressure at older female ages, all related to social and medical advance. At the same time, male deaths increased because of car accidents, lung cancer, and coronary artery disease, also associated with male behavior and life styles (Enterline 1961). In addition, males have greater occupational hazards and greater incidence of death by violence (Bogue 1959:197).

Up to this point, a sociological theory for female superiority has been presented. There is, however, evidence in favor of a biological basis for female superiority. First, there appears to be a general biological law regarding female superiority in every animal species that is sexually differentiated. Females have been found to outlive males in fruit flies, beetles, spiders, rats (Kallman and Jarvik 1959:231) and chickens (Landauer and Landauer 1931). There is even female superiority in the womb, with more male stillbirths than female (Dublin et al. 1949:129-130). It is believed by geneticists that the biological influence operates through genetically based female secondary sex characteristics, which produce differences in behavior, metabolism and body structure, rather than through the direct effect of harmful sex-linked genes. The reason that deleterious recessive X-linked genes would not account for shorter male life span is that they would tend to be eliminated by selection (Clark 1964:227-228).

An interesting sociological study of male and female Catholic teaching orders tends to corroborate the biological hypothesis. These orders provide equal health conditions, fairly homogeneous strains and hazards, and removal of the differential sex roles of ordinary living. Yet the female religious orders show a higher life expectancy (Madigan 1957; Madigan and Vance 1957). With the social factor somewhat controlled, one is left with a biological explanation of the finding.

On the basis of the foregoing, one may conclude that an underlying female superiority was originally overwhelmed by adverse environmental conditions which were focused particularly on the female. When this was lifted, the female was able to come into her own. Under this hypothesis, female longevity will continue to rise as her social status continues to improve, until an asymptote is reached, at the point of the optimal environment, and at a higher level than the male asymptote, the difference in levels being equivalent to the factor of female genetic superiority.

Social Class

The same question as to the interrelated operation of genetic and social factors is contained in the findings regarding social class predictors of longevity. Three measures of social class are occupation, income, and education. These may be hypothesized to be interrelated as follows: Higher education facilitates attainment of higher status jobs; and higher status jobs usually bring higher incomes. Higher status salaried positions are generally less hazardous to health. Lower status positions are more prone to occupational hazards such as fatigue, inorganic dusts (notably silica and asbestos), absorption of poisons, excessive heat, and sudden variations in temperature and dampness. For example, Whitney (1934) found the mortality rate of unskilled workers almost double that of professional workers. Higher status positions also have more liberal sick leave benefits, which make it unnecessary to stay on the job when one should be home nursing one's health.

Higher education, in addition to placing individuals in "healthier" occupational roles, also sensitizes individuals to the importance of health maintenance and the availability of health-maintaining resources.

Higher income, which also goes with higher education and healthier occupation, furthers implementation of health-maintaining resources such as food, clothing, housing and medical care. Poverty and economic status are thus powerful predictors of longevity (Stevenson 1921; Altenderfer 1947).

A complex of highly correlated factors conspire to negate the optimum environment for the attainment of maximum life span. The fact that the environmental optimum has not yet been reached in the United States despite its high standard of living, technology, and so forth, is suggested by the fact that there exist other countries of even lower mortality, notably, the Scandinavian countries and The Netherlands, and there is no reason to believe that the gene pools involved are any different with respect to longevity (National Center for Health Statistics 1964). On the basis of the latest available information from the United Nations Statistical Office, twenty-two countries have higher male life expectancy at birth than the U.S. and eight have higher female life expectancy (Population Index 1968).

Another factor in the relationship between social class and longevity is the fact that the more physically and mentally competent tend selectively to occupy the higher status occupations. There is thus a double effect: the genetically superior with respect to longevity are more likely to get into the more protected and lucrative occupational roles, which in turn augment through environmental factors their genetic predisposition to longevity. This means that the genetic factor not only favors longevity in its own right but also indirectly favors longer life by inducing a more favorable environment such as is associated with higher occupational status.

That general life styles which accompany given educational occupational status contribute to the mortality rate has been suggested by the reports of the Registrar-General of England and Wales (1938). Since the age-at-death of spouse is recorded on the death certificate, it is possible to find out whether there is any concordance in longevity between husband and wife. It was found that the mortality of husbands was similar to men of their occupation, and the mortality of wives was similar to that of their husbands. This suggested that there was a general life style factor related to an occupationally determined social class position which was responsible for mortality among husbands and wives, rather than merely the particular conditions of husband's occupation affecting husbands only.

The factor of education was shown to be a longevity determinant in an early Metropolitan Life Insurance Company study (1932). College graduates from eight eastern colleges had a better life expectancy than the general white male population, and honor men among the college graduates had an even better life expectancy. If we may assume the honor men to be an especially intelligent group, this suggests that intelligence is also a longevity determinant. Terman's gifted children at mid-life did indeed show better longevity characteristics than would be expected at their age group (Terman and Oden, 1959:29).

If we may assume that distinguished professional and business men listed in the *Who's Who in America* are intellectually superior to the general population, the finding about their superior longevity (Metropolitan Life Insurance Company 1968) is also evidence for the relationship between intelligence and longevity. The age-specific mortality of a sample of *Who's Who* listing was compared to the mortality of the general white population in similar occupations. For all ages studied (45 to 64), the mortality of the *Who's Who* group was 30 percent below that of the general population. The highest longevity within the *Who's Who* group was that of scientists, and the lowest was that of journalists. If we may assume equal intellectual endowment among the *Who's Who* scientists and journalists, we would infer that scientists have the most favorable vocationally-related environment and the journalists the least favorable. This inference can only be made for the top scientists and top journalists, however. In any case, these data are suggestive of the interplay between environmental and genetic effects. (We are assuming that intellectual endowment has a genetic component.)

Role Satisfactions

A study of 1247 Roman Catholic priests from an unnamed order (Madigan 1962) showed a lower age-specific mortality than that obtained for the United States white male population. This was interpreted as due to the superior role satisfactions of this group, particularly since on other grounds such as lack of exercise, high cholesterol diet, overweight, and life stresses alleged to be in excess of the general population, the priests would be expected either not to have a lower mortality or to have even a higher mortality. Unfortunately, the conclusion that this lower mortality is due to role satisfactions is probably not valid because social class was not controlled. The priests occupy a higher social class position and have corresponding social class life styles. Therefore, their mortality experience should not have been compared with that of the general population (of their sex, race, and age), but only with that of their social class. Such a control, for example, was exercised in the *Who's Who* study just cited. If this were done, and the priests still came out with a more favorable longevity, the role satisfactions hypothesis would indeed be supported. The weight of evidence, however, is against such a finding, since two previous studies on the longevity of priests do not bear out Madigan's findings. These were the study by the Registrar-General of England and Wales on all priests in England and Wales for 1931, and an unpublished study by the Sociology Department of Catholic University in Washington, D.C., 1951, on Redemptorist priests of the Baltimore area (cited by Madigan 1962).

Marital Status

Like social class, marital status has also been an important predictor of longevity. The married have greater life expectancy at all ages. This general finding may be ascribed to an interaction of biological and social factors. By selection, those in poor health and of unfavorable temperament are less likely to marry either because they elect not to marry or are passed by. The least healthy in the population, then, tend to remain among the unmarried. In addition, once married, the individual presumably has an environment more favorable to longevity, such as emotional support, better nutrition, and better chance for care in time of illness (by the spouse).

It is possible that the selective health factor in entering marriage has become less important with the increase in the proportion of the population who enter marriage. Thus, during the period from 1940 to 1960, there was a ten percent increase in the proportion married (Spiegelman 1963), which means that a less healthy group may now be getting married which did not before; unless, of course, there has been a general upgrading of the health of the population so that the increment getting married still falls within a healthy group. With greater supports from an improved socioeconomic system it is possible that the effects of marginal health, otherwise discouraging to marriage, are being neutralized. Perhaps a little bit of each is operating: better health in the population and better socioeconomic support to compensate for poor health.

Buttressing the life expectancy figures, there is greater mortality for the single person in each of the leading causes of death. This higher mortality is more marked for males than females (Ibid.). One might speculate that females are more hardy to begin with (note the sex differential in longevity), or that health as a selective factor for entry into marriage plays a less important role for females than males, or that single life is less dangerous for women than men. A particularly significant factor increasing mortality of the single person is the greater incidence of deaths by violence among them. This factor particularly applies to the male.

Social change may be weakening the advantage of the marital environment, because of relegation of kinship functions outside the kinship system, which facilitates adjustment outside of the marital bond. For example, single people can secure food, clothing and shelter in quite acceptable ways outside of the marital or kinship bond by resorting to bachelor apartments, restaurants, laundries, and so forth, resources which were formerly not available.

In the future then, the longevity differential to be accounted for by the marital environment may be lessened due to the convergence of marital and nonmarital environments with respect to their favorableness for longevity. Secondly, with higher marriage rates any biological selective factor for marriage or remarriage will also play a less important role. This effect is probably facilitated by medical and socioeconomic advances which bring people into marriage who otherwise would not be. These trends, if they do materialize, will make less crucial the controversy as to the relative importance of the selective factor or the protective environment in explaining marital longevity differentials (Shurtleff 1956; Berkson 1962).

Actually, any marital differentials should be viewed against a background of a host of other variables which influence longevity in addition to marriage. Secondly, any changes in marital differentials should be examined in terms of changes over time in the influence of these other variables. The same thing could, of course, be said with respect to other factors in differential mortality, particularly entities which are complex and interact in complex ways with other factors. This may be described as a multivariate approach applied iteratively in a diachronic sequence. The alternative, which is the consideration of the simple bivariate relationship, in this case that between marriage and longevity, leads to the "fallacy of misplaced concreteness" (Whitehead 1925) and dead end speculations. The multivariate approach, on the other hand, has a better chance of leading to explanatory insights.

Multivariate Approach

The use of multivariate approach in the prediction of longevity involving in addition both physical and social variables is illustrated by the current work of Palmore (Chapter 18). Essentially what this investigator did was to demonstrate how the predictive power of actuarial life expectancy tables can be improved by adding health, psychological, and social predictors in addition to age, sex, and race predictors already built into the table. The five additional predictors were arrived at by selecting the highest correlating items with years survived by zero order correlation. The number was limited in this way in order to minimize loss of cases due to missing observations.

It would have been better not to preselect the independent variables entered into the multiple regression, particularly on the basis of their low zero order correlation. The power of the regression procedure is more fully used when a larger number of variables is entered, including poorly correlating ones. The whole point of a multivariate predictive procedure such as regression is to take into consideration interactive effects while searching for the best predictors. Preselecting predictors by zero order correlation limits the regression procedure from doing its job. The justification for preselecting the items because of missing observations is tenuous because of the availability of computer routines which dub in values, usually means, for the blanks.

Another problem arises from assigning survivorship to the still living by dubbing in the actuarial expectancy. The hypothesis of the study is that the actuarial expectancy introduces error into the prediction because it leaves important variables out of consideration and, therefore, the introduction of additional variables would improve the prediction. If the author uses as the criterion variable on the living cases, which represent over one-half the cases, a survivorship into which is built the very error he is trying to correct, he may be thereby vitiating the effectiveness of his procedure. One wonders whether better prediction from a combination of living and deceased cases, as compared to decreased cases alone, may not have been at least in part because of the spurious correlation with the criterion variable introduced. The major predictor, actuarial expectancy, at the beginning of the study, is similar to the life expectancy in 1969 used in the criterion variable.

In a follow-up paper (1969a, also Chapter 18) Palmore redid his analysis, deleting the actuarial predictor from the independent variable set and constructing a new criterion, a "longevity quotient," made up of the original longevity measure divided by the initial actuarial expectancy. The purpose of this was to standardize by age, because the longevity measure varied systematically with age. The change essentially consisted of shifting the actuarial predictor into the role of denominator in the criterion. The longevity quotient thus controlled for age by showing how much longer or shorter an individual survived than did the average of his own age group. Also by deleting the actuarial variable as a predictor, he removed the spurious correlation which formerly existed between independent and dependent variables by virtue of the fact that they both contained the actuarial term. However, the quotient still had the disadvantage of using an actuarial estimate of a survivorship for those still living.

In his data, Palmore found no evidence for a relationship between parental and subject's age-at-death, and inferred that this supports an environmental rather than a genetic basis for longevity. In this connection, he cited the similar conclusions of a Soviet investigator (Chebotarev 1969). The issue, of course, is not whether the etiology of longevity is environmental or genetic, but rather what is the relative importance of each. Parental age-at-death, in any case, is not a "pure" genetic variable, but a mixture of both genetic and social effect.

One other criticism is the problem of control for the secular effect which may intrude into Palmore's sample because of the differences in birth year. Palmore feels that the use of a longevity quotient controls for the secular effect to a large extent since the actuarial life expectancy at any given time reflects secular changes in death rates. However, he concedes that if substantial declines in death rate did occur, then his use of the current life table would yield inaccurate results.

Aside from these methodological problems, Palmore's work is a revolutionary advance over the literature already reviewed since it both incorporates a multivariate approach and combines physical and social variables in the same set. In addition, it attempts to combine multivariate analysis with life table data, thus building on the life table technique.

An Experiment in Inductive Data Analysis

Finally, the writer would like to report briefly on his own work in prediction of life span, which centers on the use of multivariate methods for examining a large number of predictors. The data were obtained by interviewing next-of-kin of 500 recently deceased males from the Boston area. Seventy variables were selected for insertion into multiple regression and discriminant analyses. By this method, 15 to 25 variables were found to be adding significantly to the prediction or discrimination. In the regression equation the criterion was the continuous variable age-at-death, which ranged in the sample from 50 to 90, while in the discriminant function analysis the criterion was age-at-death below 70, and 70 and over, representing the dichotomization at the mean of the age-at-death distribution. The same variable set was also inserted into parallel factor analyses of the lower and upper age-at-death groups.

In addition, two nonlinear methods were used: (1) a nonlinear discriminant analysis, which inserts higher order terms such as cross-products into the discriminant set, and (2) a nonlinear factor analysis (Shepard and Carroll 1966), involving both clustering of variables and cases. The various procedures were used on the same data set to show how significantly findings differed based on what procedure was being used. In particular, the nonlinear clustering by cases identified those outlying cases which were in fact increasing classification error in the linear discriminant analysis. A problem, however, posed by the nonlinear procedures was that the computational state of the art limited the number of variables and number of cases that could be dealt with without incurring unreasonable machine time costs.

Aside from the issue of developing methodology for prediction of life span and obtaining substantive findings along the way, the rationale was to select predictors that could be built into the long term longitudinal design of the Normative Aging Study of the Veterans Administration (Bell, Rose, and Damon 1966). Actually, a start had been made through a hypothesis generating study on 149 Spanish-American War veterans who were octogenarians at the time (Rose 1964). These 149 living octogenarians were evaluated with respect to social characteristics which appeared to be survivor characteristics in that they deviated from demographic norms, and these variables were then tested in the study of the 500 deceased Bostonians.

In general, physical and genetic variables tended to link with each other more than with social and psychological variables. This is because variables within domains naturally tend to be more similar to each other, and this was brought out both in linear and nonlinear factor analysis. Many examples, however,

26

occurred of cross-domain variables linking together. Both the linear factors and nonlinear clusters gave abundant evidence of this. Factors referring to social class, based on occupational level, also contained intelligence, which certainly has a genetic component, physical activity variables, and various psychological traits. In the nonlinear clusters, one cluster included school performance, health, and a number of psychological traits. Another cluster linked type of job, religion, and catching colds.

In the nonlinear discriminant analysis, again, cross-products tended to be comprised of variables from the same domain. Yet, there were numerous examples of cross-products made up of cross-domain components. Two examples of cross-products composed of social and physical variables were age difference between subject and spouse times health at age 40-49, and age difference between subject and spouse times on-job physical activity age 40-49. Other cross-products coupled a physical to a psychological variable: off-job activity age 40-49 times worried, and on-job activity at age 20-29 times conserved energy.

Also, physical variables tended to be more important than social variables, both in linear regression and discriminant analysis and in nonlinear discriminant analysis. Yet, there were many examples of the reverse. In regression analysis, "worried" had a higher F than "number of illnesses, age 40-49," and "looked older than age, over 40." In discriminant analysis, marriage ranked considerably higher than "catching colds" and "illnesses, age 40-49." Also occupational level ranked higher than "health, age 30-39."

A related finding in the factor analysis (and corroborated by physical higher-order terms in the nonlinear discriminant analysis) is that in the advanced age-at-death group the special survivor characteristics are physical rather than social in nature. This may be due to the fact that genetic and physical factors account for advanced survivorship rather than do social life styles, simply because the physical factors are more important in determining longevity. This may be so, but there are two factors which militate against such a conclusion. One is that within the lower age-at-death group (in the factor analysis), the differences between the longer and shorter living groups were more prominently social than physical. Secondly, the advanced age are more homogeneous socially than younger aged groups, due to occupational retirement and physical changes which retrench social activity. Therefore, social differences by age are less present among the upper age-at-death group so that physical differences become more prominent. One might say that age is a greater leveler, socially speaking, so that what is left to account for earlier death at advanced age are physical differences.

An unsolved problem in the writer's research is the secular effect. In the design used, it was necessary for subjects to be born at different times in order to have different ages at death and still die within the same year. It was necessary for deaths to occur within the same year because, for the purpose of a reliable "one shot" data collection from a survivor, it was necessary that the death occur one to three months before the interview. Likewise, the logistics of conducting a time-constrained research made it necessary to cluster the interviews within a circumscribed period. The next major step in the writer's research is to carry out a "one shot" yet secular free design.

References

Altenderfer, M.E. "Relationship between per Capita Income and Mortality, in Cities of 100,000 or more Population," *Public Health Reports*, 62:1681, 1947.

Arvay, A. and Takacs, I. "The Effect of Reproductive Activity on Biological Aging in the Light of Animal Experiment Results and Demographical Data," *Gerontologia Clinica*, 8:36-43, 1966.

Beard, Belle Bone. "Longevity and the Never Married," in C. Tibbetts and W. Donahue (eds) *Social and Psychological Aspects of Aging*, Columbia University Press, N.Y., 1962, pp. 36-50.

Beeton, M. and Pearson, K. "Data for the Problem of Evolution in Man, II; a First Study of the Inheritance of Longevity and the Selective Death-Rate in Man," *Proc. Royal Society London*, 65:290-305, 1899.

Beeton, M. and Pearson, K. "On the Inheritance of the Duration of Life, and on the Intensity of Natural Selection in Man," *Biometrica*, 1:50-89, 1901-02.

Bell, Alexander Graham. "The Duration of Life and Conditions Associated with Longevity, A Study of the Hyde Genealogy," Genealogical Record Office, Washington, D.C., 1918.

Bell, Benjamin, Rose, Charles L. and Damon, Albert. "The Veterans Administration Longitudinal Study of Healthy Aging," *Gerontologist*, 6:179-183, 1966.

Berkson, Joseph. "Mortality and Marital Status: Reflections on the Deviation of Etiology from Statistics," *American Journal of Public Health*, 52:1318-1326, 1962.

Bogue, Donald. *The Population of the United States*, Free Press, Glencoe, Ill., 1959.

Chase, Helen C. "White-Non-White Mortality Differentials in the United States, *Health, Education and Welfare Indicators*," June 1965, pp. 27-38.

Chebotarev, D.F. "Longevity and the Role of its Investigation in the Elucidation of Aging Processes," *Proc. of 8th International Congress of Gerontology*, Vol. 1, Washington, D.C., 1969.

Clark, Arnold M. "Genetic Factors Associated with Aging," in Bernard L. Strehler (ed), *Advances in Gerontological Research*, Academic Press, N.Y., 1964, pp. 207-255.

Cohen, Bernice H. "Family Patterns of Mortality and Life Span," *The Quarterly Review of Biology*, 39:130-181, June 1964.

Curtis, Howard J. "Biological Mechanisms Underlying the Aging Process," *Science*, 141:686-694, Aug. 23, 1963.

Dublin, L.I., Lotka, A.J., and Spiegelman, M. *Length of Life*, Ronald Press, N.Y., 1949.

Dublin, L.I., and Marks, H.H. "Overweight Shortens Life," *Statistical Bulletin Metropolitan Life Insurance Co.*, 32:1, 1951.

Enterline, Philip E. "Causes of Death Responsible for Recent Increases in Sex Mortality Differential in U.S.," *Milbank Memorial Fund Quarterly*, 39:312-328, 1961.

Gruman, Gerald J. "A History of Ideas About the Prolongation of Life—the Evaluation of Prolongevity Hypotheses to 1800," *Trans. Am. Philos. Soc.*, Vol. 56, part 9, 1960.

Jalavisto, E. "Inheritance of Longevity According to Finnish and Swedish Genealogies," *Ann. Med. Internal., Fenniae*, 40:163-274, 1951.

Kallmann, Franz J. "Twin Data on the Genetics of Aging," in G.E.W. Wolsten-holme and C.M. O'Connor (eds), *Methodology of the Study of Aging*, J.A. Churchill, London, 1957, pp. 131-143.

Kallmann, F.J. and Jarvik, L.F. "Individual Differences in Constitution and Genetic Background," in James E. Birren (ed), *Handbook of Aging and the Individual*, University of Chicago Press, Chicago, 1959, pp. 216-263.

Korenchevsky, V. *Physiological and Pathological Aging*, Hafner, N.Y., 1961.

Landauer, W., and Landauer, A.B. "Chick Mortality and Sex-Ratio in Domestic Fowl," *American Naturalist*, 65:492-501, 1931.

Lansing, A.I. "The Influence of Parental Age on Longevity in Rotifers," *Journal of Gerontology*, 3:6, 1948.

Linder, Forrest E. and Grove, Robert D. *Vital Statistics Rates in the United States: 1900-1940*, Government Printing Office, Washington, D.C., 1947, p. 12.

Logan, W.P.D. "Social Class Variations in Mortality," *Public Health Reports*, Vol. 69, No. 12, Dec. 1954, pp. 1217-1223.

Madigan, Francis C. "Are Sex Mortality Differentials Biologically Caused?", *Milbank Memorial Fund Quarterly*, 35:202-223, 1957.

Madigan, Francis C. "Role Satisfaction and Length of Life in a Closed Population," *American Journal of Sociology*, 67:640-649, 1962.

Madigan, Francis C., and Vance, R.B. "Differential Sex Mortality: A Research Design," *Social Forces*, 35:193-199, 1957.

Metropolitan Life Insurance Co., "College Men Long Lived," *Statistical Bulletin*, N.Y., Vol. 13, No. 8, Aug. 1932.

Metropolitan Life Insurance Co., "Longevity of Prominent Men," *Statistical Bulletin*, Vol. 49, Jan. 1968.

National Center for Health Statistics, "The Change in Mortality Trend in the United States," *Vital and Health Statistics*, P.H.S. Pub. No. 1000, Series 3, No. 1, Public Health Service, Washington, 1964.

Palmore, Erdman B. "Physical, Mental, and Social Factors in Predicting Longevity," *Gerontologist*, 9:103-108, 1969.

Palmore, Erdman B. "Predicting Longevity: A Follow-up Controlling for Age," *Gerontologist*, 9:247-250, 1969a.

Pearl, Raymond. "Studies on Human Longevity, IV; the Inheritance of Longevity," *Human Biology*, 3:245-269, 1931.

Pearl, R., and Pearl, R.D. *The Ancestry of the Long-Lived*, The Johns Hopkins Press, Baltimore, 1934.

Population Index, "Complete Expectation of Life at Various Ages in Selected Countries," Vol. 34, Oct.-Dec., 1968, Office of Population Research, Princeton University, Princeton, N.J., pp. 513-517.

Preas, S. "Length of Life of Parents of Offspring in a Rural Community," *Milbank Memorial Fund Quarterly*, 23:180-196, 1945.

Registrar-General's *Decennial Supplement, England and Wales*, 1931, Part IIa, "Occupational Mortality," London, 1938.

Rose, Charles L. "Social Factors in Longevity," *Gerontologist*, 4:27-27, 1964.

Sawin, P.B. "The Influence of Age of Mother on Pattern of Reproduction," *Ann. N.Y. Acad. Sci.*, 57:564-574, 1954.

Shepard, R.N. and Carroll, J.D. "Parametric Representation of Non-linear Structures," in P.R. Krishnaiah (ed) *Multivariate Analysis*, Academic Press, N.Y., 1966, pp. 561-592.

Shurtleff, Dewey. "Mortality Among the Married," *J. Am. Geriatric Soc.*, 4:654, 1956.

Spiegelman, Mortimer. "The Changing Demographic Spectrum and Its Implications for Health," *Eugenics Quarterly*, 10:161-174, 1963.

Spiegelman, Mortimer. *Significant Mortality and Morbidity Trends in U.S. since 1900*, Am. Coll. of Life Underwriters, Bryn Mawr, Pa., 1966.

Stevenson, T.H.C. "The Incidence of Mortality upon the Rich and Poor Districts of Paris and London," *J. Royal Stat. Soc.*, 80:90, 1921.

Terman, Lewis M., and Oden, Melita H. *The Gifted Group at Mid-Life*, Stanford University Press, Palo Alto, 1959, p. 29.

Thomlinson, R. *Population Dynamics, Causes and Consequences of World Demographic Change*, Random House, N.Y., 1965.

Whitehead, Alfred N. *Science and the Modern World*, MacMillan, N.Y., 1925.

Whitney, J.S. "Death Rates of Occupation Based on Data on the U.S. Census Bureau, 1930," National Tuberculosis Association, N.Y., June 1934, cited by Dublin et al., 1934, pp. 213-214.

Wilson, E.B., and Doering, C.R. "The Elder Pierces," *Proc. Nat. Acad. Sci., U.S.*, 12:424-432, 1926.

Yerushalmy, J. "Neonatal Mortality by Order of Birth and Age of Parents," *Am. J. Hyg.*, 28:244, 1938.

Yuan, I-Chin. "Life Tables for a Southern Chinese Family from 1365 to 1849," *Human Biology*, 3:157-179, 1931.

van Zonneveld, R.J., and Polman, A. "Hereditary Factors in Longevity," *Acta Genet. et Statist. Med.*, 7:160-162, 1957.

Part II
Physiological Predictors

Bernard Strehler begins this section with a summary of present knowledge and recent findings on how the genes determine the maximum possible life span of all species and how the controller genes limit the extent to which cells reproduce themselves which, in turn, cause a decline in function and ultimate death in humans. Linn, Linn, and Gurel then present evidence showing the usefulness of their Cumulative Illness Rating Scale, based on assessments of examining physicians, to estimate biological age and to predict death or survival.

Some of the results of the twenty-year old longitudinal study of heart disease in Framingham, Massachusetts are reported by its director, William Kannel. This and the following chapter by Erdman Palmore show that among middle-aged and aged persons the maintenance of physical activity, weight control, and avoiding cigarettes are strongly related to better health and longevity.

Alvin Goldfarb reports on various predictors of mortality among the institutionalized aged, chief of which are incontinence, marked physical dependency, severe chronic brain syndrome, and poor mental status. He also concluded that the effect of transferring certain types of patients (such as those with severe brain syndrome) from one institution to another may increase the likelihood of earlier death because of "transfer shock."

Wang and Whanger conclude this section with a review of the available evidence and the recent findings from the Duke studies which indicate that brain impairment with relatively early onset reduces longevity.

3

Genetic and Cellular Aspects of Life Span Prediction

Bernard L. Strehler

Introduction

Relevance of Biological Mechanisms to Gerontology

The essentially universal biological phenomenon of aging causes effects on the behavior and structure of human beings that are reflected in nearly all aspects of life. The basic genetic mechanisms of living things lead, in the case of humans, to an interrelated group of phenomena that range in their complexity from changes in simple molecules to a particular kind of social structure. In each case the common element is that some pattern, whether molecule or individual, changes in a statistically predictable manner and gives rise to predictable consequences. The role of the gerontological sciences is to uncover the basic nature of these changes so that more effective means of dealing with their effects may be developed. In the development of this, as any other science, the most complete ability to modify or control the process and its effects hinges on the completeness with which the "original" causes and mechanisms are understood.

For this reason, although the conceptual tools and research methodologies of the different aspects of gerontology differ from each other, they do, in fact, constitute a continuum of concepts and phenomena which must ultimately become interrelated. This chapter is intended to outline some of the concepts and findings at the level of the genes (and of the cells whose activities they control) that have an ultimate, if not immediate, relevance to the more complex manifestations of behavior, health and predictable social interactions.

Definitions

Prediction as a Biological Property. Every aspect of the evolved functions of living systems, including man, may be viewed as a reflection of predictive processes. The ability to predict successfully confers upon a given genetic line the ability to survive in a hostile natural environment through appropriate

Bernard L. Strehler is Professor, Division of Biological Sciences and Gerontology Center, University of Southern California.

responses (reflex or purposeful actions) which further the three cardinal requirements of any persistent living system: reproduction, avoidance of destruction and acquisition of food. Prediction (i.e., the formulation of a suitable response to a given set of environmental factors or measurements) occurs even at the level of gene synthesis and action. In the very simplest case, the DNA is a special type of predicting machine, which possesses the ability to form predictably accurate copies of itself because the raw materials of which it is made are complementary in their shapes and affinities to different parts of the preexisting DNA molecule.

At the level of DNA function, its role is equally predictive in the sense that it controls (contains directions for) the manufacture of totally different kinds of substances which permit the system—from bacterial virus to man—to respond to those patterns predictably present in the future environment (because they were present in the past environment) in a manner which increases the changes of long-term survival.

These substances and structures secondarily produced under the control of DNA (the instruction carrier) include such materials as enzymes which have a shape (over parts of their surfaces) that are complementary to the shapes of molecules predictably encountered in their environments. Collections of such gene-encoded enzymes generate mutually complementary enzymes which interact with each other's products in predictable manners (metabolism).

At an early stage of evolution of living systems it became of advantage to incorporate such collections of cooperative molecules into small packages called cells which, because they possess a somewhat impervious outer coating (the cell membrane), are better able to survive in various kinds of environments. By analogy with the advantages conferred upon cooperative collections of enzymes when they were inclosed within a membrane, collections of cells evolved (higher organisms), which were better able to resist natural destructive forces, acquire food and reproduce effectively. Thus, the course of evolution has led to the survival of many kinds of biological systems which consist, as does man, of billions or trillions of cells, each derived from one single cell (the fertilized egg), and containing different parts which serve functions related to predictable events in the environment or the interior of the system.

Among the most important of these, in terms of the evolution of man, was a group of specialized cells, called neurons, derived from skin-like cells. These cells (present in the billions in the brain and central nervous system) permitted a new kind of prediction to take place, one which did not have to be imprinted directly on the DNA. Rather this prediction ability is based on the fact that certain kinds of events re-occur repeatedly during the lifetime of an individual animal. The brain, receiving sensory inputs from a variety of special sense organs, records these patterns (which correspond in some way to the patterns in the environment which generated them) and causes adaptive responses by the system as a whole, when perception of a part of a previously recorded pattern makes the prediction likely that the rest of the previous environmental pattern is also present. Thus one does not need to see the fire if one senses the smoke—because smoke and fire were part of a total pattern previously recorded. The capacity to perform this kind of predictive process (based on associative memory) and logical processing of trains of interrelated associate memories confers great survival advantages on those systems which possess them. We are the present culmination of this evolutionary process.

At an even higher level of integration, the adoption of predictable patterns of interaction between individuals within a species (as cultural patterns) permitted groups of animals, including humans, to cooperate in insuring their members' survival. Social behavior, formation of groups, cultures, political devices, and nations represent the most complex expression of the primordial tendency of molecules, which act cooperatively, to succeed while other noncooperative systems fail.

At all levels of complexity it is the capacity to predict effectively that permits the continuation of life within a species—but the selective evolutionary forces which produce species that exist perennially did not lead to the perennial existence of the individual members of most kinds of living things (i.e., immortality). Instead, certain properties of the instructions which a species contains within its DNA leads to the inevitable death of the individual DNA-carriers. Man, despite his remarkable qualities, is not immune to this aspect of genetic selection. Like most of his animal relatives he has a limit to his life span as an individual—while the species goes on and on.

Genetic Determination of Life Span. There is absolute certainty that maximum life span possible for the member of a given species is determined by the nature of the DNA that species contains. The validity of this generalization is attested to by the fact that a given life span is a characteristic of each species. From the Ephermerids (insects that live for only a few happy reproductive hours) to man (and some birds) which can last for over a century, and turtles and trees which can live for hundreds or thousands of years respectively, the maximum length of life is limited—i.e., set, by genetic factors. Further evidence that length of life is inherited is provided by the fact that the length of life of ancestral forms determines the length of life of offspring in a manner directly correlated with the degree of identity of the DNA between two individuals. It is thus possible, even within a species, to find subgroups which possess greater than average life spans and subgroups which possess less than average life spans. In the case of humans, families that have much greater than average life spans are known— conversely, some families have genetically determined, short life spans because of defects in the DNA which cause certain diseases to appear selectively within them.

The most conclusive evidence that maximum life span (as well as such disparate conditions as schizophrenia, Batten's disease, diabetes, sickle cell anemia, I.Q., etc.) is genetically based is presented by a comparison of the life spans of identical twins (which have essentially identical DNA, because they were derived from a single fertilized egg) as compared to fraternal twins and unrelated individuals. The correlation between expected length of life and closeness of genetic relationship is such as to verify what is obvious from the comparisons of life spans between species—i.e., the genes contain the information that specifies the maximum life span.

Cells and Life Span. The smallest semi-independent functional unit of a human being is the cell. It is therefore probable that aging, and the consequent certainty of death, is due to changes within cells, to changes in the number of cells and to changes in the relationships between cells according to some as yet undetermined equation. It is to events that occur within the individual cell as influenced by its DNA that one must look for the primary gene effects that lead to senescence. If the cells of which one is made are capable of long life then the individual may persist for a long time; if one's cells are fragile and impermanent and incapable of replacement once maturity has been reached, a shorter life span is a certainty.

The cells of the body fall into three classes as regards their ability to replace themselves. The first class, including cells of the skin, of the lining of the gut and of the blood are continually being replaced. Very little of the aging process seems to accrue to these cells (even though their individual lifetimes are only a few days to a few months in the human). One hardly ever dies of tired skin or tired blood, Geritol notwithstanding. The second class of cells are able to replace themselves when the "need" arises. Thus the liver can regenerate if part of it is removed. But the third class of cells, which include brain cells, many parts of the connective tissue system (muscles, vessels, tendons, etc.) are either not replaceable at all or only very poorly so.

The feature which distinguishes these three types of cells is their relative ability to produce more cells, that is, to undergo a process of cell division which is called mitosis. We do not yet fully understand the mechanisms which control whether a cell will divide or not. What is required, of course, is that the cell manufacture those materials which are specifically required if it is to divide. In the brain cell (and other fixed post-mitotic cell types) the machinery necessary for division is, it seems, irretrievably turned off. We possess the same grain cells we had during childhood and the memories that constitute our individuality are stored in this pre-set ensemble of cells. When these cells die (ca. 2000 per second appear to die in the human) or become nonfunctional, whatever part of our "selves" was recorded in them is lost. When a sufficient number of these or other irreplaceable cells is lost or defective, one's chances of overcoming a particular challenge is reduced, and when a sufficient challenge occurs, death ensues.

It is not appropriate to describe in detail the changes which are known to occur in cells as they age. Only a few changes will be mentioned, en passant. One of the most striking of these is the accumulation of small particles called "age pigments" (lipofuscin), within the cytoplasms of heart, brain, adrenal, gonadal and other cell types. These accumulations may take up as much as 25 percent of the intracellular volume. That they probably have harmful effects is shown by the occurrence of certain mutants, particularly one causing a disease known as Batten's disease. This affliction is apparently caused by the accumulation of massive amounts of "age pigments" in very young individuals. Individuals who inherit this disease, one of the ameurotic juvenile idiocies (blindness accompanied by mental degeneration in children), die in early childhood, as a rule. Another type of cellular aging may be reflected in the reduced capacity of cells which have undergone many divisions to divide further. Clonal aging of this kind may be observed in cell cultures outside of the body and may, in certain cell types such as those conferring immunity, be of importance in resisting certain environmental challenges such as those posed by invading microorganisms. Aging of cells also results in changes in their ability to retain immunological memories. During early life, an individual develops a tolerance to his own characteristic substances and fails to kill cells containing them, as he does cells possessing "foreign" substances. During aging loss of such tolerance for certain of their own proteins is observed in many individuals and a sort of self-destruction through auto-immune disease occurs. The immune system also appears to lose its ability to recognize and suppress aberrant cells that arise continually during the lifetime. This loss of immune capacity is probably the chief reason that cancer is so prominent a cause of death among the aged. The older person often cannot effectively react to the altered cancer cell.

The Gompertz Function

About 150 years ago an English insurance actuary, by the name of Benjamin Gompertz, discovered that the chances of death followed a very simple mathematical equation as a function of age. He found that the chances of dying doubled about every eight years for the human. The equation which describes this relationship is $R = R_0 e^{\alpha t}$, where R is the probability of dying at a given age, t; R_0 is the extrapolated probability of dying during very early life, e is the base of the natural logarithm system and α defines the rate of doubling. This relationship between age and chances of dying is illustrated in Figure 3-1. The interesting thing about the Gompertz equation is that the value of α and R_0 vary from species to species (and probably genetically, from subgroup to subgroup). For short-lived animals R_0 and alpha are large; for long-lived species they are small. Figure 3-2 illustrates the values of these two constants derived from the study of specific kinds of animals.

The Mechanisms of Gene Function in Determining Time of Death

Nature of Genetic Material

Genetic information takes two forms, i.e., is encoded within two types of molecules, DNA and RNA. In most species of living things, DNA, which has greater stability (and other features which favor its utilization) is the dominant

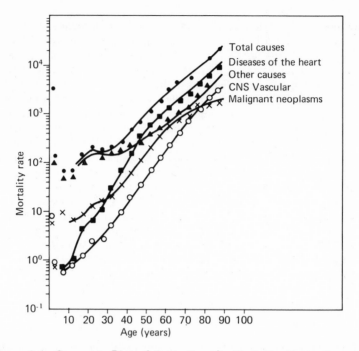

Figure 3-1. Gompertz Plot of Cause-Specific Mortality Rates. Source: Strehler, *Time, Cells, and Aging* (New York: Academic Press, 1962), p. 114. Used with permission.

form. The basic structure of DNA is a double spiral—a very long molecule. The two parts of the spiral are related to each other in a very specific way—one spiral is the chemical opposite (i.e., complement) of the other.

The basic building blocks out of which DNA is made consist of just four different kinds of molecules. Two of these are purine nucleotides, adenylic acid (A) and guanylic acid (G), and two are pyrimidine nucleotides, cytidylic acid (C) and thymidylic acid (T) (see Figure 3-3). The key feature of these molecules is that they form two complementary pairs. One pair is A-T which members have a natural affinity for each other; the other pair is G-C, which members also have a selective affinity for each other. The two strands of the DNA consist of two sequences of bases, one in each strand, which are exactly complementary to each other, as shown in Figure 3-4. It is the complementarity of G for C and of A for T which permits DNA to cause the formation of more DNA like itself. The indispensable function of DNA, the production of more DNA, is thus explicable on the basis of this complementarity between just two pairs of bases.

All of the other functions of DNA are also based on this primeval quality. This includes, in particular, the ability to cause the formation of quite different

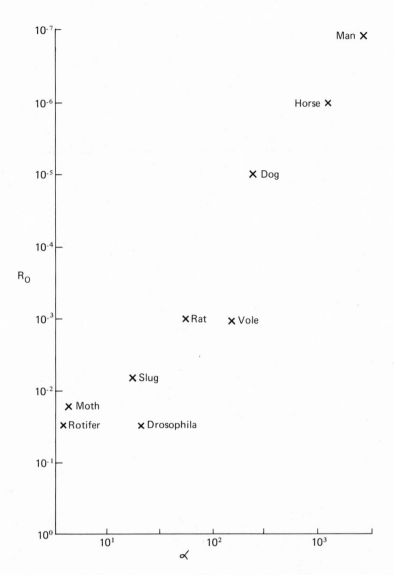

Figure 3-2. Relationship between α and R_O for Various Species of Animals. (α is slope of Gompertz plot; R_O is intercept of Gompertz plot.)

40

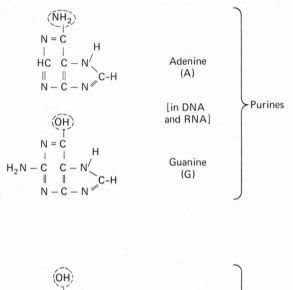

Adenine
(A)

[in DNA and RNA]

Purines

Guanine
(G)

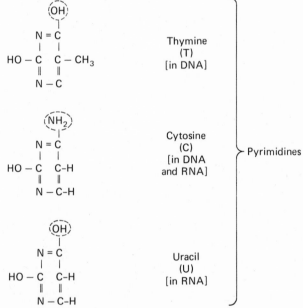

Thymine
(T)
[in DNA]

Cytosine
(C)
[in DNA and RNA]

Pyrimidines

Uracil
(U)
[in RNA]

A   Pairs with T (in DNA) or U (in RNA)
G   Pairs with C (in Both DNA and RNA)

Figure 3-3. The Structures of the Genetic Bases.

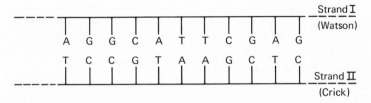

Note: Wherever one strand has an "A", the other has a "T";
also every "G" is paired with a "C".

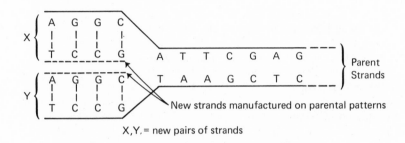

X,Y. = new pairs of strands

Figure 3-4. Complementarity of the Double Helix.

kinds of molecules called proteins, which as enzymes, act as specific accelerators
(catalysts) of only certain of the reactions a raw material might undergo, and as
specific structural elements as well. This second function of DNA, a most
remarkable one, is possible because the sequence of bases in DNA stand for
specific proteins and other structures. By "stands for" one means codes for, and
the second role of DNA is expressed through the decoding of the genetic
sequences through the intervention of special decoder devices which cause the
assembly of amino-acid chains (proteins) according to the coded instructions
present in the DNA "library."

The Products of Genetic Material

This remarkable feat is achieved approximately as follows: Under the influence
of a particular enzyme (called RNA polymerase) a copy of a specific region of
the DNA is manufactured, using the same complementarities which direct the
replication (duplication) of the DNA itself. The molecule produced, called
messenger RNA (mRNA), possesses the same information (sequence of
nucleotides) which was present in the original DNA strand copied (but in

complementary form) and this molecule (which differs in slight chemical details) is transmitted to the regions of the cell where the information it contains may be translated into proteins. The assembly of proteins also makes use of the complementarities between base pairs. But the means through which this is achieved is remarkable, to say the least.

The actors in this play include 4 different kinds of structures in addition to the m-RNA: (1) ribosomes, (2) tRNA molecules (the translator molecules); (3) enzymes which attach the correct amino acid to the correct translator and (4) the amino acids themselves. (Certain energy sources are also required.) Basically the interaction of these components is as diagramed in Figure 3-5. The mRNA is taken up at one of its ends by the ribosome; at the same time a translator molecule (which possesses a region containing just three nucleotides which region is complementary to the three nucleotides present in the message that are bound to the ribosome) becomes affixed to the ribosome. (In fact, two such tRNA molecules occupy adjacent positions as determined by the sequences present in the mRNA). At their opposite ends the tRNA molecules are attached to the amino acid (there are 20 different kinds) which corresponds to the meaning of the triplet of message nucleotides. Such triplets are called codons and only 64 different codons are possible (4 x 4 x 4 = 64). The next step is that the amino acid of one tRNA is transferred to the amino acid on the tRNA next to it. After transfer the recipient tRNA, now with two amino acids in a chain attached to it, slides over to the position previously occupied by the other tRNA, dragging with it the message for a distance corresponding to just three nucleotide positions. The new codon now present in the ribosome attracts its particular tRNA with attached amino acid and the above processes are repeated until the message has been completely translated into the amino acid sequence the message specified in coded form. The presence of specific code words in the message signal either start of message or end of message (called non-sense because they cannot usually be translated—no corresponding tRNA species are available).

The various materials that make up the synthetic and working machinery of a cell are thus manufactured one after another and in correct proportions and arrangements as the cell grows and/or differentiates into one or another specialized cell type.

The Controller Genes

Among higher forms of life a special problem presents itself. This is the fact that the DNA is really a vast library of instructions (as many as 100,000 specific genes may be present in the human) but that a given cell requires that only some of these instructions be converted into useful materials. Because the different kinds of cells that make up a complex animal or plant possess different kinds of specific proteins, but each contain identical DNA libraries, some means must exist which causes only certain genes to become expressed in some cells and

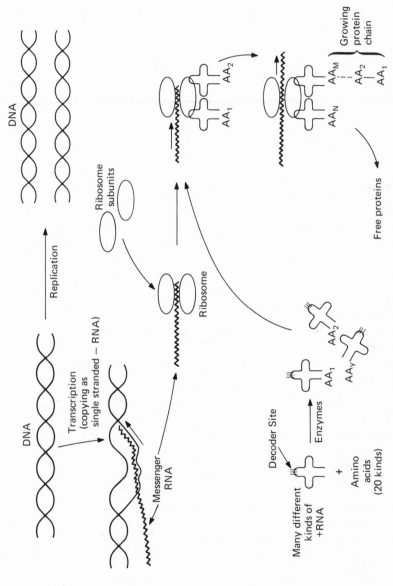

Figure 3-5. How Proteins are Synthesized.

other gene combinations to be expressed in other cell types. This function is served by a special group of genes whose products control the activities of other genes. It is in the properties of these controller genes that both the intimate mechanisms of development and of aging are to be found. For, the information which is required to produce all the products needed to maintain youthfulness is present within each cell's DNA, but the cells are prevented from doing so by the activities of the controller genes.

Several, quite different theories of the nature and effects of these controller genes have been proposed. Because such genes, in bacteria, control gene expression by directly controlling the kinds of mRNA produced, models based on this primitive group of controllers enjoyed some vogue among embryologists and gerontologists for a while. More recently, however, it has become apparent that the major site of action of controller genes in higher organisms is at the sites at which translation takes place.

One specific theory originally proposed by the author in 1965 now appears to have wide acceptance by developmental biologists because of the results of recent experiments. These experiments indicate that one cell type differs from another in its respective ability to translate different code words for the same group of amino acids. This will become understandable if one realizes that there are only twenty different amino acids to be included in the protein chains, but that different code words stand for these twenty different amino acids. In other words, the code is redundant: more than one codon (in most cases) can be used to encode for a particular amino acid (Table 3-1). This means that the same sequence of amino acids can be written down in many millions of alternative sequences of bases.

The way in which this great flexibility appears to be used during cell differentiation is that the controller genes determine which group of code words (language) a given cell can translate. Provided that the messages standing for proteins appropriate to that type of cell are written down in the language the cell can translate, it will make only those proteins belonging to that language set.

We now come to the crux of the matter as it applies to the aging phenomenon. If an animal is to make the most efficient use of its material resources (food, in this case) it will be so designed that it does not produce products it does not need for survival up to the time of reproduction. This means that devices will be selected for, which will turn off those genes which produce products that are not needed for the survival of the individual beyond reproduction. The specific way in which this is accomplished probably consists in the removal, as a cell matures, of its ability to translate one or more code words involved specifically in the manufacture of such adequately synthesized products. In other words, some of the primary controllers are turned off by a second set of controllers which ultimately limit the ability to translate messages only to those products of immediate use.

That different cell types differ in the kinds of tRNA they can use is shown in Figure 3-6.; that differentiated cells lose the ability to attach certain amino acids to specific tRNA's as they age is shown in Figure 3-7. These and other findings seem to validate the hypotheses.

Table 3-1
The Genetic Code

1st ↓ 2nd →	U	C	A	G	↓3rd
U	PHE	SER	TYR	CYS	U
	PHE	SER	TYR	CYS	C
	LEU	SER	Ochre	?	A
	LEU	SER	Amber	TRP	G
C	LEU	PRO	HIS	ARG	U
	LEU	PRO	HIS	ARG	C
	LEU	PRO	GLUN	ARG	A
	LEU	PRO	GLUN	ARG	G
A	ILEU	THR	ASPN	SER	U
	ILEU	THR	ASPN	SER	C
	ILEU	THR	LYS	ARG	A
	MET	THR	LYS	ARG	G
G	VAL	ALA	ASP	GLY	U
	VAL	ALA	ASP	GLY	C
	VAL	ALA	GLU	GLY	A
	VAL	ALA	GLU	GLY	G

The essence of the above concepts is that a highly deterministic set of instructions, that regulates where and when each gene will be active, is present in living things. During early life this set of instructions, choosing among different cell languages, causes maturation; but as maturity is approached some materials necessary for very extended life (or immortality) can no longer be manufactured. Consequently, animals age because the storehouse of materials manufactured during development gradually deteriorates. As these materials deteriorate, the functions they support also deteriorate, until a point is reached where some environmental or internal challenge can no longer be overcome and death ensues.

Conclusions

Maximum Life Span is Inherited

The length of life of an individual depends upon two factors: whether he encounters a challenge he cannot overcome and what the rate of deterioration of

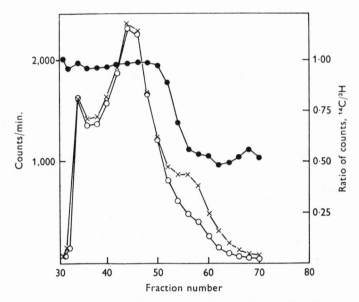

Figure 3-6. Chromatography of a Mixture of Transfer RNAs from Liver, Reticulocytes and Heart. (Labelled with (^{14}C) leucine by liver enzymes (x) and (^{3}H) leucine by reticulocyte enzyme (O). After attachment of leucine, transfer RNAs labelled by each tissue were mixed together, isolated and chromatographed. The change in ratio of ^{14}C- to ^{3}H- counts (O), corresponding to the third peak, suggests different complements of leucine enzymes.) Source: Strehler, et al., *Proceedings of the National Academy of Science*, 57:1754, 1960. Used with permission.

his irreplaceable components is. The former factor is influenced by the nature of the environment to a considerable extent and the improvements in average longevity which have accrued from public health measures and antibiotics largely result from a reduction in such environmentally derived challenges. The second factor, the time of onset and rate of decline, is determined by the nature of the genes a person inherits. If the gene products which might deteriorate are produced for an extended period, the beginning of decline will be postponed; if the products are very well-made, the rate of their deterioration will be slow and the life span after maturity is reached will be correspondingly long. What has been selected for, particularly in social animals such as humans, is both an extended period of maturation (because this is particularly useful if much learned information is to be transmitted) and an extended period of decline (because this permits the mature individual to transmit the benefits of his experience to his offspring).

Some individuals, possessing genetic abnormalities, have shorter than expected life spans, because some of the gene products they need for extended

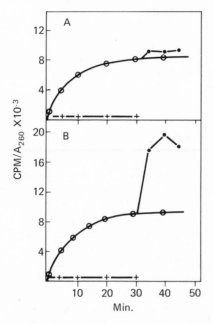

Figure 3-7. Evidence that Plant Tissues Lose Ability to Carry Out Some Steps in Protein Synthesis. (Upper curve: at beginning, open circles, "old" enzyme was used to attach amino acids to tRNA's from young plants. At 30 minutes additional "old" enzyme was added—no effect. Lower curve: same except enzyme from young plants added at 30 minutes. Note that a new group of tRNA molecules were activated.) Source: Bick and Strehler, *Proceedings of the National Academy of Science*, 68:226, 1971. Used with permission.

life are either defective or absent. The prediction of individual probable life span depends upon the particular collection of genes one has inherited and how this collection operates in a particular environment. In predicting in the individual case one can only induce correlations between the expectancy of individuals of supposedly similar inheritance or of individuals who occupy seemingly similar environments. At present, the accuracy of such predictions is limited by the extent to which these various factors can be evaluated in an individual and the accuracy with which one can predict their probable interaction with each other.

*Maximum Life Span is an Indirectly
Evolved Quality*

Because the genetic factors which determine the length of life were selected so as to improve the chances of survival up to and including the age of reproduction, some of these evolved characters, particularly those which improve the efficiency of utilization of food materials, set the stage for later decline (senescence) as "accidental" side effects. Such effects are called pleiotropic in genetic-evolutionary terminology, and while they may have permitted us to enjoy being alive in the present, they lead to the end of this joy, as we age and die.

Maximum Life Span can be Modified

That the length of life presently determined by the genes can be modified is supported by the fact that the inherited life span differs from species to species. Because all animals and plants are genetically related (descended from common ancestors), it follows that some lines, such as our species, evolved very great life spans. That man has reached the maximum possible life span is not likely, because all species are continually subject to the process of variation and selection. Positive and deliberate selection for substantially greater maximum life span is therefore feasible for the human species if it should decide that this is in its interest.

There are two additional means through which the maximum life span of individuals may be greatly extended. One of these involves the manipulation of the environment in which man or his cells exist. Obviously the avoidance of harmful foods, the avoidance of noxious chemical substances, and the practice of "ideal" living habits will add some years to life and life to years. But the major advances in controlling the rate (and perhaps reversing) of deteriorative processes lie in two directions. One of these involves the suppression of the rate of deterioration of already manufactured components. Because age pigments, at least, appear to arise from cross-linkage reactions, such chemical additives as may reduce this reaction will proportionally extend life to the extent that such reactions are determinative.

The second direction lies in the reactivation of the controller genes that affect one's ability to make specific substances or cells needed for indefinite existence. Because the nature of these controller substances may be more simple than was previously supposed and might well be inserted into cells in a very precise manner, the chance for a chemical modification of the maximum life span is probably closer to realization than most persons anticipate.

It is unfortunate that so little effort directly concerned with basic questions of this nature is being funded under present governmental priority systems. But even in the presence of the starvation diet which biological gerontology presently enjoys, some fall-out, applicable to gerontological goals (a longer happy healthy life span), will undoubtedly accrue from quite unexpected basic findings in other areas.

The Relevance of Basic Science to Applied Sciences

Man is concerned not only with the control of events that affect him in the here and now, but with the prediction of how events in the future will affect him.

This concern with the future has served the species well. Because of their very nature the applied sciences are more concerned with problems that exist in the present and there is ample justification, in view of man's mortality, for devoting a large fraction of available resources to solving problems in the here and now. But the ability to solve such problems in the future depends principally upon the extent to which the underlying rules and mechanisms that cause certain effects to occur are understood. In this context, the role of the basic biological scientist is to provide these general rules and an understanding of their genesis in the intricacies of molecular and cellular interaction. From such understanding, applied to an expanding hierarchy of complexity, will derive that better life in the future which is the object of all wise men and good.

4

Measurement of Physical Impairment and its Relationship to Aging and Death

BERNARD S. LINN, MARGARET W. LINN,
AND LEE GUREL

The almost constant force of mortality presents a powerful argument for the concept of continuous decay of vitality (Brody 1923; Loeb and Northrup 1917; Pearl 1928). Jones (1959) has stated that the process can be regarded as a growth of impairments of various kinds, proposing that death rate is a measure of physiologic age as well as that of internal impairment. This theory holds that morbidity leaves increments of impairment.

That so few devices exist for rating physical pathology is the more surprising in view of the large number for rating psychopathology, a far less concrete and verifiable area. Perhaps the most widely used instrument in the sphere of physical illness is the Cornell Medical Index, a lengthy self-report of symptomatology. Almost all research regarding clinical prediction has relied on measures of disability, that is, impairment of *function*. Little work, other than the guides prepared by the American Medical Association, has focused directly on the concept of impairment of *structure*. Impairment of structure presupposes the presence of significant disease or injury and is manifested through symptoms, signs, and laboratory findings concerning organic pathology and as such, must be evaluated by a physician. Disability, on the other hand, refers to how impairment affects the person in terms of functioning and incapacity, and may be rated by anyone familiar with the patient.

Our work on a measure of impairment began in 1964. Development of the Cumulative Illness Rating Scale (CIRS) drew on the observation that practicing physicians are involved daily in decisions which imply a quantitative estimate of organ impairment. Such assessments are at the heart of diagnosis and prognosis.

An earlier version of this chapter was read at the 14th Annual Conference of the Veterans Administration Cooperative Studies in Psychiatry, Houston, Texas, 1969.

Bernard S. Linn is Associate Chief of Staff for Research and Education, Veterans Administration Hospital, Miami, Florida, and Assistant Professor of Surgery, University of Miami School of Medicine.

Margaret W. Linn is Research Social Worker, Veterans Administration Hospital, Miami, Florida, and Clinical Assistant Professor, University of Miami School of Medicine.

Lee Gurel is Director, Psychiatric Program Evaluation Staff, Veterans Administration, Washington, D.C.

The CIRS seeks only to record the physician's everyday, reasonably accurate and uniform global assessments of organ impairment and to make explicit that aspect of his evaluative activity which continually associates disease, degree of impairment, and prognosis.

Figure 4-1 shows the present version of the scale. There are 13 items grouped by body systems, with vital organs rated separately. Ratings from 0 to 4 are recorded for each.

From the beginning, the primary interest was in a brief assessment tool applicable to the study of biologic aging. Working with the instrument, it seemed to have promise for assessing effects of treatment, predicting clinical outcome, and for screening or survey purposes. Initial studies of reliability and validity were encouraging. Using Kendall's W, and interjudge total score reliability in the 90's was obtained, the exact value varying slightly with factors such as level of experience for the physicians. Also, scores were significantly correlated with early death on follow-up, with vital organ involvement, length of hospitalization, and number of hospitalizations and illnesses.

Estimates of Biological Age

Chronological age, although it is the simplest index of aging known, is not always the most useful criterion. Some persons are old at 50, and others are surprisingly young at 80. An operational definition of biological age, which could more accurately measure a person's residual life capacity, would have numerous applications for clinical medicine and the prediction of life span.

Previous attempts to measure biological age have utilized variables such as greying of hair, vital capacity, skin changes, blood pressure, and muscular function. We began with the assumption that physiological age and bodily impairment were related and that morbidity, in fact, left increments of impairment that could be measured. We took the position that persons who lived into extreme old age were more biologically elite. It had been observed clinically that individuals who live longer represent a unique group who seem to have been born physically tough and endowed with a sound body. We believed we would find that the person who survived to old age had been physically resistant to illness, thus showing little cumulative impairment. To test this hypothesis, a comparison (Linn, Linn, and Gurel 1967) was made between 57 subjects over age 75 and two groups of living controls 10 and 20 years younger (N = 59 and 56, respectively). Comparisons of health histories and ratings on the CIRS revealed no significant differences between the groups, suggesting that older subjects, although they had lived longer, had accumulated no more identifiable pathology. However, specific kinds of illnesses were related to each group, indicating that the older subjects formed a separate population from the general aging population dying from leading killer diseases.

The relationship of past physical resistance to aging must of necessity use mortality as an outcome criteria. A second investigation (Linn, Linn, and Gurel

Instructions: Indicate for each item the term that *best* describes the degree of impairment. For illnesses that cause impairment on more than one of the items, more than one item must be rated. For example: A CVA may impair neurological, vascular, and MSI. A tumor with metastasis requires a rating on the item describing the primary site of the cancer and a rating on vascular describing the extent of the lymph node involvement. When more than one illness occurs for a given item, it is the total impairment from these illnesses that is rated.

Each system should be rated as follows:

0 - None		3 - Severe
1 - Mild	2 - Moderate	4 - Extremely Severe

CARDIO-VASCULAR-RESPIRATORY SYSTEM

1. : __: CARDIAC (heart only)
2. : __: VASCULAR (blood, blood vessels and cells, marrow, spleen, lymphatics)
3. : __: RESPIRATORY (lungs, bronchi, trachea below the larynx)
4. : __: EENT (eye, ear, nose, throat, larynx)

GASTRO-INTESTINAL SYSTEM

5. : __: UPPER GI (esophagus, stomach, duodenum, biliary and pancreatic trees)
6. : __: LOWER GI (intestines, hernias)
7. : __: HEPATIC (liver only)

GENITO-URINARY SYSTEM

8. : __: RENAL (kidneys only)
9. : __: OTHER GU (ureters, bladder, urethra, prostate, genitals)

MUSCULO-SKELETAL-INTEGUMENTARY SYSTEM

10. : __: MSI (muscles, bone, skin)

NEURO-PSYCHIATRIC SYSTEM

11. : __: NEUROLOGIC (brain, spinal cord, nerves)
12. : __: PSYCHIATRIC (mental)

GENERAL SYSTEM

13. : __: ENDOCRINE-METABOLIC (includes diffuse infections, poisonings)

Figure 4-1. Cumulative Illness Rating Scale.

1969) studied 300 subjects who had died, 100 in each age group of 55-64, 65-74, and over 75. Table 4-1 shows results of multivariate analysis of variance comparing the three groups. Although total CIRS scores were not significantly different, patterns of illness were. Ratings of cardiac, vascular, and respiratory system impairments showed differences between groups which were significantly different at the .05 level, and hepatic and psychiatric impairments which were significantly less among the older subjects at the .01 level or less. One conclusion, which may not be as facetious as it first appears, is that a person can accrue only so much impairment, regardless of age. That is, when he attains a certain pathology score of around 15 on the CIRS, his number is up, literally.

Prediction of Death

These studies led to using the CIRS as a predictor of early death. In the Veterans Administration Program Evaluation Staff's studies of patients going from 18 Veterans Administration hospitals to nursing homes, the instrument was used as a measure of impairment. Using stepwise multiple regression techniques, Table 4-2 shows the CIRS (excluding ratings on psychiatric impairment) as a predictor

Table 4-1
Mean Scores on the CIRS for Three Age Groups

Items	Age			Statistical Significance	
	55-64	65-74	Over 75	F Ratio	P Less Than
Cardiac	1.63	2.35	1.97	3.7	.02*
Vascular	2.74	3.26	2.88	3.2	.04*
Respiratory	2.76	2.15	2.29	3.0	.05*
EENT	0.44	0.60	0.47	0.6	.53
Upper GI	1.18	0.87	1.14	1.1	.33
Lower GI	0.71	0.60	0.87	1.4	.23
Hepatic	1.24	0.48	0.45	9.2	.001**
Renal	0.55	0.43	0.88	2.9	.06
Other GU	0.70	0.65	0.92	1.2	.31
MSI	1.46	1.14	1.10	1.8	.15
Neurologic	1.14	0.91	1.11	0.6	.55
Psychiatric	0.41	0.26	0.06	5.4	.005**
Endo/Metab.	0.98	1.19	0.71	2.8	.06

Note: Multivariate $P < .001$ using Wilks Lamda Criterion for differences between groups.
Total Scores of 15.9, 14.8, & 14.9 were not significantly different $P < .14$
*Significant at $P < .05$ (univariate F)
**Significant at $P < .01$ (univariate F)

Table 4-2
The CIRS (Less Psychiatric Impairment) as a Predictor of Death, with Age and Cancer Controlled, on 663 Patients Going to Community Nursing Homes

Predictor Items	r	Cumulative R	R^2	ΔR^2
Cancer	.433**	.433	.188	.188**
Age	.108*	.452	.204	.016**
Renal	.246**	.502	.252	.048**
Cardiac	.180**	.515	.266	.014**
Endo/Metab.	.167**	.525	.275	.009**
Other GU	.213**	.531	.282	.007*
Vascular	.187**	.534	.286	.004*
Additions of 7 More CIRS Items		.539	.291	.005

Note: Without age and cancer partialled out, respiratory, renal, upper GI, other GU, and vascular ratings contributed at the .01 level to an increase in R^2. An R of .384 was reached by the same 12 CIRS items.
All R values are significant at $P < .01$
*Significant at $P < .05$
**Significant at $P < .01$

of mortality six months later for the 663 patients followed (Gurel, Linn, and Linn 1969). It can be seen that, after controlling for age and cancer, ratings on renal, cardiac, endocrine-metabolic, other genito-urinary, and vascular systems all contributed at statistically significant levels to prediction of early death. Additional analyses showed that the CIRS added significantly to ability to account for variance in mortality, even after other behavioral, historical, and diagnostic data had been partialled out.

How impairment related to other behavioral and diagnostic data in these studies is also of interest in providing further information about the scale's validity. Ratings on the total sample of 845 patients going from Veterans Administration to community nursing homes (445 psychiatric and 400 medical-surgical) were correlated with other behavioral and diagnostic data. Some of the findings are shown in Table 4-3. As expected, CIRS ratings on specific items correlated significantly with related diagnoses listed on the physicians discharge summaries, such as arteriosclerotic heart disease, diabetes, emphysema, stroke, and chronic brain syndrome. For example, ratings of metabolic impairment were higher for cases of diabetes or vascular, musculo-skeletal-integumentary, and neurologic ratings were higher in cases of stroke. Cancer correlated with higher ratings on respiratory and upper gastro-intestinal systems, which one might expect knowing the sample selected.

56

Table 4-3
Correlates of Selected Behavioral and Diagnostic Data on 845 Patients Going to
Nursing Homes

CIRS Items	Levels of Nursing Care	Total Number of Diagnoses	Non-ambulatory	Self-care Dependent	Anxiety Depression	Bedfast
Cardiac	–	.29**	.11*	.12**	.11*	.13**
Vascular	.14**	.28**	.22**	.25**	–	.19**
Respiratory	–	.14**	.12**	–	–	.16**
EENT	–	–	–	–	–	–
Upper GI	–	–	.09*	–	.13**	.14**
Lower GI	–	–	–	–	–	.09*
Hepatic	–	.10*	–	–	–	–
Renal	.14**	.14**	.21**	.16**	–	.22**
Other GU	.18**	.16**	.28**	.24**	–	.27**
MSI	.18**	.14**	.51**	.26**	–	.26**
Neurologic	.28**	.22**	.46**	.48**	–	.32**
Psychiatric	.16**	–	.19**	–	.10*	–
Endo/Metab.	–	.15**	.11*	–	–	.11*

* Significant at $P < .05$ (Pearson r)
** Significant at $P < .01$ (Pearson r)

**Comparison of Disability and
Impairment Ratings**

In another sample of 268 males from the Veterans Administration hospital in Miami, ratings by nurses on a disability scale were compared with ratings on the impairment scale in predicting death within six months (Linn, Linn, and Gurel 1968). Both regression and discriminant function techniques were applied to the data. Table 4-4 shows results of the regression. It can be seen that a useful and different share of variance is predicted by each kind of information (impairment and disability). A multiple R of .418 was reached by impairment, with disability adding uniquely to bring this up to an R of .511. However, three items, two from the impairment measure and one from the disability scale, accounted for almost 80 percent of the predictable variance in early death. Discriminant function analyses of each death indicated a classification accuracy with impairment ratings of 74 percent as compared with 68 percent for the disability items. We were not able to predict successfully other outcomes such as readmission or discharge from nursing homes, but we believe this related to nursing home criteria of discharge and readmission being less well defined than discharge and readmission in hospitals.

Table 4-4

Prediction of Death Using Impairment Items First and Adding Disability Items on 268 Medical-Surgical Patients Going to Nursing Homes

Predictor Items	r	Cumulative R	R^2	ΔR^2
Impairment Items				
Respiratory	.314**	.314	.099	.099**
Vascular	.288**	.395	.156	.057**
EENT	.112	.403	.163	.007
Lower GI	.084	.411	.169	.006
Neurologic	−.045	.415	.172	.003
All 13 Items		.418	.174	
Adding Disability Confused	.188**	.471	.222	.048**
All 16 Items		.511	.261	

Note: Impairment items listed are those selected by Stepdown Discriminant Function as the best set of predictors, multivariate P<.0001.When analyzed separately, impairment yields 74% predictive accuracy and disability yields 68% accuracy.

All R values are significant at the .01 level

*Significant at P < .05

**Significant at P < .01

The latest work with the CIRS explores the possibility of using ratings obtained from medical records in place of in vivo ratings (Linn, Linn, and Gurel, unpublished data). One hundred and four rather severely impaired patients were rated by their own physicians (55 doctors from medical and surgical services) and by another physician using only the records. Ratings were made at the time the patients were discharged from the hospital. Intraclass r's computed between the 13 CIRS items ranged from .19 to .66, with few items reaching anywhere near respectable reliability. One possible interpretation of this finding was that the CIRS items themselves were not reliable. Since we had tested previously only for total score reliability, we asked two physicians to rate in vivo, but independently, the same 30 patients. The resulting intraclass r's are shown in Table 4-5. This shows that the inter-judge reliability of the items was generally quite acceptable. Since reliability of the instrument did not appear to be the problem, the interpretation was made that useful ratings could not be made from records, an interpretation consistent with the common view that medical records are poor sources for research data.

However, to determine the validity of the two types of ratings (in vivo and records), the two sets of ratings were used to predict death at a six months' follow-up. Thirty-seven percent of the 104 subjects had expired by that time.

Table 4-5
Reliabilities of Ratings Made In-Vivo by Two Physicians on 30 Patients

Items	Intraclass r
Cardiac	.92
Respiratory	.91
Upper GI	.91
Psychiatric	.89
Vascular	.86
Endocrine-metabolic	.85
EENT	.82
Other GU	.79
Renal	.78
Neurologic	.75
Lower GI	.70
MSI	.67
Hepatic	.56

Using discriminant function techniques, we found that both sets of ratings were significantly and almost equally related to death on follow-up. Accuracy of the CIRS from records was 85 percent, while the in vivo CIRS had a 79 percent predictive accuracy. On further examination of the discrepancy between the in vivo CIRS and the CIRS from records, what seemed to be occurring was that the physician doing in vivo ratings concentrated on the condition for which the patient was being treated. Although the in vivo CIRS was reasonably accurate, it often did not take into account some of the impairments the patient had accumulated in the past. Neither were ratings from records perfect. For example, details needed to rate musculo-skeletal-integumentary impairment, such as the degree of paralysis, were often missing from the records. What seemed to emerge was that both in vivo and recorded knowledge of the patient were needed to most effectively rate impairment.

In comparing ratings of disability and impairment, we are not condemning disability scales. In fact, they have proved quite satisfactory for many purposes in the past. We only stress that the quantification of impairment has been almost totally neglected, as evidenced by the dearth of impairment rating scales. It is our contention that, where the interested physician's evaluation is available, this can be painlessly and profitably recorded for research. In our experience, some physicians have commented that rating their patients on the CIRS has helped them organize their thinking about the patient as a "whole" person. Physicians routinely make these required observations as a part of diagnosis and treatment;

quantifying them could lead to significantly better classification and prediction in clinical medicine and in longevity research.

References

Brody, S. The kinetics of senescence. *J. Gen. Physiol.*, 6:245-257, 1923.

Gurel, L., Linn, B.S., and Linn, M.W. Predicting mortality in a sample of nursing home patients. Paper presented at the 8th International Congress of Gerontology, Washington, D.C., 1969.

Jones, H.B. The relation of human health to age, place, and time; in *Birren Handbook of Aging and the Individual*, pp. 336-363, Chicago, University of Chicago Press, 1959.

Linn, B.S., Linn, M.W., and Gurel, L. Physical resistance and longevity. *Geront. Clin.*, 11(6):362-370, 1969.

Linn, B.S., Linn, M.W., and Gurel, L. *Impairment and disability as predictors of clinical outcome*. Paper presented at the 21st Annual Meeting of the Gerontological Society, Denver, Colorado, 1968.

Linn, M.W., Linn, B.S., and Gurel, L. Physical resistance in the aged. *Geriatrics*, 22:134-138, 1967.

Linn, M.W., Linn, B.S., and Gurel, L. Unpublished data.

Loeb, J., and Northrup, J.H. On the influence of food and temperature on the duration of life. *J. Biol. Chem.*, 32:103, 1917.

Pearl, R. *The rate of living*. New York, Knopf, 1928.

5 Habits and Heart Disease

WILLIAM B. KANNEL

There is mounting evidence to suggest that man, by altering his environment, has promoted an increasing incidence of coronary heart disease. The replacement of muscle power with machines, enrichment of the diet with hard fat, cholesterol and calories, and manufacture and promotion of the ready made cigarette appears to have exacted a toll in increased mortality from cardiovascular disease. Possibly as a result, the cardiovascular sequelae are now the chief force of mortality in affluent nations. About half of all deaths in the U.S. are from cardiovascular causes and coronary disease; a cerebrovascular accident, a congestive failure is all too frequently the reward for achieving an advanced age. Most of these deaths arise from atherosclerotic or hypertensive disease. The dominance of cardiovascular diseases as a force of mortality is largely a tribute to the revolution in our understanding of the epidemiology and consequent control of infectious and nutritional deficiency diseases. This has produced a radical alteration in the pattern of disease and forces of mortality acting on the population. Mortality early in life dropped sharply and as more people survived to older ages they have become increasingly subject to the influence of the chronic and "degenerative" diseases. Thus, the chronic cardiovascular diseases, like some bedrock of mortality have emerged as the layers of infectious and nutritional disease was removed.

In a long-term prospective epidemiological study underway since 1949 at Framingham, Massachusetts, 5,127 men and women aged 30-62 years at entry have been examined every two years for the development of coronary heart disease. The rate of development of disease in subjects classified according to antecedent habits was observed for over twelve years.

The results of this study have demonstrated that certain physical habits are associated with excess risk of developing coronary heart disease. The findings provide clues to possible causes of coronary heart disease and suggest means of prevention, since habits and environment are susceptible to change. For example, excessive cigarette smoking, obesity, and sedentary living are among suspect factors associated with increasing the chances of developing coronary heart disease. It is worthwhile, therefore, to direct attention to the findings concerning such habits and the potentials for health improvement that may lie in their alteration.

William B. Kannel, M.D. is Director, Heart Disease Epidemiology Study, National Heart Institute, Framingham, Mass.

Energy Balance

Although controversy still continues concerning which components of diet are of paramount importance in atherosclerosis and coronary heart disease, it is generally agreed that energy balance is important, regardless of the nutrient make-up of calories consumed. Detailed examination of the components of energy balance in Framingham subjects indicates its prominent role in coronary heart disease.

Assessment of the risk of disease using various possible indices of habitual energy expenditure indicated that sedentary males were more susceptible to lethal episodes of coronary heart disease (such as myocardial infarction and sudden death) than were physically active males. The risk of death from heart attacks in men was sharply increased in those with sedentary living habits. "Less active" males had more than three times the risk of "most active" males (Figure 5-1). The risk of less lethal manifestations of coronary disease—angina pectoris or coronary insufficiency—in men was not appreciably affected by their habitual level of physical activity.

The association between sedentary living habits and increased coronary heart disease mortality is also revealed using various other possible indicators of physical activity status (Figure 5-2). Those physically inactive sedentary living habits, with a weak hand grip, a low vital capacity, those ever overweight by more than 23 percent and those with high pulse rate all had two or three times the coronary mortality rates relative to those by these indicators more physically active. While no precise valid method for measuring habitual energy expenditure in general population samples has yet been devised, the fact that all of those possible indicators point in the same direction is highly suggestive.

In males, sustained high levels of physical activity may confer protection against severe manifestations of coronary heart disease by (a) stimulating the development of collateral circulation when the coronary blood flow is impaired by atherosclerosis; and (b) helping prevent overweight, with attendent benefits of lower serum lipid levels, lower blood pressure, and reduced cardiac work load.

Weight Patterns

Whether caused by over-eating, inadequate exercise, or both, excess weight increased the individual's risk of developing angina pectoris and of sudden death, but not of non-fatal myocardial infarction. Risk of angina pectoris rose progressively with increasing relative weight. Individuals more than 20 percent overweight had almost three times the risk of those more than 10 percent underweight (Figure 5-3).

Grossly overweight individuals had an increased risk of sudden death. More than three times as many sudden deaths occurred in those 20 percent or more overweight than in the general population.

Obesity may increase coronary heart disease risk by (a) increasing blood levels

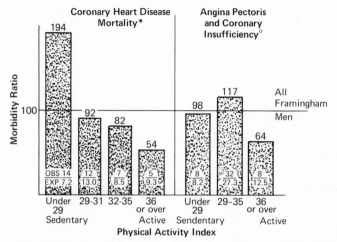

Figure 5-1. Physical Activity Index Related to Coronary Heart Disease Mortality, Angina Pectoris, and Coronary Insufficiency. Source: Kannel, "The Framingham Heart Study: Habits and Coronary Heart Disease," Public Health Service publication no. 1515, U.S. Department of HEW, PHS, NHLI.

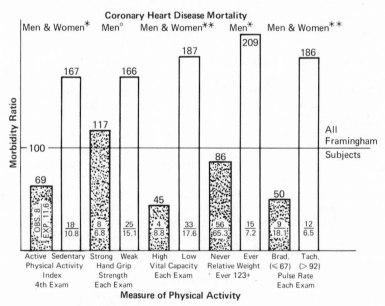

Figure 5-2. Physical Activity Related to Coronary Heart Disease Mortality. Source: Kannel, "The Framingham Heart Study: Habits and Coronary Heart Disease," Public Health Service publication no. 1515, U.S. Department of HEW, PHS, and NHLI.

of cholesterol and other lipids; (b) increasing the blood pressure; and (c) increasing the work load of the heart.

Diet

Controversy continues to rage concerning the influence of the nutrient composition of the diet on atherogenesis and coronary morbidity and mortality. While an impressive amount of evidence from epidemiologic studies, animal investigation, and manipulative metabolic studies in humans has accumulated to incriminate the saturated fat, cholesterol and refined carbohydrate in the diet as hyperlipidemia promoting and atherogenic, the uncomfortable fact remains that within the free-living population samples little relationship has been demonstrated between what people appear to be eating and either their blood cholesterol content and their coronary disease status. This apparent paradox requires explanation.

Areas in which the population exhibits high cholesterol values characteristically have diets different in composition and calories from those where low values are the rule. Migrants from "low cholesterol" areas to "high cholesterol" areas are often subsequently found to have higher cholesterol levels and to have changed their dietary pattern. Manipulation of the diet can alter serum cholesterol values in predictable fashion in humans, and in animals, can produce atherosclerotic deposits or cause established lesions to regress.

It is therefore a mistake to infer from the studies of free-living populations on high intake fat, cholesterol and refined carbohydrate which show no correlation between what people say they eat and their blood cholesterol levels, that diet plays no role in the evolution of atherosclerosis within populations. There is much evidence to suggest that it plays an important if not key role in determining the average blood cholesterol values in a population. The trouble is that in studies of free-living affluent populations there are not enough people who are habitually consuming the kind of diet characteristic of those where low cholesterol values are spontaneously found; or those which must be fed in metabolic studies in order to produce lower lipid values; to allow a demonstration of an association between diet and serum cholesterol. Evidently at the high intakes characteristic of affluent populations, the variation in cholesterol values from one person to the next depends on other factors including possibly innate ability to cope with the overload, energy balance, and state of health, among others. Lipid values within affluent populations, while apparently not proportional to the degree of overload may still be primarily set at a high level as a consequence of the composition of the diet. We may simply not have a biologically correct range of values to allow a demonstration of the influence of diet on blood lipids *within* the population. For example, Connor has convincingly shown that in the range of dietary cholesterol intakes between zero and 400 mg. per day, blood cholesterol is proportional to intake. Beyond this range there is no further association between the two. The bulk of persons in affluent population samples are above this range for cholesterol and evidently above the threshold for saturated fat and refined carbohydrate as well, particularly since they are often storing calories.

Cigarette Smoking

Cigarette smoking clearly increased the risk of severe manifestations of coronary heart disease, such as myocardial infarction and sudden unexpected death, but not risk of developing angina pectoris.

The rate of development of coronary heart disease was related to the *number* of cigarettes smoked each day, but not to the *duration* of the smoking habit. When the individual gives up cigarettes, his risk of coronary heart disease appears to be reduced towards the low level of those who never smoked. These observations suggest that cigarette smoking does not accelerate the development of atherosclerosis, but rather may act as a trigger factor for such dangerous complications as thrombosis or arrhythmias, especially in persons with an already compromised coronary circulation.

The risk of coronary heart disease other than angina pectoris among heavy cigarette smokers was about twice of that of nonsmokers. The low risk among pipe and cigar smokers suggests that tobacco smoke must be inhaled to produce its baneful effect. When an individual gives up the cigarette smoking habit, his risk quickly reverts to the low risk level of those who have never smoked or who smoke only a pipe or cigar.

A marked excess of sudden deaths occurred among cigarette smokers (possibly three fold) compared to nonsmokers (Figure 5-4). Furthermore, risk of sudden death increased with the number of cigarettes smoked. The risk of sudden, unexpected death among heavy cigarette smokers may be as high as five times that of nonsmokers. Mortality from coronary heart disease is clearly increased with the number of cigarettes smoked daily (Figure 5-5). However, the duration of the cigarette smoking habit was unrelated to coronary heart disease risk.

The contribution of cigarette smoking to risk of coronary heart disease appears to be independent of other demonstrated risk factors. At any level of blood pressure, vital capacity, or serum cholesterol, cigarette smokers had an excess risk and in multivariate analysis virtually none of the increased risk associated with cigarettes can be attributed to be associated among risk factors.

In subjects predisposed to heart attacks by high blood pressure or elevated cholesterol level, cigarette smoking appeared to be an extremely dangerous habit (Figure 5-6). Persons with any one of these three abnormalities had a risk of heart attacks about 50 percent greater than those with none of these risks, while persons with any two of these abnormalities had a risk of heart attacks about three times as great as those with none of these abnormalities. Those with all three abnormalities have a risk almost eight times as great as those with none of these abnormalities.

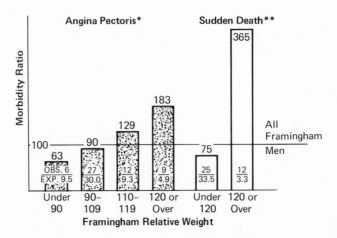

Figure 5-3. Relative Weight Related to Angina Pectoris and Sudden Death. Source: Kannel, "The Framingham Heart Study: Habits and Coronary Heart Disease," Public Health Service publication no. 1515, U.S. Department of HEW, PHS, NHLI.

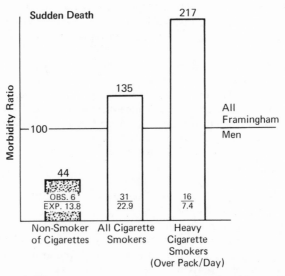

* Unusual difference

** Highly unusual difference

Based on 12 years Biennial Follow-up Experience

Figure 5-4. Cigarette Smoking Related to Sudden Death. Source: Kannel, "The Framingham Heart Study: Habits and Coronary Heart Disease," Public Health Service publication no. 1515, U.S. Department of HEW, PHS, NHLI.

67

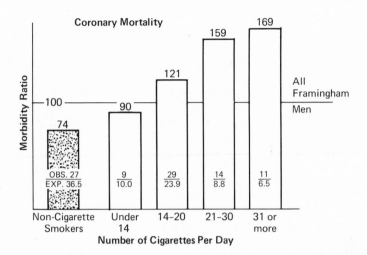

Figure 5-5. Number of Cigarettes Related to Coronary Mortality. Source: Kannel, "The Framingham Heart Study: Habits and Coronary Heart Disease," Public Health Service publication no. 1515, U.S. Dept. of HEW, PHS, NHLI.

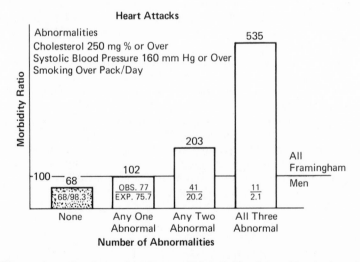

Figure 5-6. Number of Abnormalities Related to Heart Attacks. Source: Kannel, 'The Framingham Heart Study: Habits and Coronary Heart Disease," Public Health Service publication no. 1515, U.S. Department of HEW, PHS, NHLI.

Unrelated Living Habits

Among the factors found not to influence the individual's risk of developing clinical coronary heart disease were the use of alcohol and coffee, hours of sleep, marital status, and family size.

Consumed in moderation, alcohol apparently had no harmful effects on the circulation. However, neither did it protect the blood vessels against the consequences of atherosclerosis. Nor was coronary heart disease risk affected by moderate amounts of coffee despite the temporary effects of caffeine on the cardiovascular system.

Habitual lack of "adequate sleep" (six hours or less sleep per night) did not appear to increase coronary heart disease risk, despite the possibilities that lack of sleep may indicate some emotional stress. Similarly, marital status was unrelated to risk of coronary heart disease, even though changes in marital status through separation, divorce, or death would be regarded by many as evidence of long-standing emotional upheaval. Finally, family size also appeared unrelated to risk of developing coronary heart disease, even though some married couples with very large families might be construed as living under stressful conditions.

Summary

There is increasing evidence that certain habits or modes of life not only increase an individual's risk of premature and accelerated development of coronary heart disease, but may also adversely affect his chances of surviving a heart attack when it occurs. However, pernicious habits and environmental influences are often susceptible to change.

Although controlled scientific studies altering such factors have not been carried out, there are grounds for optimism that with the aid of his physician the highly susceptible individual may substantially reduce his heart-disease risk by: giving up cigarettes, achieving and maintaining desirable weight through prudent eating habits, and improving his physical fitness with a sensible program of exercise. Such measures are especially indicated in persons who have such atherogenic coronary precursors as hypertension, high cholesterol levels, diabetes or electrocardiographic abnormalities such as left ventricular hypertrophy.

For further information on these and other findings of the Framingham Heart Study, the reader may consult the articles in the bibliography.

References

Damon, A., Damon, S.T., Harpending, H.C., and Kannel, W.B.: Predicting coronary heart disease from body measurements of Framingham males. *Journal of Chronic Disease*, 21:781-802, 1969.

Doyle, J.T., Dawber, T.R., Kannel, W.B., Heslin, A.S., and Kahn, H.A.: Cigarette smoking and coronary heart disease. *New England Journal of Medicine*, 266:796-801, 1962.

Friedman, G.D., Kannel, W.B., and Dawber, T.R.: The epidemiology of gallbladder disease: observations in the Framingham study. *Journal of Chronic Disease*, 19:273-292, 1966.

Friedman, G.D., Kannel, W.B., Dawber, T.R. and McNamara, P.M.: Comparison of prevalence, case history and incidence data in assessing the potency of risk factors in coronary heart disease. *American Journal of Epidemiology*, 83:366-378, 1966.

Kannel, W.B.: Cigarette smoking and coronary heart disease. *Internal Medicine*, 60:1103-1106, 1964.

Kannel, W.B.: Coronary heart disease epidemiology: implications for practice. *Epidemiologie Kardiovaskularer Krankheiten*, 82-97, 1970.

Kannel, W.B.: The epidemiology of coronary heart disease: methodologic considerations the Framingham study. *Epidemiologie Kardiovaskularer Krankheiten*, 25-42, 1970.

Kannel, W.B., Dawber, T.R., and McNamara, P.M.: Vascular disease of the brain—epidemiologic aspects: the Framingham study. *American Journal of Public Health*, 55:1355-1365, 1965.

Kannel, W.B., Castelli, W.P., and McNamara, P.M.: Cigarette smoking and risk of coronary heart disease. Epidemiologic Clues to Pathogenesis. In *Toward A Less Harmful Cigarette*, National Cancer Institute Monograph No. 28, Washington, D.C.: U.S. Government Printing Office, 1968, 9-20.

Kannel, W.B., Castelli, W.P., and McNamara, P.M.: Serum lipid fractions and risk of coronary heart disease. *Minnesota Medicine*, 52:1225-1230, 1969.

Kannel, W.B., Castelli, W.P., McNamara, P.M., and Sorlie, P.: Some factors affecting morbidity and mortality in hypertension. *Milbank Memorial Fund Quarterly*, 47:116-142, 1969.

Kannel, W.B., Gordon, T. and Offutt, D.: Lift ventricular hypertrophy by electrocardiogram. *Internal Medicine*, 71:89-105, 1969.

Kannel, W.B.: Gordon, T., Castelli, W.P., and Margolis, J.R.: Electrocardiographic left ventricular hypertrophy and risk of coronary heart disease. *Internal Medicine*, 72:813-822, 1970.

Kannel, W.B., LeBauer, J.E., Dawber, T.R., and McNamara, P.M.: Relation of body weight to development of coronary heart disease. *Circulation*, 35:734-743, 1967.

Kannel, W.B., and McNamara, P.M.: The evidence for excess risk. *Minnesota Medicine*, 52:1197-1201, 1969.

Kannel, W.B., McNamara, P.M., Feinleib, M., and Dawber, T.R.: The unrecognized myocardial infarction. *Geriatrics*, 25:75-87, 1970.

Kannel, W.B., Skinner, J.J., Schwartz, M.J., and Shurtleff, D.: Intermittent clausication. *Circulation*, 41:875-883, 1970.

Kannel, W.B., Schwartz, M.J., and McNamara, P.M.: Blood pressure and risk of coronary heart disease: the Framingham study. *Diseases of the Chest*, 56:44-52, 1969.

Moriyama, I.M., Dawber, T.R., and Kannel, W.B.: Evaluation of diagnostic information supporting medical certification of deaths from cardiovascular disease. In *Study of Cancer and other Chronic Diseases*, National Cancer Institute Monograph No. 19, Washington, D.C.: U.S. Printing Office, 406-419.

6

Health Practices, Illnesses, and Longevity

ERDMAN PALMORE

Regardless of the associations of certain physiological measures and longevity, a more practical question is, "What health practices contribute to longer life?" There is widespread agreement that inactivity, obesity, and cigarette smoking are usually associated with a higher incidence of various illnesses and higher mortality rates (Mayer 1968; Metropolitan Life Insurance Company 1960; Morris 1958; Society of Actuaries 1959; U.S. Public Health Service 1967 (see also Chapter 5)). There is corresponding evidence that the health care practices of exercise, weight control, and avoiding cigarettes contribute to the lower incidence of several illnesses and to greater longevity. Recently the question has been raised as to whether these health practices are associated with such lower rates of illness and mortality among the aged as to justify lower health and life insurance premiums for persons who exercise, have moderate weights, and avoid smoking. This chapter presents the evidence from the Duke Longitudinal Study of Aging which indicates that such health practices to contribute to lower rates of illness and mortality.

Methods

The data came from an on-going longitudinal interdisciplinary study of 268 community volunteers, aged 60-94 at initial examination during 1955-59 (Palmore, 1970). All subjects were ambulatory, noninstitutionalized residents of the central North Carolina area. The initial panel did not constitute a random sample, but were chosen from a larger number of volunteers so that their sex, race, and occupational distribution approximated that of the area. Nevertheless, analysis of selection and attrition factors indicates that the panelists were a social, psychological, and physical elite among the aged and became more so through time. Thus, the present findings may not apply in the same way to a less elite sample of aged.

The health practices of exercising, keeping a moderate weight, and avoiding

Revision of a paper originally titled "Health Practices and Illness among the Aged," *Gerontologist* (Winter) 10:4:313-316, 1970. Research supported in part by NICHD Grant HD-00668.

71

smoking, were recorded at the initial interview while the measures of illness were derived from interviews and examinations conducted three or four years later, except for the information on operations which was collected about ten years later. Since the health practices preceded the illnesses, there are better grounds for inferring a causal relationship than in cross-sectional studies when data on health practices and illness refer to the same point in time.

The measure of exercise was the number of locomotor activities recorded in response to the question "What do you do in your free time?" Locomotor activities were defined as involving physical mobility either in its performance or in getting to the place to do it. This was in contrast to sedentary activities such as listening to the radio or TV, writing letters, playing cards, reading, etc. This is not an ideal measure of the actual amount of exercise, because it does not indicate either the strenuousness nor the amount of time spent in such exercise, nor does it ask about locomotor activities at work. However, this was the best measure available from the initial interviews. On the whole, it is probably a safe assumption that most of those reporting more locomotor activities tend to get more exercise than those reporting less locomotor activities.

The measure of overweight and underweight was the ratio of body weight to the square of body height in inches. Careful statistical analysis of various indices of overweight show that this index is more closely related to the amount of excess fat than is the simple ratio of weight to height (Khosla and Lowe 1967).

The indicator of tobacco use is a composite classification based on responses to two questions: "How often do you use tobacco?" and "In what form do you use tobacco?" The responses to the first question were coded into five categories: never used; not used in last year; slight present use (cigarettes 1-4 a day, cigar and/or pipe 1-2 a day, occasional snuff or tobacco chewing); moderate present use (cigarettes 5-10 a day, cigar and/or pipe 3-4 a day, frequent snuff or chewing tobacco); and heavy present use (cigarettes 11 or more a day, cigar and/or pipe 5 or more a day, constant use of snuff or chewing tobacco). The responses to the second question on type of tobacco were coded in five categories: never used, cigarettes, cigar, pipe, snuff or chewing tobacco. Various ways of classifying subjects according to their responses to these questions were tried and the following three-way classification was found to give the clearest results: persons not using tobacco or using only slight amounts; persons using non-cigarette tobacco in moderate or heavy amounts; and persons smoking cigarettes in moderate or heavy amounts. It was found that relatively few women (about 25 percent) used tobacco in moderate or heavy amounts and this use showed little relationship to illness. Therefore, the data on tobacco in this paper is for men only.

There were several measures of illness recorded in the second wave of examinations. The number of days spent in bed during a year was based on the subjects' response to the question, "How many days did you spend in bed last year because of not feeling well?" The number of operations since the initial interview was also based on subjects' reports and physicians' examinations. There were so few operations reported in the first three or four year interval that we cumulated the operations reported over the approximately ten year span between initial interview and the fourth wave of the study. Subject attrition between the second and fourth waves reduced the numbers in the base by 46 percent for these tabulations. The hospitalization measure is also based on the physician interview with the subject in which he recorded all hospitalizations and operations since the initial examination. The number of doctors' visits per year is based on the subjects' response to the question, "In the past two years have you seen a doctor: once, 1-5 times, 6-10 times, 10-20 times, or more than 20 times?"

The Longevity Quotient is the observed number of years the subject lived after the initial examination (or the estimated number of years for those still living) divided by the actuarily expected number of years remaining after the examination based on the age, sex, and race of the subject (see Chapter 18). Thus an LQ of less than 1.0 would mean that a person lived fewer years than expected. The LQ has the advantages of controlling precisely for the effects of age at initial examination and of providing a continuous variable indicator of longevity.

We also used two subjective indicators of illness based on responses to the question, "Would you say your health has changed since you were here last time?" (the proportion who said their health had become worse was used in this analysis) and the question, "How would you rate your health at the present time?" (the proportion who said very poor or poor was used in this analysis). It was found that these subjective self-evaluations of health were even more closely related to actual functioning and use of medical care than the more objective physician's ratings.

Findings

Of the three health practices examined, the amount of exercise was most closely related to more of the illness and mortality indicators than the other two health practices (Table 6-1). The proportion who had spent two or more weeks in bed per year was two and a half times greater among those with few locomotor activities than the others. The proportion who had three or more physician visits per year was about one and a half times as great among those with few locomotor activities as among the others. The percent who were hospitalized and the percent with operations were substantially greater among those with a few locomotor activities, although these two relationships were not statistically significant at the .05 level. The proportion rating their health as becoming worse since the last examination was about half as large among those with the most locomotor activities as among the others and the proportion rating their health as poor was more than four times as large among those with few locomotor activities died sooner than actuarily expected compared to between a fourth and third of those with more locomotor activities. Thus, even though some of the relationships were not statistically significant and several of the relationships are

Table 6-1
Locomotor Activities are Followed by Less Illness

Illness Indicator	# Locomotor Activities:			Kendall Tau C	
	0-5	6-7	8 or more		
% in bed 2+ weeks per year	26	11	10	.1	p<.01
% with 3+ Dr's visits per year	44	31	33	.09	p<.05
% hospitalized	32	31	24	.07	NS
% with 1+ operations	30	20	19	.09	NS
% rating health as worse	38	39	21	.16	p<.01
% rating health as poor	18	6	4	.11	p<.05
% with LQ of less than 1.00	54	28	33	.17	p<.01
Numbers in base	50	64	67		

not monotonic, regardless of which indicator is used, those who reported more locomotor activities at the initial interview had substantially less illness and lived longer than those with less locomotor activities.

Those overweight or underweight had more illness according to most of the indicator (Table 6-2). We found these relationships to be clearest when we used cutting points which separated out the tenth with the lowest weight/height^2 ratio (.030 or less), and the tenth with the highest weight/height^2 ratio (.046 or more). Using these cutting points, those underweight compared to the normal weight had almost twice as large a proportion who spent two or more weeks per year in bed and those overweight had almost three times as high a proportion with illness compared to those with normal weight. Similarly, those underweight had 10 percent more who had been hospitalized and those overweight had 14 percent more hospitalized compared to those of normal weight. Those underweight did not have a larger proportion rating their health as worse but those overweight had 21 percent more rating their health as worse. Both those underweight and those overweight had three times as large percentages who rated their health as poor. They also had substantially larger percentages who died earlier than actuarily expected. The other indicators of illness did not seem to be related to weight.

Cigarette smoking had relationships with fewer of the illness indicators than did the other two health practices (Table 6-3). Only the proportion dying sooner than expected had a statistically significant relationship to cigarette smoking. Two-thirds of those who were moderate or heavy cigarette smokers died sooner than expected, compared to less than 40 percent of the others. The moderate or heavy cigarette smokers also had somewhat more with operations and more with three or more doctor's visits per year than the others. Those with no use or slight

T able 6-2
Overweight and Underweight are Followed by More Illness

Illness Indicator	Weight/Height^2			Kendall Tau C	
	.031-.045	<.031	.046+		
% in bed 2+ weeks per year	12	21	33	.09	p<.05
% hospitalized	26	36	40	.07	NS
% rating health as worse	32	21	53	.04	NS
% rating health as poor	7	21	20	.08	NS
% with LQ of less than 1.00	36	44	42	.05	NS
Numbers in base	145	14	15		

Table 6-3
Cigarette Smoking is Followed by More Illness Among Men

Illness Indicator	Tobacco Use:			Kendall Tau C	
	None or Slight	Mod. or Heavy Non-cigarette	Mod. or Heavy Cigarette		
% with 1+ operations	26	25	33	.04	NS
% with 3+ Dr's visits per year	33	24	38	.01	NS
% rating health as worse	23	29	29	.06	NS
% with LQ of less than 1.00	39	38	67	.19	p<.01
Numbers in base (men)	48	21	21		

use of tobacco had a somewhat lower proportion who rated their health as having become worse compared to the moderate or heavy tobacco users. The other indicators of illness did not seem to be related to tobacco use.

When we combine the health practices, we see that there tends to be an additive effect on health (Table 6-4). Persons having all three positive health practices had about a third the percentage spending two or more weeks in bed per year compared to those with one or none of the health practices. (There was only one person with none of the positive health practices.) Similarly, those with all three positive health practices had substantially lower percentages who saw physicians frequently, were hospitalized, had operations, rated their health as becoming worse, rated their health as poor, and lived fewer years than actuarially expected. Four out of these seven relationships were statistically significant at the .05 level or below.

Table 6-4
More Health Practices are Followed by Less Illness

Illness Indicator	Number of Health Practices			Kendall Tau C	
	0-1	2	3		
% in bed 2+ weeks per year	30	18	11	.12	p < .05
% with 3+ Dr's visits per year	50	30	36	.02	NS
% hospitalized	40	32	25	.10	p < .05
% with 1+ operations	25	29	17	.10	NS
% rating health as worse	45	32	33	.04	NS
% rating health as poor	20	12	5	.10	p < .05
% with LQ less than 1.00	59	42	29	.22	p < .01
Numbers in base	20	57	91		

Conclusions

Despite the small or moderate levels of these associations and the lack of statistical significance for about half the indicators, the consistent relationship of health practices to less illness and greater longevity, which was found with most of the indicators, supports the conclusion that positive health practices did contribute to better health among this group of elderly persons. The fact these health practices were usually most strongly related to longer life indicates that they have a long-term effect on health which is greater than in the short run effect on any one of the illness indicators. We believe that the lack of statistical significance shown by several of the associations is due to the small numbers in some of the base groups and the gross nature of some of the measures.

When an association is found in a cross-sectional, that is, the one-point in time study, there is the chicken-and-egg problem of which came first and which caused the other. In the present study this is less of a problem because it was a longitudinal study and the health practices were measured at the beginning of the study while the illness and mortality indicators were measured later. This does not eliminate the possibility that greater illness occurred both before and after the beginning of the study among those without the positive health practices and that these illnesses may have contributed to fewer locomotor activities, less weight control, and more cigarette smoking. There is also the possibility that both the health practices and health itself are caused by some third set of uncontrolled variables such as greater education, higher intelligence, healthier environments, etc. It is difficult, if not impossible, to assess the importance of these possibilities without tightly controlled experiments, which, of course, are very difficult and expensive in this area. Lacking such experiments one has to rely on findings from related studies and generally accepted theories to interpret the meaning of these findings. We believe that most other studies and theories of the relation of health practices to health support our interpretation that exercise, weight control, and avoiding cigarettes contribute to better health and longevity.

It would be interesting to know which of these health practices had the strongest effect on health. Unfortunately, the complex multivariate analysis necessary to answer this question satisfactorily does not appear feasible due to the size of the sample and nature of the indicators used in this study. However, the cross-tabulations do suggest that exercise may have the strongest effect, because it usually shows the highest level of association and statistical significance. Also it is important to note that regardless of relative importance, all three health practices tend to have an additive effect: each additional health practice tends to reduce the proportions of those with illness and with early death.

References

U.S. Public Health Service: The health consequences of smoking. A Public Health Service review. Washington, D.C. U.S. Dept. of HEW, Public Health Publication No. 1696, 1967.

Khosla, T. and Lowe, C.: Indices of obesity derived from body weight and height. *British Journal of Preventive and Social Medicine*. 21:122-128, 1967

Marzen, J.: *Overweight: Causes, Cost, and Control.* Englewood Cliffs, N.J. Prentice-Hall, Inc., 1968.

Morris, J. and Crawford, M.: Coronary heart disease and physical activity c work. *British Medical Journal*, 2:1485, 1958.

Society of Actuaries: *Build and Blood Pressure Study*. 1959.

Metropolitan Life Insurance Co.: *Overweight: Its Prevention and Significance.* 1960.

Palmore, E. (ed.): *Normal Aging*, Duke University Press, Durham, N.C., 1970.

Palmore, E.: Predicting longevity, *Gerontologist* 9:247-250, 1969.

7
Predictors of Mortality in the Institutionalized Aged

ALVIN I. GOLDFARB

The death rate of old people in institutions is, age for age, higher than that of the general population. This is particularly true in the first few months after their admission for the first time to a state hospital. The higher death rate probably reflects the physical and mental disabilities which led to their need for institutional care, treatment, or protection.

Among the psychiatric characteristics that have been reported as predictive of death in the aged is the presence of organic mental syndrome, and the absence of associated schizoid or affective disorder. Conversely, aged patients with persistent or recurring nonorganic mental disorder, or disorders of affect or content without organic syndrome, appear to have a good outlook for survival. Roth and Kay suggested that the differential death rates of affective psychosis, "late paraphrenia," senile psychosis, cerebral arteriosclerosis with psychosis, and acute confusion not only attest to the predictive value of such classifications, but are evidence of the distinctive character of the processes they represent (Goldfarb 1966; Post 1951, Roth 1953, 1955, 1956, 1960; Kay and Roth 1955; Kay 1962).

Kay, Norris, and Post further emphasized that the outlook for survival in patients with purely functional disorder—chiefly affective—is best; a mixed syndrome of the organic and functional type has an intermediate prognosis; mild intellectual impairment does not appear to affect the outcome; and "definite dementia renders recovery unlikely." In one study they stated: "Serious physical illness, acute organic-confusional states, and age over 80 were the main conditions associated with death within the year; 40 percent of cases with acute confusion died within 3 months" (Kay, Norris, and Post 1956). It should be noted here that the outlook for those who recover from acute confusional states may be good, contingent upon the illness behind the acute condition. Similar findings were reported by Guze and Cantwell, and more recently by Simon and his group in San Francisco (Guze and Cantwell 1964).

In a study of older persons referred for psychiatric care in a home for the aged, 60 percent were found to have an organic mental syndrome. Of 59 such patients followed from 4-7 years, over 50 percent died by the end of the fourth year (Goldfarb 1958). Mortality rates in the group declined with the passage of time as the "weaklings" were eliminated and only the "stalwarts" survived.

Alvin I. Goldfarb, M.D. is Associate Clinical Professor of Psychiatry, Mt. Sinai Hospital and Medical School, New York, N.Y.

Institutionalization and Longevity

It has been contended that institutionalization *per se* tends to shorten life; and that the processes of investigation into the individual's need for care, and of assistance in finding and utilizing care facilities, in themselves are conducive to earlier death than might otherwise occur. The hypothesis that some institutions presumably designed to offer prosthetic and protective services to the aged actually shorten their lifespan warrants testing.

Investigation of this and other hypotheses relating institutionalization to mortality is made possible by information accumulated in a special study conducted in 1958-65 in the New York City metropolitan area. Data derived from this seven-year study of 1,279 persons over age 64 residing in three different types of institutions permit examination of the relationship of a number of characteristics—physical, mental and social—to longevity, and to the effect upon the individual's lifespan of the type of institution in which he resides (Goldfarb 1969).

Our sample was drawn from a representative group of nine voluntary homes for the aged (553 subjects), thirteen small proprietary nursing homes (482 subjects), and three state hospitals (244 subjects). Females outnumbered males 2-1 in each setting. The sample consisted of all aged persons in these institutions at a specific time, rather than consecutive admissions. In the case of the state hospitals, only patients admitted after age 65 were included in order to eliminate the effects of early hospitalization. Also persons in residence less than three months were excluded, thus weeding out those admitted with brain syndrome related to acute illness or to terminal conditions.

Vital statistics and historical information regarding the subjects were obtained from institutional records. Each subject also received medical, psychological, and psychiatric examinations. Due to the complexity of these procedures, and the fact that the examinations were conducted at different times, the data are not complete for all subjects. Nevertheless, no fewer than 1,016 subjects received the full battery of tests and were followed for the full period of seven years.

The medical examination, in addition to rating pathologic conditions in the various organ systems, rated over-all physical condition and functional status. After examination, the internist made a prognosis in each case of the patient's likelihood of survival for one year. New admissions to the State hospitals were in the poorest physical condition; about 40 percent of those who survived the first three months required active medical care. The nursing home population was the worst from the standpoint of physical functional status, patients in the State hospitals were intermediate, those in homes for the aged functioned best (Pollack, Kahn, Gerber, and Goldfarb, 1960).

The psychological examination included two special tests for brain syndrome: the Mental Status Questionnaire (MSQ), and the Face-Hand Test (F-HT). The MSQ consists of 10 simple questions which test the subject's orientation in time and place; his memory, both recent and remote; and his ability to recall general and personal information. In the F-HT the subject, his eyes closed, is touched simultaneously on one cheek and the dorsum of one hand for a total of 10 trials—4 contralateral (for example, right cheek and left hand) and 4 ipsolateral (for example, right cheek and right hand), with 2 symmetric combinations (face=face and hand=hand) as teaching trials. Failure after the teaching trials to designate the stimuli correctly is indicative (in adults) of brain damage. About 90 percent of persons who made mistakes with eyes closed also made them in trials with their eyes open.

The psychiatric examination included assessment of the presence and degree of chronic brain syndrome (CBS), of associated psychosis or other type of psychiatric disorder, as well as the extent of management problems and the psychiatrist's prognosis of one-year survival.

The subjects in this sample fell into the following psychiatric categories: no mental disorder, 10 percent; mental disorder but no brain syndrome, 5 percent; brain syndrome, 85 percent. Evidence of brain syndrome was found in 79 percent of the residents in old age homes, 88 percent of those in nursing homes, and 94 percent of first admissions in old age to state hospitals (Goldfarb 1962).

There was remarkable concordance between the psychiatric evaluation and the psychologist's rating of CBS on the basis of the two tests. About 94 percent of subjects making no MSQ errors were found to have no or mild CBS; some 95 percent of those who made 10 MSQ errors were found to have moderate or severe CBS. The results were similar for the F-HT: some 70 percent of those negative on this test were rated as having no or just moderate CBS. There was also a high correlation in mental and physical functional status. The great majority (67 percent) of subjects making 2 or less MSQ errors were found to be in relatively good physical functional condition; in contrast, only 19 percent of those making 9-10 errors had good physical functional status. This was true of all age groups and in all three types of institutions (Kahn, Goldfarb, Pollack, and Peck 1960; Goldfarb 1964).

Since old age homes, nursing homes, and state hospitals presumably admit patients for social, medical, and psychiatric reasons respectively, they might be expected to have different populations and different mortality rates (Figure 7-1). Actually, their populations had overlapping characteristics and very similar death rates, when these rates were calculated on the basis of the subject's physical and mental condition rather than in terms of age or sex.

Clinical Prognoses and Death Rate

Nearly one-fourth of the entire sample (23 percent) died within one year. This was considerably less than predicted by psychiatric and medical examiners (32 and 35 percent respectively) at the start of the study. Survival of the aged subjects remained higher than predicted by the examiners throughout the seven-year follow-up (see Table 7-1). Their prognoses for individual subjects proved even less accurate. In 322 cases internist and psychiatrist disagreed as to projected survival; even in the 176 cases where they did agree, only 40 percent died within the year. And when they agreed on a favorable prognosis, there still was a 12 percent death rate the first year.

A breakdown by age group showed, as anticipated, a linear relationship between the death rate and the chronological age of the subjects at the start of the study (Figure 7-2).

Functional Status and Death Rate

Such high proportions of such groups are affected with, and die from arteriosclerotic cardio-vascular and renal disease that simple medical diagnoses are not sufficiently precise (Figure 7-3). In a search for more precise predictive features, medical examination data were summarized on a number of scales. The characteristic most clearly related to mortality, in this category, was impairment of physical function. Subjects with little or no impairment had the lowest death rate each year; those with severe impairment of function had the highest. As previously indicated, a high correlation existed between physical and mental impairment in all subjects in the sample.

There was one clear-cut factor consistently and unequivocally associated with high mortality every year at all ages in both sex groups and in all three institutions: incontinence of urine or feces. It was found in 21 percent of the subjects in this study. Their death rate within one year was 38 percent; at the end of three years it was 75 percent; after seven years it was 87 percent. As good a predictor of mortality as any single variable in this study, it is particularly useful since its detection requires no special training, scoring system, or rating scale.

All in all, the four characteristics found to correlate most significantly and consistently with high mortality in aged institutionalized persons were (1) incontinence, as noted above; (2) marked physical dependency (need for assistance in getting in and out of bed, moving about, dressing, washing, and bathing); (3) a psychiatrist's impressions of severe CBS; and (4) 9-10 errors in MSQ responses. These were termed "high mortality indicators" because the afflicted subjects had the highest death rates each year of the study. Each of them reflects brain damage, and is tantamount to a diagnosis of severe CBS. The relationship of the four high mortality indicators to the death rate of aged patients in each of the three types of institutional settings is shown in Table 7-2. When none of these indicators is present, the death rate is 40 percent below average the first year, and 30-10 percent lower the remaining years. When any one indicator is present, the death rate is 40 percent *above* average the first year, and slightly higher than average subsequently. When two indicators are present, the death rate is 70 percent higher the first year, and 28-10 percent higher the rest of the period. With three indicators, the death rate is 87 percent higher the first year, 52-21 percent higher later. And with all four indicators, the death rate is 120 percent higher the first year and 67-22 percent higher subsequently. More than half (52 percent) of the subjects with all four characteristics died within the first year.

When none of the high mortality indicators is present, likelihood of death is lowest in all three types of institutions. It is highest in state hospitals during the

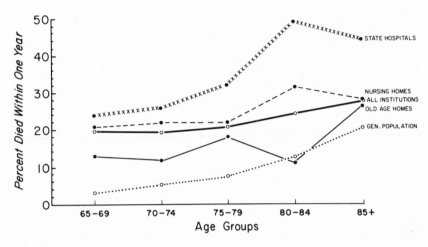

Figure **7-1**. Mortality within One Year by Age Groups and Type of Institution, Compared with the General Population.

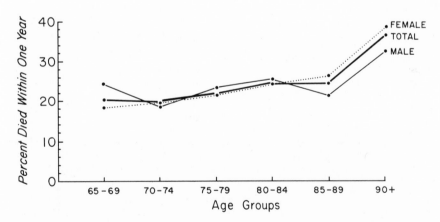

Figure **7-2**. Mortality Within One Year by Age Groups and Sex. Source: Goldfarb, et al., "Predictors of Mortality in the Institutionalized Aged," *Diseases of the Nervous System*, 27:21, January 1966. Used with permission.

Table 7-1

Death Rate Over a Seven-Year Period for Selected Categories of Aged Institutionalized Persons

	#	Total	1 yr.	2 yrs.	3 yrs.	4 yrs.	5 yrs.	6 yrs.	7 yrs.
					Percent Who Died Within:				
All Persons		1280	23	42	54	65	73	79	82
Sex: Male	426	1279	25	44	58	69	78	83	87
Female	853		23	41	53	63	71	77	80
Age: 65-74	345	1268	19	37	46	58	66	72	76
75-84	633		24	41	52	62	72	77	81
85+	290		28	52	68	79	85	90	92
Old Age Home	553	1279	17	33	45	56	67	73	76
Nursing Home	482		26	49	60	72	79	85	89
State Hospital	244		35	52	64	71	76	81	83
Res: under 1 year	493	1266	30	49	61	71	77	82	85
1 to 2 years	265		20	38	51	65	75	81	83
2 to 5 years	304		19	38	51	60	69	75	81
5+ years	204		19	37	47	57	69	74	77
Mobility: Good	799	1168	18	36	49	61	69	75	79
Fair	157		25	45	55	65	78	82	87
Poor	192		27	48	61	72	81	89	90
Physical Dep: Mild	786	1176	15	31	45	57	67	73	77
Mod.	133		26	49	61	69	80	86	89
Severe	257		37	63	74	82	88	93	95
Continent	919	1163	16	34	47	58	67	74	78
Incontinent	244		38	61	75	84	92	95	97
Brain Syn.: None-Mild	476	1136	10-12	25-27	36-39	48-49	61-58	67-66	71-71
Mod.	355		23	44	57	70	78	84	88
Severe	305		37	60	75	84	90	93	94
M.S.Q. errors 0-2	334	1166	11	23	34	45	58	65	71
3-8	408		17	36	51	63	71	77	81
9+	424		35	60	73	83	89	93	94
Prog. for Life Und. 1 yr. (P)	424	1122	32	54	68	77	83	89	91
(I)	317	1160	35	59	72	82	89	92	95
(P. & I.)	176	1057	40	66	80	89	93	95	96
Prog. for Life Over 1 yr. (P)	698	1122	15	32	45	56	67	73	77
(I)	843	1160	15	32	45	57	67	73	77
(P. & I.)	549	1057	12	28	41	53	64	72	76
Py. Funct. Imp: None-Mild	416	1167	10	23	33	48	58	65	69
Mod.	419		20	43	59	69	77	83	86
Sev.	332		35	58	70	78	86	91	94

Table 7-2
The Relationship Between Mortality and Four High Indicators of Mortality

Four High Indicators of Mortality	#	Total	Percent Who Died Within:						
			1 yr.	2 yrs.	3 yrs.	4 yrs.	5 yrs.	6 yrs.	7 yrs.
OAH									
None	309	100	11	21	34	46	59	66	71
Any 1	70	100	28	44	59	69	81	86	89
Any 2	42	100	35	55	81	95	98	98	100
Any 3	19	100	41	63	79	89	100	100	100
All 4	14	100	64	86	100	100	100	100	100
Total	454	100	17	32	46	58	69	74	78
NH									
None	146	100	17	34	45	60	68	77	84
Any 1	87	100	28	44	59	71	78	84	87
Any 2	76	100	33	54	63	75	79	88	89
Any 3	54	100	33	59	76	85	96	100	100
All 4	33	100	38	58	70	85	100	100	100
Total	396	100	26	45	58	71	79	86	89
SH									
None	39	100	18	18	31	41	51	59	62
Any 1	42	100	41	40	60	64	71	76	79
Any 2	38	100	51	53	68	74	84	89	89
Any 3	24	100	59	75	88	88	88	96	96
All 4	23	100	61	78	87	96	96	100	100
Total	166	100	35	48	63	69	75	80	83
Total									
None	494	100	14	25	37	50	61	68	74
Any 1	199	100	32	43	58	69	78	82	86
Any 2	156	100	39	54	69	80	85	91	92
Any 3	97	100	43	64	79	87	95	99	99
All 4	70	100	52	70	81	91	99	100	100
Total	1016	100	24	40	53	65	74	80	83

first year; thereafter it is lowest there and highest in nursing homes. When one or more indicators is present, death rates generally are highest in the old age homes except during the first year, when they invariably are highest in state hospitals.

Psychiatric Syndromes and Death Rate

Because of their importance as predictors of mortality, careful analysis was made of the diagnostic categories of CBS—the psychiatric reflection of brain cell loss, hence brain damage.

The National Conference on Nomenclature of Disease in 1933 recommended categorization of old people with organic mental syndrome under two general headings: "Senile Psychosis" and "Psychosis with Cerebral Arteriosclerosis." When the psychiatrist is in doubt, it suggested, he should give preference to the second classification (National Conference on Nomenclature of Disease 1933). In 1952 the A.P.A. revised its recommendations and suggested that mental disorders of the senium in which there is evidence of brain damage (as reflected by disorientation, memory loss, and intellectual deficit) be categorized as "Brain Syndrome": acute when it appears to be reversible, chronic when it appears even in part to be irreversible. CBS was further subdivided according to presumed etiology and associated mental conditions, such as disorders of affect or content (American Psychiatric Association 1952).

In analyzing the data of our study, one of our principal aims was to determine what method of diagnostic classification is most highly predictive of mortality and survival. Therefore we rated the subjects in three ways: (1) according to the diagnostic nomenclature popular in 1933; (2) according to the recommendations of 1952; and (3) according to the degree of CBS present: none, mild, moderate, or severe, as determined independently by psychiatric examination and by the two special tests—the MSQ and the FHT.

It is of interest that individuals categorized as having associated disorders of affect or content almost invariably had at most only mild or moderate degrees of brain syndrome; and conversely, persons rated as having severe brain syndrome had no associated disorders of affect or content. These latter were not infrequently called—in the old nomenclature—presbyophrenic, delirious, and confused, or psychiatric with senile deterioration. The differences in death rate of persons categorized in this way are shown in Figure 7-4. Obviously, psychiatric classification is highly predictive of death rate. These categories, however, appear to be related to defects of cognition which can be more directly identified.

When patients are classified according to the degree of intellectual defect measured irrespective of their behavioral disturbance, then prediction is even more precise. Subjects with *mild* CBS exhibited virtually the same age-related mortality as those with no brain syndrome (Figure 7-5). Together, they comprised 43 percent of the sample, and their death rate was substantially below the average, ranging from 10 percent the first year to 71 percent at the end of seven years. Subjects with *moderate* CBS, 31 percent of the sample, had a mortality rate slightly above average. Subjects with *severe* CBS had the highest

87

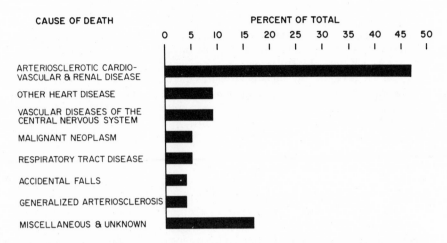

CAUSE OF DEATH · PERCENT OF TOTAL

Figure 7-3. Leading Causes of Death One Year after Examination. Source: Goldfarb, et al., "Predictors of Mortality in the Institutionalized Aged," *Diseases of the Nervous System*, 27:22, January 1966. Used with permission.

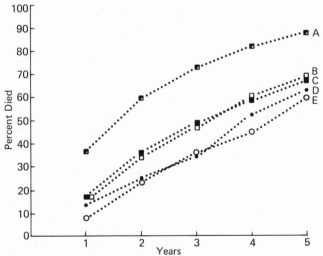

A. Traditional Organic = Presbyophrenic psychosis, delirious and confused and senile deterioration categories, combined
B. Senility or cerebral arteriosclerosis
C. Senility or cerebral arteriosclerosis with disorder of affect or content
D. Disorder of affect or content
E. No psychiatric disorder

Figure 7-4. Psychiatric Category and Mortality.

death rate in the entire sample: 37 percent died during the first year, 60 percent were dead by the end of the second year, only 10 percent survived five years, and just 6 percent were still alive at the end of seven years. These patterns were similar for each type of institution.

As shown in Figure 7-6, the Mental Status questionnaire is a reliable predictor of longevity in old age homes. Similar patterns are shown in the other types of institutions. These patterns vividly demonstrate the usefulness of careful estimate of the degree of CBS in aged persons.

Other Characteristics and Mortality

In Table 7-1 is noted the relationship of a variety of personal characteristics to death rate over the seven-year period. In addition, one factor not listed in the table—nutritional status—was found to be strongly related to mortality. Some 42 percent of the subjects rated "poor" on a three-point nutrition scale were dead within one year. In contrast, when nutritional status was "good" or "fair," the respective death rates within one year were 12 and 30 percent.

Curiously enough, at first glance obesity appeared to be a favorable prognosticator. Subjects rated as obese showed a one-year mortality rate of only 11 percent—essentially the same as those whose nutrition was rated "good." This, however, turned out to be a statistical artifact, which illustrates the necessity for careful evaluation of the kind of data reported here. The obese subjects were few in number and all of them were female; they probably represented the few hardy survivors of a notoriously lethal condition.

Degree of mobility was also related to mortality, although not as strongly. Mobility was classified into three levels: normal or good; fair, decreased, or reduced; and poor, limited, or restricted. The corresponding one-year death rates were 18 percent, 25 percent, and 30 percent.

Blood pressure appeared to be associated with life expectancy, but the many facets of this item and the complexities of the relationships which developed preclude clear-cut conclusions. We can say, however, that in no case was high blood pressure an indicator of poor prognosis; on the contrary, persons with high blood pressure, systolic or diastolic, had a lower than average mortality in each age and sex group examined. Low blood pressure, on the other hand, was associated with a higher than expected mortality, but this relationship was observed only in females, where it was rather strong. Furthermore, the disparity between over-all mortality and mortality of those with low blood pressure increased with advancing age, so that those over 85 years of age with low blood pressure had a mortality rate approximately 50 percent higher than the norm for that age group. Prognosis was worse if both systolic and diastolic pressures were low—less than 140 and 70, respectively—than if only one or the other was below the designated figure. Thus, while hypertension is an unfavorable sign in the general population, the opposite appears to be true in this aged and infirm group. Low blood pressure in this context is probably a sign of general debility, and therefore a harbinger of relatively immediate peril.

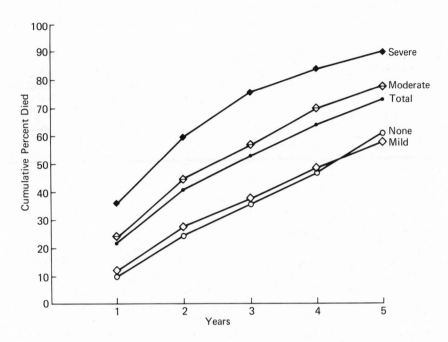

Figure 7-5. Degree of Brain Syndrome and Mortality.

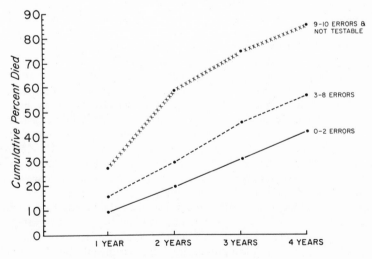

Figure 7-6. MSQ Score and Mortality.

Discussion

In general, the data in this study indicated that evaluation of physical and mental functional status, based on quantifiable methods of examination, may be useful predictors of mortality in institutionalized old people. They also suggest that the lifespan of severely impaired and disabled patients is related more to their physical condition or "viability" than to the type of institution where they reside or to its program, provided, of course, that it provides them with basically adequate shelter, food, and medical care.

Mortality rates by category are not uniform within each of the three types of institutions, however. This may be because (1) the measures of impairment are too gross to differentiate residents who actually differ; or (2) disability rather than impairment is measured—and the latter appears to be greater in nonsupportive milieus than where optimal functioning is encouraged; or (3) because functionally impaired persons fare better or worse in different milieus.

With respect to the last possibility, despite wishes to the contrary, it appears doubtful that giving extra services to aged persons who need protective and supportive care because of marked brain damage, as indicated by severe chronic brain syndrome, materially prolongs their lives. Such services may, however, add immeasurably to their comfort and dignity. On the other hand, old people who are relatively unimpaired mentally may actually live longer in shelters with programs and services which contribute to their pleasure and maintenance of dignity while protecting them from danger and self-neglect.

Three important factors that we have not been able to control for adequately must be taken into account in judging the effectiveness of specific institutions and their programs and services in promoting longevity. These have to do with points in time at which the patient's need for institutionalization is identified and met. How long was he ill? How long has he waited for admission? How long has he been under care?

It often is difficult to determine how long a patient has been ill or impaired. The mentally disturbed individual cannot provide the facts, and families usually are unreliable informants except under skilled and careful questioning. People who apply to old age homes for help must wait the longest for admission. This may account for the higher death rate of some persons in old age homes as compared to seemingly similar patients in nursing homes and state hospitals, where they are promptly admitted in a crisis. Conversely, many "immediately" admitted patients have a high death rate because of acute illness. The death rate in institutions appears to be related, under some circumstances, to the speed of admission; it is low for survivors of long waiting periods which have weeded out the weak, but high for persons admitted rapidly with critical illness.

Length of residence, on the other hand, was related inversely to mortality in all types of institutions. Recent admissions had the highest death rate, when matched for age, compared to those longer in residence. This was particularly true of older subjects. In all age groups, in all institutions, the death rate among residents of less than three months was 35 to 40 percent; but the death rate is related more clearly to age for residents of longer periods as shown in Figure 7-7. These rates probably reflect the fact that many admissions to institutions are precipitated by accidents, exacerbation of illness, or threat of imminent death. Those who weather the initial crisis have a much more favorable outlook.

Nevertheless, some observers feel that institutionalization itself, as a shift from one home and social group to another, often provokes feelings of rejection and resignation and thereby hastens death (Bloom, Blenkner, and Markus 1969; Aldrich and Mendkoff 1963). Attempts to explore the effect of shift from one institution to another (transfer shock) in this study proved difficult and complex. The results strongly suggested that transfer might actually increase the likelihood of earlier death, not so much for psychological reasons as because of the physical condition of the patient. Thus the death rate of persons with severe brain syndrome increased on transfer, while that of individuals with little or no brain syndrome was somewhat lower than expected (Goldfarb, Shahinian, and Turner 1966).

An important finding in this study was the discovery that severity of brain syndrome in the institutionalized aged was closely related to years of education, except in the very old (85 and over). Education has been identified as an excellent index of socioeconomic status, and our data verified the close relationship of occupation and income or financial dependency to both years of education and severity of brain syndrome (Pollack, Goldfarb, and Kahn 1962).

It may be that adverse socioeconomic conditions may contribute to the development of brain damage and the emergence of measurable brain syndrome relatively early in old age, and that longevity is in this way affected by early socioeconomic conditions. This leads to a stimulating hypothesis:

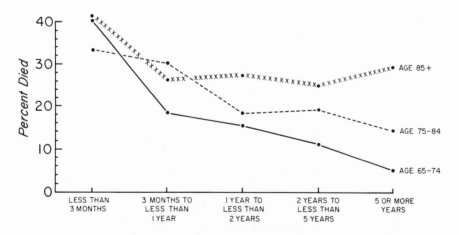

Figure 7-7. Length of Institutional Residence Prior to Examination and Death Rate One Year after Examination, by Age Groups.

In our society, good education early in life may act as a protection against geriatric decline in mental and physical functioning. The sequence may be as follows: poor education makes for socioeconomic deprivation, which contributes to physical illness, which results in chronic invalidism or impairment of function (physical or mental), which ultimately leads to a shorter lifespan. Conversely, good education leads to socioeconomic advantages and protection against illness, accidents, invalidism, and excessive disability.

Thus, while heredity may be an important determinant of longer lifespan, interaction with environment early in life is obviously important if inherited potential is to be achieved. As with other factors, nature is affected by nurture, and each is significant. Longevity may be more closely related to social factors than to medical care. Efforts to prolong human life may, in the long run, depend more on social change than on medical advance.

Viewed in this light, while adequate or excellent institutions can do much to provide for the dignity, comfort, and optimal opportunities for pleasure and self-realization in old age, longevity is more closely related to the relatively early acquisition, and the continual reinforcement through social opportunity, of efficiently adaptive patterns of psychological, social, and emotional functioning. These patterns of adjustment usually become established early in life and usually make the difference between maximum possible life span and premature death.

References

Aldrich, C. and Mendkoff, E.: Relocation of the aged and disabled; a mortality study. *Journal of the American Geriatrics Society*, 11:185-194, 1963.

American Psychiatric Association: Diagnostic and statistical manual of mental disorder. *Manual of Mental Disorder*, Mental Hospital Service, Washington, D.C., 1952.

Bloom, M., Blenkner, M., and Markus, E.: Exploring predictors of the differential impact of relocation on the infirm aged. *Proceedings*, Annual Convention of the American Psychological Association, 1969.

Goldfarb, A.: Seven-year follow-up of fifty-nine patients in a home for the aged. Presented at Annual Meetings of the American Psychiatric Association, May, 1958. (unpublished)

Goldfarb, A.: Prevalence of psychiatric disorders in metropolitan old age and nursing homes. *Journal of the American Geriatrics Society*, 1962.

Goldfarb, A.: The evaluation of geriatric patients following treatment. *In Evaluation of Psychiatric Treatment*, Paul H. Hoch and Joseph Zubin (eds)., Grune and Stratton, 1964, pp. 271-207.

Goldfarb, A., Shahinian, S. and Turner, H.: Death rate in relocated aged residents of nursing homes. Read before the Gerontological Society Annual Meeting in New York, November, 1966. (unpublished)

Goldfarb, A., Fisch, M. and Gerber, I.: Predictors of mortality in the institutionalized aged. *Diseases of the Nervous System*, 27:21-29, 1966.

93

Goldfarb, A.: Predicting mortality in the institutionalized aged, a seven year follow-up. *Archives of General Psychiatry*, 21:172-176, 1969.

Guze, S. and Cantwell, D.: The prognosis in organic brain syndrome. *The American Journal of Psychiatry*, 120:9, March, 1964.

Kahn, R., Goldfarb, A., Pollack, M. and Peck, A.: Brief objective methods for the determination of mental status in the aged. *American Journal of Psychiatry*, 117:326-328, 1960.

Kay, D., and Roth, M.: Physical accompaniments of mental disorder in old age. *Lancet*, pp. 740-745, October 8, 1955.

Kay, D., Norris, V., and Post, F.: Prognosis in psychiatric disorders of the elderly. *Journal of Mental Science*, 102: no. 426, 1956.

Kay, D.: Outcome and cause of death in mental disorders of old age: a long-term follow-up of functions and organic psychoses. *Acta Scandinav.*, 38:249-276, 1962.

National Conference on Nomenclature of Disease: *A Standard Classified Nomenclature of Disease*, H.B. Logie (ed.), New York: Commonwealth Fund, 702 pp., 1933.

Pollack, M., Vahn, R., Gerber, I., and Goldfarb, A.: The relationship of mental and physical status of institutionalized aged persons. *American Journal of Psychiatry*, 117:120-124, 1960.

Pollack, M. Goldfarb, A., and Vahn, R.: Social factors and mental illness in the institutionalized aged person: role of education. *Social and Psychological aspects of aging*, Clark Tibbitts and Wilma Donahue (eds.), New York: Columbia University Press, pp. 606-614, 1962.

Post, F.: The outcome of mental breakdown in old age. *British Medical Journal*, 1:436, 1951.

Post, F.: Mental Disorders in old age; differential diagnosis and management. *The Medical Press*, Modern Treatment in General Practice, Twenty-Fourth Series—Article No. 29, 1957.

Roth, M.: *Proceedings of the Royal Society of Medicine*, 46:963-964, 1953 (Section of Psychiatry, pp. 29-30).

Roth, M.: The natural history of mental disorder in old age. *Journal of Mental Science*, 101, no. 423, 1955.

Roth, M.: Geriatric problems in psychiatry. *Proceedings of the Royal of Medicine*, 48:243-244, 1956. (Section of Psychiatry, pp. 11-12).

Roth, M.: Problems of an aging population. *British Medical Journal*, 1:1226-1230, 1960.

Simon, A., and Tallery, J.: The role of physical illness in geriatric mental disorders. *Psychiatric Disorders in the Aged*, report on the symposium of the World Psychiatric Association of the Royal College of Physicians, London: Geigy Ltd. pp. 154-170, 1965.

8

Brain Impairment and Longevity

HSIOH-SHAN WANG, and ALAN WHANGER

In senescence the brain tends to undergo many changes, of which one common finding is the loss of neurons, the functional cells of the nervous system. It is believed that the total number of neurons in the brain declines almost steadily after the age of 30, in an average person at a rate of 0.8 percent per year (Vogel 1969). There are, however, considerable individual variations. Some elderly may show an abnormally rapid loss of neurons while others may develop different types of histopathological abnormalities in the brain, such as senile plaques or neurofibrillary degeneration, in addition to the neuronal depopulation.

Brain impairment is probably the most prevalent clinical problem in the elderly population. The magnitude of this problem, though difficult to determine exactly, can be illustrated to a great extent by the statistical data that are currently available in the literature. It is estimated that in 1966, 30 percent of the 466,146 resident patients and 17 percent of the 214,493 new admissions to all public and private mental hospitals in the United States were 65 years of age or over (U.S. National Institute of Mental Health, 1968 a and b). Among these elderly, the diagnosis made most commonly was organic brain syndrome, which accounted for 48 percent of the elderly resident patients and 78 percent of the elderly new admissions to these psychiatric facilities. There are also many elderly with brain impairments residing in institutions other than mental hospitals. A survey on the prevalence of chronic conditions and impairments among nursing and personal-care homes in the United States estimated that in 1964, 554,000 were living in these homes and 88 percent of them were over 64 years old (U.S. National Center for Health Statistics 1967). Of these elderly residents, 36 percent were considered to have vascular lesions affecting the central nervous system and 30 percent to have a disorder attributable to senility. Based on these data from mental hospitals and nursing and personal-care homes, it is estimated that 2.3 percent of elderly people in the United States are suffering from brain impairment of sufficient severity to require institutional care (Wang 1969a).

Many elderly with acute cerebral vascular disease are not included in the data from the above mentioned sources. These elderly may die shortly after the onset of the attack, or may remain in the community. Based on data from two

Hsioh-Shan Wang is Assistant Professor of Psychiatry, Duke University, Durham, N.C.

Alan Whanger, M.D. is Associate in Psychiatry, Duke University, Durham, N.C.

population studies for stroke, Kurtzke (1969) demonstrated that the age-specific incidence or attack rates per 1000 elderly population for stroke are approximately twice the respective mortality rates. These stroke rates vary from 8.4 for age 65 to 74, 20.3 for age 75 to 84, to 43.9 for age over 84.

Brain impairments, though of lesser severity, may also be present in elderly persons who have relatively good health and are leading an active life in the community. About one-third of a group of healthy elderly community volunteers studied in a longitudinal project at the Duke Center for the Study of Aging and Human Development were found to have EEG abnormalities and cognitive impairments (Wang 1969b 1970). Some of these elderly also showed neurological evidence of a central nervous system disorder and a reduction of cerebral blood flow.

It is well documented that mortality rates increase with advancing age and that they are dependent on a number of factors. The patterns of extra mortality associated with different medical diseases and impairments have long been an area of interest for life insurance companies. Knowledge about the prognosis and life expectancy of people with various types of diseases or impairments is clearly vital to the physician who treats, to the patient who suffers, to the patient's family, and to those who plan and develop medical services. Many diseases commonly associated with aging, such as myocardial infarction, diabetes mellitus, hypertension, obesity, pulmonary disease, etc., are known to shorten the life span and to increase the mortality rate (Metropolitan Life Insurance Company 1969). In this chapter the relationship between brain impairment and longevity will be discussed.

Longevity in Elderly Persons with Organic Brain Syndrome

Organic brain syndrome is a clinical syndrome characteristically resulting from diffuse impairment of the brain tissue function from whatever cause. Its basic manifestations are memory loss, disorientation, impairment of intellectual function and judgment, as well as shallowness and lability of affect (American Psychiatric Association 1968).

Moderate and severe organic brain syndromes can be readily recognized by the clinical examination in which the patient's behavior and responses toward some questions and tests are evaluated. It is also possible to make a rough estimate of the severity of brain impairment on the basis of such a clinical examination, and such an estimate generally agrees with the histopathological findings (Wang 1971). The usefulness and reliability of the clinical examination becomes rather doubtful, however, in the evaluation of mild brain impairment.

The literature is full of reports on the prognosis of brain impairment in the elderly population. Because many different criteria were employed for both brain impairment and prognosis, the comparison and interpretation of these data are rather difficult. Table 8-1 is a summary of several studies in which the criteria of brain impairment were close to the basic criteria of organic brain syndrome. The survival rates in elderly persons with organic brain syndrome are clearly and consistently lower than those in elderly persons with so-called functional or psychogenic mental disorders at every different point of observation. The decline of survival rate over time is also greater in the organic group than in the functional one. The survival rate of the organics is 92 percent of that of the functionals at three months. It is 71 percent at one year and only 59 percent at the end of three years.

Organic brain syndromes are known to occur frequently in advanced age. That many of these studies did not control for age raises the question whether the differences in survival rates observed between the organic and functional group might be due to age differences. In Corsellis' study, for example, the mean age of onset was estimated to be 45 years for the functional group and 63 years for the organic (1962). Although the mean duration of illness (that is, the

Table 8-1
Survival Rates (in Percent) in Elderly with Organic Brain Syndromes and Functional Psychiatric Disorders

Observation Time (after diagnosis)	Survival Rate in Percent	
	Organic Brain Syndromes Mean (range)	Functional Disorders Mean (range)
1 month (1,2)*	85 (84-86)	94
2 months (1)	81	92
3 months (1,2,7)	76 (75-77)	82.5 (75-90)
6 months (1,7)	67.5 (64-71)	82 (75-89)
1 year (1,2,3,4,7)	56.2 (43-64)	78.7 (65-87)
2 years (1,2,4,5)	49.5 (43-56)	76
3 years (2,4,6)	42.7 (34-54)	73
4 years (2,4)	37.0 (23-51)	
5 years (4)	16.5	
6 years (4)	11.8	
7 years (4)	9.2	

*References 1. Trier 1966
2. Guze 1964
3. Kay 1956
4. Goldfarb 1969
5. Himler 1955
6. Post 1951
7. Isaac 1965

interval from onset to death) was markedly longer in the functional than in the organic (23 years vs. 8 years), the age at death actually was lower in the former than in the latter (68 years vs. 71 years). In order to clarify this issue, Trier (1966) compared two age-matched subgroups from his organic and psychogenic patients. Both subgroups had a mean age of 72.6 years, with an identical standard deviation of 6.1 years. He found that, on measures of outcome, when matched by age, the subgroups generally showed slightly smaller differences than when not matched by age. These two age-matched subgroups were not statistically different in terms of outcomes in the initial period but their outcomes did show statistically significant differences at all subsequent points in time: i.e., the functional disorders had move favorable outcome.

Longevity in Elderly Persons with Different
Types of Brain Impairment

Many disorders or diseases can cause brain impairment in aged persons. The most important ones are (1) cerebral vascular disease, (2) degenerative disease primarily involving the brain, and (3) metabolic disorders that originate outside the brain.

Cerebral vascular diseases, based on their clinical picture, can be classified as focal or generalized. The focal form is characterized by its acute onset and the presence of rather discrete neurological symptoms and signs indicating a disturbance of those functions that are directly dependent on the activity of the brain tissue involved. In the generalized form of cerebral vascular disease, there is a relatively insidious development of a diffuse reduction of cerebral blood flow which leads to an extensive impairment of the brain tissue. Its clinical picture is basically the same as that of some of the cerebral degenerative diseases, such as senile dementia. The clinical differentiation between the generalized cerebral vascular disease and senile dementia, though possible, is rather difficult and unreliable. Not infrequently both may occur in the same individual.

Traditionally, the degenerative diseases that primarily involve the brain in senescence are grouped into senile or presenile dementia. In the latter, the two most important clinicopathological entities are Alzheimer's and Pick's disease. The clinical differentiation of these three types of brain disease is rather difficult. As a rule, the onset of presenile dementia is earlier, usually in the fities, than that of senile dementia, which as a rule begins in the seventies. Many authors consider Alzheimer's disease to be a severe and earlier variety of senile dementia that tends to follow a rapid course. Focal neurological findings, such as aphasia, apraxia, agnosia, etc., are more frequent in presenile than in senile dementia. Because of the similarity in focal neurological findings and age of onset, the differentiation between Alzheimer's and Pick's disease is extremely difficult. In Pick's disease, in which the brain impairment is generally circumscribed to the frontal lobe or temporal lobe, symptoms typifying a lesion of this area are more common than in Alzheimer's disease. Pick's disease, especially in its early stage, is usually associated with a relatively well-preserved memory, while in Alzheimer's disease there is a rapid and global deterioration (Ferraro 1959). A more reliable differentiation of these common degenerative diseases in senescence has therefore to depend on pneumoencephalographic or histopathological examination.

Many metabolic disorders originating outside of the brain may adversely affect the function of brain tissue. These include, for example, diabetes mellitus and many diseases of the heart, lung, kidney, and liver. The prominent clinical manifestations related to the brain are disturbance of consciousness and disorientation, with or without concurrent impairment of cognitive functioning. This syndrome is commonly called acute confusional state or acute brain syndrome, due to its reversibility when the causative disorder is corrected. Nonetheless, it is widely believed that the acute confusional state in elderly persons usually represents a beginning of a reduction in reserve capacities of the brain and may subsequently lead to permanent structural alteration in the brain.

There are numerous studies on prognosis after stroke. The data from these studies vary considerably due, to a great extent, to a difference in the demographic and pathological characteristics of the sample studied and the time of observation after the onset of stroke. In an extensive review of the literature related to this issue, Ford and Katz (1966) stated that mortality from stroke during the first two weeks after the onset probably exceeds 25 percent and may approach 50 percent for unselected major stroke. They also showed that the mortality of those who survive the initial episode is 7 to 35 percent for the first year, and increases steadily to 38 to 66 percent by the end of five years. Only a few studies have compared the mortality of patients with stroke with that of others of the same age. Adams and Merrett (1961) and Robinson and his co-workers (1959) showed that the mortality rate in stroke patients is greater than that in the general population of comparable ages while, in contrast, Pincock (1957) and Eisenberg and his co-workers (1964) failed to find any significant difference between these two rates.

There are very few studies on the longevity of elderly persons with generalized cerebrovascular brain disease, probably due to the difficulty in confirming such diagnosis clinically and to the frequent concurrence of this condition and senile dementia. Based on the work by Roth (1955) and Kidd (1962), it is estimated that there are about 50 percent more survivals in cerebral arteriosclerosis than in senile dementia during the first two years of the illness. The survival rate for cerebral arteriosclerosis is about one-half of that for affective disorders. It is greater than that for confusional state at six months and one year, but is only one-half of the confusional state survival at the end of two years. This finding suggests that among elderly persons with acute confusional state, those surviving the first year may have a relatively good prognosis.

Several studies in which the ages at onset and at death were reported and the type of pathology was determined by clinical and/or histopathological examination are summarized in Table 8-2. The expected years remaining were derived according to the age of onset in each subgroup from the 1968 Life Table

Table 8-2
Longevity in Different Brain Diseases

Brain Disease	Source	N	Age at Onset	Age at Death	Remaining Years Observed	Remaining Years Expected
I. Senile Dementia	Larsson, 1963	377	74.5	79.6	5.2	9.6
	Epstein, 1964	12	72.0	78.0	6.0	10.6
	Corsellis, 1962	35	71.0	77.0	4.6	11.1
Total		424	74.1	79.3	5.1	9.6
II. Presenile Dementia						
Alzheimer's Disease	Sjogren, 1952	18	53.1	60.2	7.1	23.1
Pick's Disease	Sjogren, 1952	18	54.5	61.2	6.7	22.3
Pick-Alzheimer Syndrome	Sjogren, 1952	29	56.4	62.4	5.7	20.6
Pick-Alzheimer Syndrome	Sjogren, 1952	15	56.1	65.2	8.3	20.6
Total		80	55.2	61.8	6.8	21.5
III. Arteriosclerotic Brain Disease	Epstein, 1964	11	66.0	69.0	3.0	14.0
	Corsellis, 1962	46	67.0	72.0	4.0	13.4
Total		57	66.8	71.4	3.8	14.0

(Metropolitan Life Insurance Company 1970). There are no significant differences among the four subgroups in presenile dementia. The ages of onset and death are youngest in presenile dementia, while the years remaining are least among those with arteriosclerotic brain disease and are only 27 percent of the expected duration. In other words, at the onset of illness, the expected life span of a patient is shortened by 73 percent in arteriosclerotic brain disease, 68 percent in presenile dementia, and 47 percent in senile dementia. This is in contradiction to Roth's and Kidd's observation.

Longevity in the Community Elderly with Brain Impairment

Although brain impairments of different types and severity are common among elderly persons who are living an active life in the community, there has been almost no report on the relationship of brain impairment and longevity in these community elderly. This is obviously due to a lack of measures for the evaluation of mild brain impairment. The clinical syndrome resulting from such mild brain impairment is difficult to detect by clinical examination. Most measures that are available for evaluation of brain status are rather traumatic and involve considerable risk. They are therefore not practical nor medically justified for use routinely on elderly persons who are apparently in good health. These traumatic methods include histopathological examination of brain tissue by biopsy, pneumoencephalographic evaluation of the brain structure, determination of cerebral oxygen consumption, angiographic study of the cerebral vascular system, and determination of cerebral blood flow by the nitrous oxide inhalation method or by the carotid injection method using a radioisotope. Many psychological tests may help to detect the cognitive impairment associated with brain impairment, but their relationships with longevity will be discussed in other chapters of this book.

The only nontraumatic method which has been established as reliable and sensitive in the evaluation of brain status and which can be used routinely is electroencephalography (EEG). It has been documented that abnormal EEG, usually characterized by a slowing of the dominate alpha rhythm and by the presence of slow waves in the theta or delta range, are very common among elderly patients with various brain diseases, including senile or presenile dementia, arteriosclerotic brain disease, and brain disturbance secondary to a variety of metabolic disorders originating outside the brain (Busse and Wang 1965). Several investigators found that patients with such EEG diffuse slowing had a higher mortality and/or a shorter life span than patients with normal EEG or only focal abnormality limited to the anterior temporal region (Obrist and Henry 1958; Cahan and Yeager 1966; McAdam and Robinson 1957).

However, EEG slowing can also occur in some elderly community residents having excellent health (Wang 1969b). Its value in predicting prognosis in a community group, particularly their longevity, is almost unknown. In a longitudinal study on a group of residents in a home for the aged, Obrist and his co-workers (1961) did find that the decline of occipital alpha frequency over time was greater in those who died earlier.

At the Duke University Center for the Study of Aging and Human Development, a group of community elderly volunteers was recruited to participate in a longitudinal project in which they were given a two-day examination by a multi-disciplinary team every two to three years. Many of these subjects recently completed the sixth examination, which occurred twelve to fifteen years after the initial one. Over half of the initial group had died during this interval.

Two indicators of longevity were employed. The Longevity Index (LI) is the total number of years from initial study to death (Chapter 18). For living subjects, the LI is the number of years from initial examination to the sixth examination, plus the expected number of years remaining at the sixth examination, obtained from the actuarial life expectancy table. The Longevity Quotient (LQ) is the ratio between LI and the actuarially expected number of years remaining after the initial examination. An LQ of greater than one means that the elderly person lived longer than expected, and an LQ of less than one means that he lived shorter than expected.

Based on findings from the clinical neurological examination, the 258 subjects were grouped as follows: (1) no central nervous system disorder (N=221), (2) cerebral disorder only (N=15), (3) extracerebral disorder only, i.e., disorder of diencephalon, brain stem, or cerebellum (N=18), and (4) both cerebral and extracerebral disorder (N=4). The normal group (1) had a mean LI of 13.5 years and a mean LQ of 1.16. As compared with the normal subjects, those having extracerebral disorder, with or without a concomitant cerebral disorder (groups 3 and 4) had a small LI (7.9) and a low LQ (0.71), while those with only cerebral disorder (group 2) had a LI of 8.5 (because they were older), but a LQ of 1.21, which is about the same as for group 1.

Two-hundred and twenty-five of these subjects had measurable rhythms in their EEG occipital tracings. The mean frequency of these EEG rhythms (i.e., dominant frequency) for each individual was measured manually (Wang 1969b). The correlation between dominant frequency and LI, as anticipated, was equal but in the opposite direction to that between dominant frequency and age (r=0.367 and −0.371 respectively). Both were much greater than the correlation between dominant frequency and LQ (r=0.172).

The slowing of EEG dominant frequency generally indicates the presence of a cerebral disorder. The findings from the Duke longitudinal project suggest that elderly persons having evidence of cerebral disorder on EEG or neurological examination can be expected to die sooner than those with no evidence of any central nervous system disorder. However, because the former individuals tend to be older than the latter, the difference in survival may largely be due to their greater age rather than to their brain disorder. This hypothesis is supported by the finding that elderly persons with such a cerebral disorder may live as long as those of comparable age in the general population. Extracerebral disorders are clearly associated with a short survival and a short life span.

Discussion

Brain impairments are clearly common among elderly persons living in institutions as well as those having relatively good health in the community. Although the data from the literature consistently demonstrates that brain impairments are usually associated with a decreased longevity, the interpretation of these data requires extreme caution. One should not expect such an association in every old person having evidence of brain impairment, because variations are common among different types of brain impairment and among individuals having the same type of impairment.

Brain impairments in old age seem to fall into two groups. One group consists of those with the cerebral disorders commonly seen among older community residents and among most senile dementia. This group is characterized by its relatively late onset. Old persons having these brain impairments probably will live about as long as other persons their age. These brain impairments can therefore be considered to be closely related to physiological aging. The other group is characterized by its early onset and includes those with presenile dementia, disorders of the diencephalon, brain stem, or cerebellum and probably generalized arteriosclerotic brain disease and acute confusional state. These brain impairments are clearly pathological conditions of old age because they are usually associated with a shortened survival (LI) as well as a shortened life expectancy (LQ). The chronological age at the onset of brain impairment as a rule can therefore serve as an indicator of its prognosis.

Another important question is *why* brain impairments affect longevity. The literature provides no clear explanation of this matter. It is speculated that the general health of elderly persons having brain impairment may be an important factor. It has been shown that there is a close association between physical illness and brain impairment (Kahn, Pollack, and Goldfarb 1961; Trier 1966). Physical illness may be the cause of, or may only be the concomitant of brain impairment. It is also possible that various systems of the body, such as the cardiovascular system may be adversely affected by an impairment or lesion of the brain (Hoff, Kell, and Carroll 1963). Elderly persons with brain impairment also usually show intellectual deterioration that may lead to inadequacy of personal care (such as nutrition, hygiene, self-protection) which, in turn, leads to physical illness or injury. The fatalistic attitude and palliative approach that commonly prevail among many laymen and professionals who serve and care for elderly patients with brain impairment or marked dementia in certain institutions may also play an important role. Many elderly patients in these institutions do not have as adequate treatment, care, and/or socialization as they could have. In contrast, some patients may be "over-treated" with too many and too large doses of sedatives or psychotropic drugs in order that they can be managed easily. Many of these drugs are known to be capable of depressing brain function or lowering blood pressure, which may in turn lead to a further reduction of cerebral blood flow, particularly in the presence of severe cerebral arteriosclerosis. More careful studies are clearly needed to clarify the role of these and other related factors in order to have a clearer understanding of the relationship between brain impairment and longevity.

References

Adams, C., and Merrett, J.D.: Prognosis and survival in the aftermath of hemiplegia. *Brit. Med. J.*, 1:52222, 1961.
American Psychiatric Association: Diagnostic and Statistical Manual of Mental Disorders (2d ed.) Washington, D.C.: American Psychiatric Association, 1968.
Busse, E., and Wang, H.: The value of electroencephalography in geriatrics. *Geriatrics*, 20:906, 1965.
Cahan, R. and Yeager, C.: Admission EEG as a predictor of mortality and discharge for aged state hospital patients. *Journal of Geront.*, 21:248, 1966.
Corsellis, J.: *Mental Illness and the Aging Brain*. London: Oxford University Press, 1962.

Eisenberg, H., Morrison, J., Sullivan, P., and Foote, F.: Cerebrovascular accidents, incidence and survival rates in a defined population, Middlesex County, Connecticut. *J.A.M.A.*, 189:883, 1964.

Epstein, L., Simon, A., and Mock, R.: Clinical neuropathologic correlations in senile and cerebral arteriosclerotic psychoses. In Hansen, P. (ed.), *Old Age With A Future*. Copenhagen: Munksgaard, pp. 272-275, 1964.

Ferraro, A.: Presenile psychoses. In Arieti, S., (ed.), *American Handbook of Psychiatry*. Vol. 2, New York: Basic Books, pp. 1046-1077, 1959.

Ford, A. and Katz, S.: Prognosis after strokes, part I. A critical review. *Medicine*, 45:223, 1966.

Goldfarb, A.: Predicting mortality in the institutionalized aged. *Arch. Gen. Psychiat.*, 21:177, 1969.

Guze, S. and Cantwell, D.: The prognosis in "organic brain" syndromes. *Am. J. Psychiat.*, 120:878, 1964.

Himler, L.: Factors influencing prognosis in psychiatric illness of the aged. *In Old Age in the Modern World*, Edinburgh: Livingstone, pp. 466-472, 1955.

Hoff, E., Kell, J., Jr., Carroll, M., Jr.: Effects of cortical stimulation and lesions on cardiovascular function. *Physiological Reviews*, 43:68, 1963.

Issac, B.: Prognostic factor in elderly patients in geriatric institution. *Geront. Clin.*, 7:202, 1965.

Kahn, R., Pollack, M. and Goldfarb, A.: Factors related to individual differences in mental status of institutionalized aged. Hoch, P. and Zubin, J. (eds.), *Psychopathology of Aging*, New York: Grune & Stratton, pp. 104-113, 1961.

Kay, D., Norris, V. and Post, F.: Prognosis in psychiatric disorders of the elderly. *J. Ment. Sci.*, 102:129, 1956.

Kidd, C.: Old people in mental hospital: a study in diagnostic composition and outcome. *Irish J. Med. Sci.*, 6:434, 1962.

Kurtzke, J.: *Epidemiology of Cerebrovascular Disease*. New York: Springer-Verlag, 1969.

Larsson, T., Sjogren, T. and Jacobson, G.: Senile dementia, a clinical sociomedical and genetic study. *Acta Psychiat. Scandinav.* suppl. 167, 1963.

McAdam, W. and Robinson, R.: Prognosis in senile deterioration. *J. Ment. Sci.*, 103:821-823, 1957.

Metropolitan Life Insurance Co.: Patterns of extra mortality for the common impairments. *Statistical Bulletin*, November, 1969.

Metropolitan Life Insurance Co.: American Longevity in 1968. *Statistical Bulletin*, August, 1970.

Obrist, W. and Henry, C.: Electroencephalographic findings in aged psychiatric patients. *J. Nev. Ment. Dis.*, 126:254, 1958.

Obrist, W., Henry, C. and Justiss, W.: Longitudinal study of EEG in old age. *Excerpta Medica*, International Congress Series No. 37: 168, 1961.

Pincock, J.: The natural history of cerebral thrombosis. *Annals Int. Med.*, 46:925, 1957.

Post, F.: The outcome of mental breakdown in old age. *Brit. Med. J.*, i:436, 1951.

Robinson, R., Cohen, W., Higano, N., Meyer, R., Lukowsky, G., McLaughlin, R. and MacGilpin, H., Jr.: Life-table analysis of survival after cerebral thrombosis-ten-year experience. *J.A.M.A.*, 169:1149, 1959.

Roth, M.: The natural history of mental disorder in old age. *J. Ment. Sci.*, 101:281, 1955.

Sjogren, T., Sjogren, H. and Lindgren, A.: Morbus Alzheimer and Morbus Pick. *Acta Psychiat. Nerol. Scandinav.* Suppl. 82, 1952.

Trier, T.: Characteristics of mentally ill aged: a comparison of patients with organic brain syndromes. *J. Geront.*, 21:354, 1966.

U.S. National Center for Health Statistics: *Prevalence of Chronic Conditions and Impairments Among Residents of Nursing and Personal Care Homes–United States*, May-June, 1964. P.H.S. Publication No. 1000, Series 12, No. 8, Washington, D.C.: U.S. Government Printing Office, 1967.

U.S. National Institute of Mental Health: *Patients in Mental Institutions*, 1966, Part II, State and County Hospitals, P.H.S. Publication No. 1818. Washington, D.C.: U.S. Government Printing Office, 1968a.

U.S. National Institute of Mental Health: *Patients in Mental Institutions*, 1966, Part III. Private Mental Hospitals and General Hospitals with Psychiatric Service, P.H.S. Publication No. 1818, Washington, D.C.: U.S. Government Printing Office, 1968b.

Vogel, F.: The brain and time. In Busse, E. and Pfeiffer, E., eds. *Behavior and Adaptation in Late Life* Boston: Little, Brown, pp. 251-262, 1959.

Wang, H.: Organic brain syndromes. In Busse, E. and Pfeiffer, E., eds. *Behavior and Adaptation in Late Life*, Boston: Little, Brown, pp. 263-287, 1969a.

Wang, H. and Busse, E.: EEG of healthy old persons—a longitudinal study. I. Dominant background activity and occipital rhythm. *J. Geront.*, 24:419, 1969b.

Wang, H., Obrist, W. and Busse, E.: Neurophysiological correlates of the intellectual function of elderly persons living in the community. *Amer. J. Psychiat.*, 126:39, 1970.

Wang, H.: The brain and intellectual function in senescence. In Jarvik, L. and Rhudich, P. eds., *Aging: Psychological and Somatic Changes*, 1971 (in press).

Part III
Psychological Predictors

Samuel Granick begins this section by surveying the available evidence that cognitive functioning is a strong predictor of longevity, particularly among the aged and the institutionalized. He suggests that declines in cognitive functioning may be early warnings of declines in biological functioning and a direct cause of health deterioration.

Bartko, Patterson, and Butler report that among a group of healthy aged males, who have been studied for over eleven years, the two strong and significant predictors of survival were highly organized behavior and the avoidance of smoking. Another behavioral variable of significance was that of mental status.

In a longitudinal study of normal aged persons in Germany, Klaus Riegel found that the most persistent predictors of longevity among the younger aged (55-64 at the beginning of the study) are subjective health ratings, while for the older age group (65 and over) the most consistent predictors are ratings of physical activities. He concludes that chances for survival among older aged persons are dependent upon the opportunities and engagement in activities which, in turn, might guarantee a good maintenance of intellectual abilities. He also finds strong evidence for a "terminal drop" in performance and behavior within five years prior to death.

Baer and Gaitz report that among elderly psychiatric patients, survival is most closely related to physical functioning capacity, with the second most important predictor being cognitive impairment. They also present evidence that the greater mortality among patients who became institutionalized was primarily due to the fact that they were less healthy, rather than to the effects of institutionalization itself. In another study of institutionalized aged and of aged awaiting entrance into homes for the aged, Morton Lieberman found that a combination of 15 psychological indices yielded a discriminate function that correctly classified 90 percent of the persons awaiting institutionalization into "survivors" and "non-survivors." He found that the four strongest predictors were cognitive malfunction, self-care ability, time extension, and passive-aggressive personality traits, even when other factors were statistically controlled. Among those already institutionalized, attitudes toward life, attitudes toward the future, and the interviewer ratings on transactions with the subjects were the three strongest predictors of survival.

David Gutmann found evidence that a passive-dependent type personality was related to greater illness and shorter life span among the Navajo and the Druze. Jarvik and Blum conclude this section with evidence from a unique study of twins (which controls for heredity), that a "critical loss" in cognitive functioning is a powerful predictor of mortality; but that decreasing scores on speeded motor tasks do not predict mortality.

Cognitive Aspects of Longevity

SAMUEL GRANICK

The recognition of a possible relationship between longevity and cognitive functioning is a fairly recent matter. No references to this subject, for example are contained in Cowdrey's (1942) extensive collection of papers which summarize and discuss the gerontological research and clinical literature. Later reviews also, such as those by Lorge (1944), Granick (1950), Shock (1951), and Lorge (1956), which focus particularly on the psychological research of later maturity, fail to deal with this area. Similarly, the several chapters in Birren's *Handbook of Aging and the Individual* (1959) which explore intellectual, perceptual and psychomotor functioning of the aged, do not mention it.

Systematic treatment of cognitive processes in relation to survival and the life span appears first to have been presented by Botwinick (1967). His discussion is quite brief, reflecting the very limited amount of research and consideration given to the subject up to that point. He provides some additional references in a later review (1970), but all told less than a dozen reports are involved, and only about half a dozen actual research studies. A further search of the literature by the present author has not brought to light any other attempt to organize the available information or to analyze and discuss it in a systematic fashion. Some additional research evidence, however, is available, along with related considerations of its significance in understanding the behavior and adjustments of the aged.

The presentation below aims to provide an up to date review of available research evidence on the relationships between cognitive functioning and survival. An effort will also be made to relate the results to other areas of functioning of the elderly, such as their medical status and psychosocial adjustments. In addition, an attempt will be made to suggest the kinds of research which would be desirable in order to broaden as well as to deepen our knowledge and understanding of this aspect of gerontology.

Cognition and Biological Status

The basis for survival of the human organism rests, of course, in the biological integrity of the individual and his continued ability to resist and avoid pathology

Samuel Granick is Director of Research, Community Mental Health Program, Philadelphia Psychiatric Center.

and varied destructive circumstances. Within the framework of his genetic makeup, which may be responsible for his rate of aging and eventual breakdown of vital processes, the ability to avoid disease and suppress factors which may cause premature death is of crucial importance. In this respect cognitive functioning is a central factor in enabling the individual to live intelligently, handle his experiences realistically and constructively, and take advantage of all that is known and available to him to maintain his health, growth, and favorable life circumstances. He might thus be successful in carrying on effectively throughout his normal life span.

Cognitive functioning is also particularly significant in revealing much that is vital about the status of an individual's central nervous system. Psychological tasks calling for perceptual operations, analytic and synthetic thinking, new learning, use of stored information, visual-motor productions of varied geometric concepts, and effective demonstration of other types of intellectual skills, test the integrity and efficiency of the CNS. These tasks are sensitive to many kinds of dislocations in brain functioning and tend to reflect the deleterious effects of advanced aging, as well as of pathological conditions on brain functioning. In view of the central importance of the CNS in maintaining and operating the vital systems within the organism, its relationship to longevity is self-evident. Cognitive functions may, thus, serve as significant indicators of the relative health of the individual and provide a basis for gauging the probable extent of his continued survival.

A third feature of cognition in relation to longevity is the possible association of level of intellectual endowment in the organism with a comparable genetically determined life span. This is an intriguing feature of scientific investigation which is related to studies in child development on the intercorrelations between mental and biological capabilities. Particularly relevant are the studies by Terman (1943) and Terman and Oden (1959). They demonstrated significant positive correlations between mental and physical abilities in children of superior intelligence which were well maintained as they grew up and moved into adulthood. A lower mortality rate than for the general population was noted for these subjects also. The hypothesis thus suggests itself that the cognitive capacities of the individual may be related to his physical survival potential, leading one to anticipate that the longevous portion of the population is likely to be the most intellectually gifted.

Mental Ability and Survival

One of the earliest indications of the possibility that length of life might be related to cognitive capabilities and functioning is suggested by the widely recognized and reported relationship between longevity and occupational level (Spiegelman 1966; Guralnick 1959; Quint and Cody 1970). The more intellectually demanding occupations, such as the professions, administrative and technical work, were found consistently to be associated with higher survival rates than the semiskilled, laborer, and agricultural areas. Until recently, this was not attributed to cognitive factors, however, but rather to socioeconomic status, and the extra health hazards imposed on individuals who work at physically strenuous jobs and who live within relatively limited financial means.

As working and economic conditions have improved for blue collar and unskilled workers, on the other hand, mortality among individuals in these occupations have dropped considerably and moved closer to those of people in the white collar occupations. Although the inverse relationship between mortality and social class continues to be demonstrated in statistical reports, the possibility now presents itself that factors other than financial and varied environmental conditions may, in part at least, be involved.

Quint and Cody (1970) call attention to a Metropolitan Life Insurance Company study (1932), which is apparently one of the earliest reports relating longevity to intellectual capabilities. This investigation found college graduates as a group to have a greater life expectancy at age 47 by somewhat over a year than white males in the sample surveyed during the years 1919-1920. Quite significantly, moreover, college "honor men" at this age showed a life expectancy of a year and a half above that of the college graduate group. This difference between the college "honor men" and all the college graduates was maintained with advancing years until age 67, when it narrowed to less than a year. The question was raised by the investigators as to whether "mental and physical fitness tend to go together."

This matter was pursued much further by Quint and Cody (1970) in their investigation of longevity among men listed in the 1950-1951 edition of *Who's Who in America*. A twelve-year follow-up study of 6,329 distinguished professional business and professional men, representing a one-sixth sample of the total group listed in the volume, demonstrated that they outlived white men of comparable age in the American population by a considerable extent. Moreover, their survival ratio was also significantly higher than that reported by insurance companies for their standard ordinary life insurance policy holders. Further comparisons between these eminent men and their occupational colleagues also showed them to have a relative mortality rate which was remarkably low. Thus, for the period 1950 to 1961 the mortality ratio was only 57 percent for the *Who's Who* sample of ages 45 to 64, as compared to all white men in the same occupations in the United States in the year 1950.

Within the *Who's Who* sample there was much variability of relative mortality rates. Correspondents and journalists showed the lowest life span; business executives were average; educators were among the longer lived of the group; and the highest longevity was experienced by the eminent scientists. It is not certain as to whether one group of eminent men was superior to any other in their cognitive capacities. Yet it does seem reasonable to suggest that in comparison with their occupational colleagues, the men of the *Who's Who* sample were probably of higher intellectual capacities. Some support is thus provided for the hypothesis of a positive relationship between cognitive endowment and survival or life span.

A somewhat related bit of evidence is provided by a recent investigation by Hinkle and his co-workers (1968) on the relationship between education and the incidence of coronary heart disease in men engaged in similar occupations. The subjects for this study were the 270,000 men employed in the Bell System Operating Companies throughout continental United States. Incidence or rate of disabling coronary heart disease (thus decreasing their survival potential) was found to be consistently lower for managers and executives than for workmen and foremen. Particularly significant also was the discovery that men who entered the organization with a college degree had a lower coronary attack rate, disability rate, and death rate "at every age, in every part of the country, and in all departments of the organization" than the men of lesser education. The researchers interpret these differences in terms of probable better biological make up of the higher educated group which is "related to, but not necessarily the result of, differences in social and eocnomic background from which they originated."

This appears to be a valid evaluation of the significance of the results, but it may not represent the full story. The probability of relatively higher general intellectual endowment on the part of the better educated men would seem to be a reasonable additional factor to be considered. An association is thus suggested between level of cognitive capacities and biological integrity, with a consequent related effect on life span.

Several research investigations provide somewhat more direct, though not definitive evidence of a positive correlation between cognitive capacities and longevity. Earlier mention was made of the study by Terman and Oden (1959) of the relatively lower mortality rate of their intellectually gifted subjects by the time they reached middle age as compared to the general population. In a longitudinal study of 134 twin pairs starting when they were 60 years of age or over, the more intellectually capable subjects at the initial testing survived after a six year period (Falek, Kallmann, Lorge and Jarvik 1960; Jarvik, Kallmann and Falek 1962). Riegel, Riegel and Meyer (1967) noted related results in their study of a group of 380 male and female subjects of age 55 and above, drawn from a representative sample of the north German population (see also Chapter 11). Five years after the initial examinations, 62 subjects were deceased. For the group which ranged in age between 55 and 64 years, the survivors had scored significantly higher on verbal type tests such as antonyms and analogies. This was not evident, however, for the group of subjects above age 64. Also no differences were found between survivors and the deceased on their general intelligence test scores.

Evidence, based on an extensive sample of subjects from the New England population, supporting a positive correlation between cognitive capabilities and life span is provided by Rose (1964). The characteristics of a group of 149 surviving veterans of the Spanish-American War as of 1959, ranging in age from 72 to 92, were studied with respect to their possible relevance to longevity. Among the striking findings was the relatively high level of intelligence, education and occupational status of the group as compared to their contemporaries. It was noted particularly that the educational level of the veterans was equivalent to that of all others of their age group in the United States population, according to the 1950 Census. They were, however, much higher than the average of the population in 1890, thus reflecting a positive relationship between education and their own longevity, as well as for that of the aged population in general in 1950.

Palmore provides additional impressive evidence along the above lines in his analysis of data from a longitudinal study conducted at Duke University with a group of 268 men and women noninstitutional residents of central North Carolina (Chapter 18). The group ranged in age from 60 to 94, with a median of 70. Evaluation of their longevity status was made thirteen years after the initial examination of their cognitive, physical, and social-personal functioning. For the survivors after the thirteen-year span, longevity was estimated by adding that period to the expected survival period based on actuarial tables. For the nonsurvivors, of course, longevity was the actual number of years lived after the initial examination. Unlike other studies, the two groups were not directly compared on the various cognitive and other measures, since the purpose of the statistical analysis was to derive a basis for predicting longevity from the patterns of functioning shown by the examination results. (This will be further discussed below.) The correlation analysis, however, demonstrated that level of cognitive functioning, particularly as measured by the performance section of the Wechsler Adult Intelligence Scale (WAIS), was significantly associated with longevity. Of the 38 variables selected for the correlation study, the weighted performance score proved to be the "third highest factor related to longevity."

Data from the same study were used by Pfeiffer (Chapter 17) to compare the mental functioning of a relatively long-lived group of 37 men and women, matched for age and sex, with a group of 37 subjects who were among the earliest to die after the initial examination. On both the verbal and performance sections of the WAIS the group of relatively long-lived subjects scored significantly higher than the subjects with a shorter life span. It was noted also that the more intelligent group had a significantly higher mean level of schooling.

All of the above studies allude to the probability that intellectual endowment may be positively related to general biological or physical capacity. This is quite clearly noted in the Terman (1943) study of intellectually gifted children and the followup investigation 35 years later by Terman and Oden (1959). The report by Hinkle and his co-workers (1968) also supports this notion, thus favoring the hypothesis that longevity and cognitive capacities are correlated. In the comparative studies of the cognitive functioning of the short- versus the long-lived subjects, however, control of physical health was not reported as being closely or clearly achieved. This was not actually attempted or considered in some of the investigations. In the Duke University study Palmore reported the physical functioning rating (based on a medical examination and history) to have the second highest correlation with longevity, the actuarial life expectancy tables being the most highly correlated of all the variables studied (Chapter 18).

Pfeiffer did compare his two study groups directly on the objective measure of physical status and found them incompletely matched (Chapter 17). For the females the matching was good, there being no difference in physical status between the long- and short-lived subjects. The long-lived males, on the other hand, were rated as somewhat healthier than the males of shorter life span. Accordingly, despite the considerable consistency in the results on the relationship between cognitive functioning and longevity, a reasonable doubt remains. Health may be the responsible factor for both extended life span of the subjects as well as their relatively superior cognitive performance or achievement over their shorter lived contemporaries.

One investigation is available which does cast some clarifying light on the matter, since a definite and careful effort was made to control the variable of medical status. The investigation by Birren and his co-workers (1963) on a group of 47 men, mean age 71.5 and ranging between 65 and 91 years, focused particularly on controlling the factor of physical health in their study of biological and behavioral functioning in the aged (see also Chapter 10). All subjects were selected on the basis of very careful and extensive medical examinations and judged to be free of significant physical pathology. A variety of tests was then administered covering the biological, psychological, social psychological and psychiatric areas. In the psychological area an extensive array of cognitive and perceptual tests was included. Since two follow-up studies were conducted on the subjects, it was possible to compare the survivors versus the nonsurvivors, matched for health status when originally tested, at each period for their relative performances on the initial testing. Birren (1964) reported the first follow-up five years after the initial testing at which time 34 were still alive and 13 had died. In comparing the scores of these two groups on the WAIS and the Raven Progressive Matrices Test of Intelligence, the survivors were uniformly and significantly superior. A set of five factors had been derived in the original investigation by an Hotelling Principal Component analysis of 32 intercorrelated scores on cognitive and perceptual tests. On two of these factors, labeled "Information Achievement" and "Concept and Stimulus Orientation," the survivors were found to be significantly higher than those who had died within the five-year span. No differences between the groups were found on the factors labeled "Eumeration Speed," "Set Flexibility," and "Speed Association."

At the time of the second follow-up study, after eleven years, the surviving group consisted of 23 men; and 24 were no longer alive. Reports by Granick and Birren (1969) and Granick (1971) confirmed and extended the above findings. Results on the WAIS and the Raven Progressive Matrices were in the same direction. Only the Information Achievement factor was significantly superior for the surviving group, however, on this occasion. The other factor differences favored the survivors, but they were not large enough to attain statistical significance. On the other hand, an array of other cognitive tests also showed higher quality functioning by the group which survived after the eleven years. These included the Draw-a-Person Test (scored according to the Goodenough criteria), Rorschach (rating of responses as to quality of formal characteristics, mainly of a cognitive and perceptual nature), Wisconsin Card Sorting (number of concepts achieved) and the Mill Hill Vocabulary Test.

Cognitive Functioning in the Prediction of Mortality

Awareness on the part of clinicians and researchers of the intimate relationship between cognitive functioning and the integrity of the CNS appears to have led to studies on prediction of longevity in two areas: (a) the association of mortality in the aged with a short term significant decline in cognitive performance, and (b) the estimation of life span by means of formulas derived from the relationships between longevity and various functional characteristics of middle aged and older adults, cognition being one of these characteristics.

A number of investigators have noted that in carrying through longitudinal studies on the aged, the initially less capable or less intelligent subjects tend to drop out and cannot be retested because of death and severe physical disability. Associated with this has been the recognition that some elderly subjects decline considerably in their intellectual functioning whereas others display little or no decline. Kleemeier (1961; 1962) appears to have been the first to be sufficiently impressed by these considerations to focus on the possibility of a meaningful relationship between a deterioration of intellectual abilities and the nearness of mortality, particularly when this deterioration is of fairly rapid and significant proportions. He studied a small group of 13 elderly men who had been tested on four occasions over a twelve-year period with the Wechsler Bellevue Intelligence Scale. No difference was found between the scores on the first and second test administration, but there was a statistically significant decline for the third and fourth testing. Not expecting such a high rate of decline he went on to study the rates of decline of the individual subjects and discovered considerable variability independent of age. Four of the subjects declined quite extensively after the second testing and to a far greater extent than the other 9 subjects. Since these men were the first to die, Kleemeier (1962) reasoned "that factors related to the death of the individual cause a decline in intellectual performance, and that the onset of this decline may be detected in some instances several years prior to the death of the person." He investigated this matter further on a group of 70 men who had been tested at least on two occasions, and of whom, 37 were living on a specific given date and 33 had died. In comparing these two groups, equated on intelligence test scores at the initial testing, he found the survivors to have a significantly lower mean annual rate of decline on the performance section or on the full scale score. He went on to argue for the validity of his hypothesis, referring also to the findings by Jarvik, Kallmann, Falek, and Klaber (1957) in their study of senescent twins as providing indirect support.

This anticipated the report by Jarvik and Falek (1963) who calculated the rate of decline on three intelligence subtests (Digit Symbol Substitution, Similarities, and Vocabulary) on the part of 34 of the senescent twins who had been tested on three occasions over a twelve-year period. A group of 11 died within five years after the last testing, whereas a group of 23, matched with the deceased group for age, had survived the five years. It was noted that only one of the survivors declined to a critical extent on more than one of the tests, whereas 7 of the 11 nonsurvivors declined on at least two of the tests. This significant difference was related by the investigators to Kleemeier's findings, as well as to results reported by Sanderson and Inglis (1961).

In this latter study a group of 15 elderly psychiatric patients who showed a memory disorder were matched for age and verbal intelligence with another group of 15 patients without a memory disorder. Both groups were tested for memory and for paired associate learning, with the memory disorder group scoring clearly lower than the other group. After sixteen months 6 of the memory disorder subjects had died but none died from the control group. Also noted was a statistically significant relationship between mortality and relatively poor functioning on the learning tests. It may be inferred from these results that there is a likelihood of mortality in individuals following fairly shortly (perhaps within two or three years) upon the heels of a memory disorder.

Associated with this is the research by Goldfarb (1969) on the prediction of mortality in institutionalized aged on the basis of the presence of four characteristics, namely, (1) severe chronic brain syndrome as determined by psychiatric examination; (2) a relatively large number of errors—nine to ten—on a brief mental status questionnaire; (3) marked physical dependency; and (4) incontinence (see also Chapter 7). Since two of these measures are related to cognitive functioning, it is of interest that the existence of two of the four characteristics was predictive of death within three years for 85 percent of the sample of 1280 subjects over sixty-four years of age.

A more direct test of Kleemeier's hypothesis on the association of imminent mortality with a sharp decline in cognitive functioning is reported by Berkowitz (1965). He had 184 aged males in a Veterans' Administration Domiciliary tested a second time five or more years after the initial administration of the Wechsler Bellevue Intelligence Scale. Within forty-two months after the second examination there were 141 survivors and 43 deceased subjects. In studying the changes in performance between the two test administrations, the subjects who had died within ten months of the second testing showed both the greatest amount and highest rate of decline. The data, however, failed to support the hypothesis that the relationship between rate or extent of decline and mortality is predictive for a period of several years. A period of only up to twenty months was found to be associated with the "imminence-of-death factor." Moreover, this study also failed to support the results of Jarvik and Falek (1963) regarding the relative instability of cognitive test scores for nonsurvivors as compared to survivors.

Further useful and significant data on the cognitive aspects of death imminence are provided by Lieberman (1965) in his report on a systematic testing program with 25 institutionalized aged subjects (see also Chapter 13). Four tasks providing six scores, some of which may be regarded as reflecting cognitive functioning, were administered every three to four weeks to the subjects during a two-and-a-half-year period. They consisted of the Bender Gestalt figures, Draw-A-Person Test, estimation of the passage of a sixty-second interval, and a projective response test to 12 line drawings of the human figure. A total of 8 subjects died during the study interval and thus served as a "death-imminent" group which could be compared to the 17 subjects making up a "death-delayed" group. They were similar in their scores at the onset, but over the time span the "death-imminent" group displayed significantly lowered performance in the quality of their reproductions of the Bender figures; made smaller Bender figures; and reduced the complexity of their human figure drawings. In contrast, the "death-delayed" group showed improvement over the time period. Of significance also are the findings that the decline in performance occurred as late as six to nine months prior to death; that change, rather than absolute level of performance correlated with mortality; and that serious nonterminal illness did not affect performance.

The consistency with which the research evidence points to a relationship between cognitive capacities and life span, as well as the association between significant intellectual decline in the aged and the probable imminence of mortality, clearly suggests the possibility that cognition may serve as at least one factor in the prediction of longevity. This, along with observations of similar relationships with longevity of such factors as physical health, social adaptation and morale have led to attempts at the development of predictive formulas or equations.

Riegel, Riegel and Meyer (1967) used a multiple regression analysis to discover which of the 32 variables measured by their examination battery administered to 380 subjects of ages 55 and above were the most significant predictors of death (see also Chapter 11). They found a distinct difference in the number and kinds of variables which were predictive for the subjects aged 55 to 64, as compared to those over 65. For the former group there were 13 variables, whereas there were only 5 variables for the older group whose relationship to mortality was statistically significant. It was noted also that the kinds of predictive variables were essentially different for both groups, but that they did have intellectual measures in common. Even though these cognitive variables entered "strongly into the regression equations," they were not as significant as "physical health" for the 55- to 64-year-old group, and "amount of physical activity" for the above 65-year-old subjects.

Specific equations relating the various factors associated with longevity were not provided in the above noted report. The possibility of such equations, however, is suggested with definite weights for each factor to enable one to predict the life span of individuals from a knowledge of such variables as their age, physical status, cognitive functioning, attitudes, activities, and social adjustments. This matter was more directly dealt with by Palmore (Chapter 18). On the basis of a multiple regression procedure the three factors found to correlate most highly with longevity (physical functioning, work satisfaction, and performance intelligence) were combined and found to improve the predictability of actuarial life expectancy by a significant amount (about one-third of the variance). This made it possible to develop a set of formulas, using those factors which most efficiently predicted longevity for the total and for each of the various subgroups of the population sample of the investigation, namely, men aged 60 to 69, men of 70 and over, women aged 60 to 69, women of 70 and above, whites, and blacks. Of the seven formulas provided in this fashion, four include the factor of intelligence as contributing significantly to the prediction. These formulas are for the total sample, the men over 70 years, the women over 70 years, and the whites. For the other groups the cognitive factor did not contribute enough to improve the prediction value over what the actuarial life expectancy, combined with one of the other factors provided.

Another kind of approach to the problem of prediction was attempted by Bartko and Patterson (1971) through the application of the linear discriminant function (LDF) to a group of 14 variables found to be positively associated with survival in the sample of 47 aged subjects from the study by Birren and his co-workers (1963, also Chapter 10). The 14 variables were among the most discriminating between the survivors and nonsurvivors eleven years after the original examinations, and included several which represent, in part at least, cognitive functioning, namely: WAIS vocabulary, Rorschach score (based on formal aspects of the responses, such as organization and quality), Raven Progressive Matrices, organization of behavior rating, and mental status test. A fifteenth variable, actuarial prediction, was also included in the LDF analysis. Unlike Palmore's approach, noted above, which sought to forecast the number of additional years a person might be expected to live, the LDF approach evaluated "the probability of an old man's surviving eleven years." Whereas Palmore (1969a) found the actuarial prediction of age of death to be the most significant variable, the LDF approach relegated it to a relatively inferior position. In fact, there was no significant difference between the survivors and the nonsurvivors on actuarial prediction. From among all the 15 variables, the combination of 2 of them, rating on organization of behavior and the presence or absence of smoking, classified about 80 percent of the subjects correctly, a result which was as high as when all the variables were taken together. For the 8 behavioral variables alone, the analysis showed the combination of "Organization of Behavior" and "Mental Status Test score" to be the most discriminating, classifying the survival status of 70 percent of the subjects correctly. Presented also by the authors are graphs reflecting the nonsurvival risk of subjects based on combinations of scores on the discriminating variables. For example, "a person with a Mental Status score of 55 (the lowest in this study) had between .98 and .74 risk of not surviving, depending on his Organization of Behavior score. Contrastingly, with a score of 182 (the highest in the study) the risk of not surviving was between .59 and .06. This represents a clear illustration of the significant relationship between level of cognitive functioning and the probability of continued survival up to a specific number of years.

Discussion

The consistency with which the cognitive factor has been found in the available research to be related to longevity is striking. It is, of course, not the only factor, nor apparently even the predominant one in defining the survival status of the aged individual. Health and psychosocial functioning seem to play prepotent roles in predicting longevity, according to the statistical calculations by Riegel, Riegel and Meyer (1967), and Palmore (1969a; 1969b). Even when the subjects do not differ in health status, as noted by Bartko and Patterson (1971), the combination of a psychosocial factor (Organization of Behavior) and a physical condition (smoking) is more effective than other behavioral and physical variables in distinguishing between survivors and nonsurvivors. Yet, the cognitive factor cannot be bypassed since it is pervasive in human behavior and very much a part of psychosocial functioning. It also is exceedingly significant in the physical status of the individual, determining in large measure how he will deal with his environment and organize his life for the maintenance of his health. Moreover, it reflects a good deal of what is happening to the CNS and consequently to the vital functions of the human organism.

Accordingly, it would seem that the various kinds of cognitive tests may be regarded as instruments which are sensitive enough to the internal operations of the individual so as to provide important clues to his survival potential. The investigations which have focused on the rates of decline in intellectual functioning in relation to mortality highlight this concept. Particularly noteworthy in this respect is the study by Lieberman (1965) which found that even severe nonmortal illness did not cause deterioration of performance in the aged subjects (see also Chapter 13). On the other hand, those who did decline significantly in their test results died fairly soon thereafter. Kleemeier (1961; 1962) emphasized this matter in his research results and stressed his impression that a sharp drop in intelligence test performance in the aged signaled imminent mortality. Some of the evidence available suggests that similar declines in learning ability may also represent the nearness of death.

Thus far the data on cognitive decline and mortality are of limited scope and only suggestive. They seem impressive enough, however, to make this an area worthy of further investigation. It would be valuable to delineate the types of tests and cognitive functions which are most sensitive to the approaching total breakdown of functioning. Similarly, much research is called for in the areas of learning, thinking and problem solving both with respect to how the aged function, as well as on how they relate to survival.

The sum of available data and research-based conclusions to date seems sufficiently impressive to warrant some confidence in the hypothesis that there is a significant positive correlation between level of intellectual capacity and life span. Implied by this is the probability that a genetic factor may be the primary basis for longevity and that intelligence is linked to this factor. This would seem to be a worthy and fertile field for research. One approach would be the assembly of data on the intellectual capacities of individuals from families of long-lived parents and grandparents. Keeping track of the life spans of these people would contribute to the delineation of the nature of the relationship between cognition and longevity. In this regard it would be important to establish controls for a variety of variables related to longevity such as physical and mental health, education, socioeconomic status and environmental conditions, particularly nutrition.

The longitudinal developmental studies which were begun when the subjects were children, such as the Terman (1943) study of intellectually gifted children, and the Berkeley child development investigation (Macfarlane, Allen, and Honzik 1954), represent a very promising basis for clarifying the relationships between longevity and the developmental characteristics of individuals in the cognitive, psychosocial, affective and physical areas. In view of the results already available on the 35 year re-study of the intellectually gifted children by Terman and Oden (1959), it would be of very considerable interest and value for gerontology to continue this investigation so as to chart the functioning of these subjects as they move into middle and old age. This would go a long way toward clarifying the extent to which cognition, combined with other factors, could be used to predict life span. It could also contribute significantly to our understanding of the genetic relationship between longevity and cognitive endowments.

On the whole, approaching the prediction of life span in mature adults points to the importance of viewing the human organism from an interdisciplinary standpoint, involving as a minimum the genetic, physiological, environmental, psychosocial, and general psychological factors. It may be that the cognitive side of an individual's functioning is one of the key aspects of gauging his overall status since it is so intricately related to his daily behavior and the operations of his body. Perhaps also the fact that higher level intellectual processes, such as abstraction and problem solving, are probably among the latest facets in the evolution of the human species, cognition is in a position to be particularly sensitive to the integrity of the organism. It is, consequently, a delicate source of cues as to the aging process and approaching breakdown of vital functions. We seem to be at the beginning of knowledge and understanding of these matters. Some valuable and exciting research awaits us in gaining a fuller and more definitive grasp of this aspect of human functioning and gerontology.

References

Bartko, J.J. and Patterson, R.D.: Survival among healthy old men: A multivariate analysis. In: Granick, S. and Patterson, R.D. (ed.): *Human Aging II: An Eleven Year Followup Biomedical and Behavioral Study*. Washington, D.C., Govt. Printing Office, 1971. (In press)

Berkowitz, B.: Changes in intellect with age: IV. Changes in achievement and survival in older people. *J. Genetic Psychol.*, 107: 3-14, 1965.

Birren, J.E. (ed.): *Handbook of Aging and the Individual: Psychological and Biological Aspects*. Chicago, U. of Chicago Press, 1959.

Birren, J.E., Butler, R.N., Greenhouse, S.W., Sokoloff, L., and Yarrow, M.R.: *Human Aging: A Biological and Behavioral Study*. Washington, D.C., Govt. Printing Office, 1963.

121

Birren, J.E.: Neural basis of personal adjustment in aging. In: *Aging With a Future*. Copenhagen, Munksgaard, 1964.

Botwinick, J.: *Cognitive Processes in Maturity and Old Age*. New York, Springer, 1967.

Botwinick, J.: Geropsychology. In: *Annual Review of Psychology*, vol. 21. Palo Alto, Calif., Annual Reviews, 1970.

College honor men long-lived. *Statis. Bull. Metrop. Life Insur. Co.*, 13, 8: 5-7, 1932.

Cowdry, E.V. (ed.): *Problem of Aging*. Baltimore, Williams and Wilkins, 1942.

Falek, A., Kallmann, F.J., Lorge, I., and Jarvik, L.F.: Longevity and intellectual variation in a senescent twin population. *J. Gerontology*, 15: 305-309, 1960.

Goldfarb, A.I.: Predicting mortality in the institutionalized aged. *Arch. Gen. Psychiat.*, 21: 172-176, 1969.

Granick, S.: Studies in the psychology of senility—a survey. *J. Gerontology*, 5: 44-58, 1950.

Granick, S. and Birren, J.E.: Cognitive functioning of survivors versus non-survivors: A twelve-year follow-up of healthy aged. Paper presented at Eighth International Congress of Gerontology, Washington, D.C., 1969.

Granick, S.: Psychological test functioning. In: Granick, S. and Patterson, R.D. (ed.): *Human Aging II: An Eleven Year Followup Biomedical and Behavioral Study*. Washington, D.C., Govt. Printing Office, 1971. (In press)

Guralnick, L.: *The Study of Mortality by Occupation in the U.S.* Washington, D.C.: National Center for Health Statistics, P.H.S., Govt. Printing Office, 1959.

Hinkle, L.E., Jr., Whitney, L.H., Lehman, E.W., Dunn, J., Benjamin, B., King, R., Plakun, A. and Flehinger, B.: Occupation, education and coronary heart disease. *Science*, 161: 238-246, 1968.

Jarvik, E.F., Kallmann, F.J. and Falek, A.: Intellectual changes in aged twins. *J. Gerontology*, 17: 289-294, 1962.

Jarvik, L.F., Kallmann, F.J., Falek, A., and Klaber, M.M.: Changing intellectual functions in senescent twins. *Acta genet.*, 7: 421-430, 1957.

Jarvik, L.F., and Falek, A.: Intellectual stability and survival in the aged. *J. Gerontology*, 18: 173-176, 1963.

Kleemeier, R.W.: Intellectual change in the senium or death and the I.Q. Presidential Address, American Psychological Association, Div. 20, 1961. (Mimeograph)

Kleemeier, R.W.: Intellectual change in the senium. *Proceedings of the Social Statistics Section of the American Statistical Association*: 290-295, 1962.

Lieberman, M.A.: Psychological correlates of impending death: Some preliminary observations. *J. Gerontology*, 20: 181-190, 1965.

Lorge, I.: Intellectual changes during maturity and old age. *Rev. Educ. Res.*, 14: 438-445, 1944.

Lorge, I.: Gerontology (later maturity). In: *Annual Review of Psychology*, vol. 7. Stanford, Calif. Annual Reviews, 1956.

Macfarlane, J.W., Allen, L., and Honzik, M.P.: *A Developmental Study of the*

Behavior Problems of Normal Children Between 21 Months and 14 Years. Berkeley, U. Calif. Press, 1954.

Palmore, E.B.: Physical, mental and social factors in predicting longevity. *Gerontologist*, 9: 103-108, 1969a.

Palmore, E.B.: Predicting longevity: A follow-up controlling for age. *Gerontologist*, 9: 247-250, 1969b.

Pfeiffer, E.: Survival in old age: Physical, psychological and social correlates of longevity. *J. Amer. Geriatric Society*, 18: 273-285, 1970.

Quint, J.V. and Cody, B.R.: Preeminence and mortality: Longevity of prominent men. *Amer. J. Public Health*, 60: No. 6, June 1970.

Riegel, K.F., Riegel, R.M. and Meyer, G.: A study of the dropout rates in longitudinal research on aging and the prediction of death. *J. Personality and Soc. Psychology*, 5: 342-348, 1967.

Rose, C.L.: Social factors in longevity. *Gerontologist*, 4: 27-37, 1964.

Sanderson, R.E. and Inglis, J.: Learning and mortality in elderly psychiatric patients. *J. Gerontology*, 16: 375-376, 1961.

Shock, N.W.: Gerontology (later maturity). In: *Annual Review of Psychology*, vol. 2. Stanford, Calif. Annual Reviews, 1956.

Spiegelman, M.: *Significant Mortality and Morbidity Trends in the U.S. Since 1900*. Bryn Mawr, Pa., American College of Life Underwriters, 1966.

Terman, L.M.: Mental and physical traits of a thousand gifted children. In: Barker, G., Kounin, J.S. and Wright, H.F. (ed.): *Child Behavior and Development*. New York, McGraw-Hill, 1943.

Terman, L.M. and Oden, M.H.: *The Gifted Child Grows Up. Genetic Studies of Genius, Vol. IV*. Stanford, Stanford U. Press, 1959.

10 Biomedical and Behavioral Predictors of Survival Among Normal Aged Men: A Multivariate Analysis

JOHN J. BARTKO, ROBERT D. PATTERSON
and ROBERT N. BUTLER

This study is based on data collected from 47 male subjects during an intensive interdisciplinary study of normal aging which began at the National Institute of Mental Health in 1955 (Birren, et al. 1963). Over 600 variables were measured on each individual in the areas of medicine, cerebral physiology and psychiatry as well as experimental, clinical, and social psychology.

The subjects were community residents over 65 years old (average age 71) who responded to an appeal for volunteers in a study of normal aging. To be included in the study they were required to be free of any significant physical diseases or psychosis. On the basis of all of the data collected, 20 of the subjects were found to have mild asymptomatic medical abnormalities which were most frequently but not exclusively related to arteriosclerosis. Thus, for many further analyses two groups were distinguished. Group I consisted of 27 subjects free of any significant physical symptoms or abnormalities, and the 20 subjects of group II had mild asymptomatic abnormalities.

Factors Related to Survival at Follow-ups

At a five year follow-up the number of survivors among the subjects was slightly greater than predicted by actuarial tables. Nonsmokers and those without arteriosclerosis survived very significantly more often than smokers or those with minimal arteriosclerosis (Butler 1967). There were suggestive relationships between survival and four psychologically important variables, e.g., marital status, psychological adaptation, outlook on life and maintenance of life goals. All of the associations were in the expected direction. At the eleven year follow-up the first two were significantly related to survival but the latter two were not.

At the eleven year follow-up, which was conducted at the Philadelphia

John J. Bartko is Mathematical Statistician, National Institute of Mental Health, Bethesda, Md.

Robert D. Patterson is Fellow in College Psychiatry, Medical Department and Educational Research Center, M.I.T., Cambridge, Mass.

Robert N. Butler is Research Psychiatrist, Wasnington School of Psychiatry, Washington, D.C.

123

Geriatric Center, 23 subjects had survived and 24 had died. This was significantly more survivors than were predicted by actuarial tables and confirmed the initial impression that the subjects were an unusually healthy group of men. A comprehensive report of this follow-up has been presented elsewhere (Granick and Patterson 1971). Consistently, the survivors were healthier or more normal on the variables, measured eleven years earlier, than the nonsurvivors. This was true for measures of physical health such as blood pressure, arteriosclerosis, serum cholesterol, overall health status, and cigarette smoking. Those who survived also consistently performed better on psychological and psychomotor tests (see Chapter 9). Survivors were also healthier on two psychiatric measures (adaptation and mental status) and two psychosocial measures (organization of behavior and psychosocial losses). A morale index which was obtained from a detailed content analysis of interviews also showed a trend toward greater survival among those with higher morale.

Two unexpected relationships were found. First, men of greater weight survived more often even though all were of normal weight. This is surprising because among younger men the heavier survive less frequently. However, a similar positive relationship between weight and survival among elderly men has been reported before (Society of Actuaries 1959). A puzzling association was found between lower serum albumin and death from carcinoma. The carcinoma in all five deaths from carcinoma happened to be in the gastrointestinal tract. If future studies substantiate this relationship, serum albumin might become an early indicator of carcinoma.

In contrast, measures of cerebral physiology such as cerebral blood flow and cerebral matabolic rate of oxygen measured by the nitrous oxide method (Kety and Schmidt 1948) did not differentiate between survivors and nonsurvivors.

Multivariate Analysis

The above is a cursory description of the univariate characteristics of several of the variables. However, in order to assess the interdisciplinary nature of the various factors relating to survival a statistical multivariate analysis was performed. A linear discriminant function was used to obtain the risk or probability of a subject's not surviving eleven years after the first study. Analyses were performed on a set of 15 variables as well as subsets of behavioral and physical variables alone.

A more detailed discussion of the statistical analyses, the variables and the outcome of the study can be found in Bartko and Patterson (1971). These variables[1] were submitted by the investigators representing each area and were

[1]The variables selected are only a very small proportion of the more than six hundred measurements made on the subjects at their initial examination. Since the total 600 x 600 correlation matrix of variables was not an input feature of the multivariate technique, no statistical assurance is given that the variables selected were the "best" statistical subset (in the multivariate sense) from the 600 available. There may be other variables whose

Table 10-1
Variables Used in Multivariate Study

Behavioral Variables	Physical Variables
1. Adaptation	1. Actuarial prediction
2. Mental status test	2. Average systolic blood pressure
3. Organization of behavior	3. Cerebral metabolic rate of oxygen
4. Psychosocial losses	4. Chronic cigarette smoking†
5. Raven Progressive Matrices Test	5. Electroencephalogram modal frequency
6. Rorschach*	6. Group I, II (Health status)
7. Speed of copying words	7. Weight
8. WAIS vocabulary subtest	

*Scored for formal characteristics of responses rather than projective content.
†Coded 0 for pure nonsmokers, former smokers, and cigar and pipe smokers.
Coded 1 for chronic cigarette smokers.

selected as those most highly related to survivorship or, in a few instances, were included because they were of considerable theoretical interest. The meaning of most of the variables is self-explanatory; however, an exception is the rating of organization of behavior (Behv) which was obtained from interview data and was intended to measure the level of planning, complexity and variation characteristic of the men's daily lives (Yarrow et al. 1963). The following five-point scale was used:

1 Activities are few. These are chores, routines, as necessity requires. Little variation.
2 Predominantly routines but some little "puttering" attempt to break through routine and chores.
3 Sporadic or spotty attempts at planned activities and absorptions. Some slight direction, mainly things to fill-in.
4 Structured and planned, some variation but not elaborate. Some "direction" to his activities.
5 Many activities. Structured, planned, varied, involved, new, complex, self-initiated activities and involvement.

performance is better than those presented here. However, the results are quite good. Further, while not passing through a statistical multivariate sieve, the 600 variables have passed through eleven years of statistical as well as clinical analyses. Many univariate analyses as well as smaller scaled cross-disciplinary multivariate studies have been performed. Hence the variables selected have a sound clinical and statistical foundation. They represent the best judgment of the investigators, most of whom were participants in the initial as well as the follow-up examinations.

Data reduction techniques were not used in the study since it was felt important to use variables which other investigators could measure directly as opposed to linear functions of variables, e.g., factor scores.

The classical linear discriminant function (LDF) for two groups is a weighted linear function of multivariate variables. The coefficients of the LDF are derived following the criterion of maximal separation (distance) between the groups (Fisher 1936). Associated with the LDF is a classification problem. Given a sample object on which measurements are made, an LDF value is obtained. It is a single value, namely the sum of weighted measurements made on the object. If the LDF is greater than some value (usually zero) then the sample object is classified into the first group say, otherwise the second.

Classical Approach

We have applied this technique to the 47 subjects of whom 23 were survivors (S) at the 11 year follow-up, and 24 were nonsurvivors ($\overline{S}$). The discriminant analysis program that was utilized, operated in a stepwise fashion on the 15 variables. The variables with a significant contribution at $p \leq .05$ were included in the linear discriminant function (LDF). They were organization of behavior (Behavior or Behv) and smoking. The LDF obtained was:

$$LDF = -2.88 + 1.07(Behv)^2 - 1.60(Smok)^3 . \qquad (1)$$

To illustrate the use of the LDF, suppose a subject were a nonsmoker (0) and had a behavior rating of 5; his LDF value is then $-2.88 + 1.07(5) - 1.60(0)$ = 2.47. This subject in the classical sense would be classified as a survivor (S), because for this particular LDF (equation 1) the boundary value is zero with the mean LDF for survivors positive while the mean LDF for nonsurvivors is negative.

The variables behavior and smoking yielded the same classification matrix, i.e., 4 misclassifications out of the 23 survivors (S) and 5 misclassifications out of the 24 nonsurvivors ($\overline{S}$), as did all the variables when included in the LDF.

Our main interest is not in illustrating the use of the LDF for classification purposes, but rather in the use of the LDF to study the quantitative nature of the dependence of risk (probability) of not surviving eleven years on behavior and smoking.

Risk Approach

The classification process using an LDF assigns an individual to a group depending on his value of the LDF. Greater certainty in assignment is felt the

[2] $p < .01$

[3] $p < .05$

farther the LDF value is from the decision value or dividing point. There are intermediate values about which one might feel uncertain, i.e., values in the region of overlap of populations, and hence one is tempted in consequence to construct a doubtful region, i.e., one in which no judgment or group assignment is made. This mode of thinking can be formalized by requiring a probability of belonging to a population rather than a classification procedure. Such a technique is a natural outgrowth of a desire to know the risk of not surviving (P), rather than the assignment of a subject to a class of survivors or nonsurvivors.

In Table 10-2 the risk of not surviving is computed for each of the 47 subjects using

$$P = 1/[1 + ([1-p]/p) e^{LDF}] \qquad (2)$$

where $p = 24/47$, $(1-p) = 23/47$ and the LDF is given by equation (1).

Since smoking was coded as a (0.1) variable and behavior was a five point scale variable, it was possible to group the subjects by their smoking and behavior values. All of the combinations were represented except for a smoker with a behavior rating of 1 (Table 10-2). The risk of not surviving for eleven years depends very heavily upon the organization of behavior.

As an illustration of the use of the risk of not surviving column, consider a nonsmoker with a behavior rating of 4; his LDF value is $-2.88 + 1.07(4) - 1.60(0) = 1.40$, and his risk value via equation (2) is .208.

Note the higher risk in general for the smokers and higher risk for subjects with low behavior scores. A nonsmoker with a 1 (least organized) on the behavior scale has an 86 percent chance of not surviving, while another nonsmoker with a 5 (most organized) has an 8 percent chance of not surviving. The risk for smokers exceeds that for nonsmokers for all levels of behavior rating. The difference in risk ranges from 10 percent (behavior rating of 1) to 36 percent (behavior ratings 3 and 4). For smokers the risk of not surviving is less than 50 percent only for the case where the behavior rating is most favorable, i.e., a 5 rating.

The number of subjects in each class is shown as well as the number misclassified. There is quite good agreement between the number of observed and expected nonsurvivors (24 vs. 24.06).

The last column (Comments) of Table 10-2 can be compared to the misclassified subjects mentioned above. Of the 23 survivors, 4 were misclassified as nonsurvivors. Of the 24 nonsurvivors, five subjects were misclassified as survivors.

Behavioral Variables

The risk approach was run for all subjects on the behavioral variables (Table 10-1) alone. The only variables of statistical significance $p \leqslant .05$ entering the LDF were behavior and the mental status (Ment) score. The LDF obtained was:

Table 10-2
Risk of Not Surviving: Smoking and Behavior Variables (N = 47)

	Behavior Rating	Observed No. Survivors (S)	Observed No. Nonsurvivors (S̄)	Total at Risk	Risk* of Not Surviving	Expected No. Nonsurvivors	Comments
Non-smokers	1	0	1	1	.866	.866	
	2	0	7	7	.689	4.823	
	3	8	1	9	.432	3.888	one S̄ called a S
	4	4	1	5	.208	1.040	one S̄ called a S
	5	5	1	6	.083	.498	one S̄ called a S
Total		17	11	28		11.115	
Smokers	1	0	0	0	.970		
	2	1	5	6	.916	5.496	one S called a S̄
	3	1	4	5	.791	3.955	one S called a S̄
	4	2	2	4	.565	2.260	two S called S̄
	5	2	2	4	.309	1.236	two S̄ called S
Total		6	13	19		12.947	(Total of 9 misclassifications)
Total		23	24	47		24.062	

*Risk = $1/[1 + 23/24\, e^{LDF}]$; LDF from equation (1).

$$\text{LDF} = -6.40 + .76(\text{Behv})^4 + .03(\text{Ment})^5. \qquad (3)$$

The LDF (equation 3) was utilized as discussed above and risk values were obtained using an equation of the form of equation (2). Figure 10-1 illustrates the risk values. The behavior measure is numbered 1 through 5 on the chart. The abscissa is the mental status score and the ordinate is the risk of not surviving.

The contributions of mental status and organization of behavior to the risk prediction gives a unique opportunity to speculate about the role of organic mental factors vs. social and emotional factors in survival.

The mental status test score which measured mental abilities and organic mental impairment, appeared to reflect two major influences: 1) the degree of any organic mental decline and; 2) life long intelligence.

Organization of behavior reflected the subject's social and emotional state. Those with higher scores were more involved with others, better adapted, had higher morale and less psychosocial losses. These factors might have an effect on survival. However, behavior was also associated with organic mental decline and this could be the reason for its association with greater survival.

The effect of organic mental changes on behavior is to some extent controlled if we compare two subjects with the *same* mental status score and *differing* behavior scores. In Figure 10-1 we can compare two men each with a mental status score of 133 (the mean of the group). If one man had a behavior score of 1 (poorest) his risk of not surviving would be 86 percent while if the other man's behavior were structured, varied and involved self-initiated activities (score 5) his risk of not surviving would be 22 percent. With the organic state of the brain partially controlled for by the constant mental status score it seems that the impressive difference in probability of survival may in part be due to social-emotional factors.

The figure also demonstrates the strong relationship between mental ability (in this instance measured by mental status test) and the risk of not surviving. A person with a mental status score of 55 (the lowest in this study) had between a 98 percent and 74 percent risk of not surviving depending on his behavior score. Contrastingly, with a score of 182 (the highest score in the study) the risk of not surviving was between 59 percent and 6 percent. A higher mental status score meant better functioning.

Physical Variables

An analysis was performed using the physical variables alone. Average systolic blood pressure (ASBP) was the first variable (via the stepwise LDF program) to enter and weight was second. The LDF obtained was

---

[4] $p < .01$

[5] $p < .05$

130

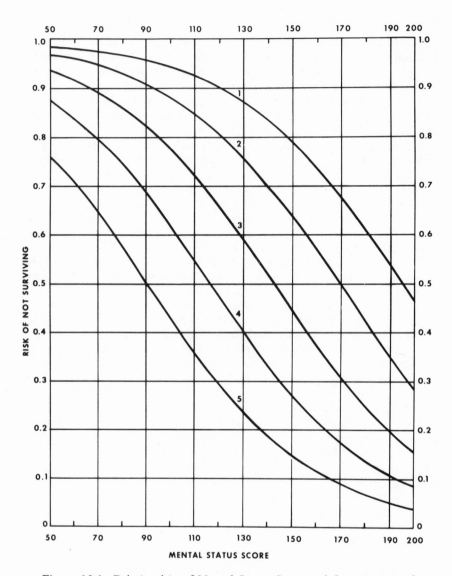

Figure 10-1. Relationship of Mental Status Score and Organization of Behavior to the Risk of Not Surviving. (Organization of behavior scores are along the curves.) Source: Bartko, in S. Granick and R. Patterson, eds. *Human Aging II* (Washington, D.C.: Government Printing Office, 1971).

$$LDF = 1.85 - .05(ASBP)^6 + .07(Wt)^7. \qquad (4)$$

The positive coefficient for weight means that greater weight is associated with a greater chance of survival as mentioned above. Lighter weight and earlier death may have been associated because of more marked catabolic processes in the non-survivors (Libow 1971).

Following previous discussions and using equation (4) and one of the form of (2), risk values were obtained. Figure 10-2 illustrates these risk values. Weight ranges from 45 to 90 Kg. and appears above the curves of the chart. The abscissa is average systolic blood pressure and the ordinate is the Risk of Not Surviving.

The figure shows the substantial influence of weight upon survival even for constant blood pressure values. If a man with a blood pressure of 133 (the mean for the group) weighed 45 Kg. his risk of not surviving would be 86 percent while if he were heavier and weighed 90 Kg. his risk of not surviving would be 16 percent i.e., his probability of surviving would be substantially greater. A similar interrelationship of weight, blood pressure and survival has been reported by the Society of Actuaries (1959).

The range of values for weight and blood pressure presented in the figure correspond to the range of values actually observed in the study. There is no justification for generalizing that obese old men (with weights greater than those shown in the figure) would also have small risks of not surviving. Indeed obese men in general have higher mortality rates than the nonobese.

A substantial association between level of systolic blood pressure (all values which are normal for aged men) and risk of not surviving is also illustrated: the higher the blood pressure, the greater the risk.

Discussion

Since the subjects of this study were in very good physical health and were free of psychotic mental disease, it may seem remarkable that measurements made on them should contribute much to predictions of whether or not they would live eleven years. The relationship between the variables and eleven year survival is more remote than the connection we recognize between a terminal illness and death. The results urge us to examine factors associated with eventual death which are not diseases in the usual sense. Having shown that some social and psychological states are associated with survival, we are faced with understanding the mechanism through which they are related.

Inferences about the meaning of the association between organization of behavior and the risk of not surviving must be made cautiously because organization of behavior is significantly correlated with many other physiological, social and psychological factors. It was also significantly correlated with the

---

[6] $p < .01$

[7] $p < .05$

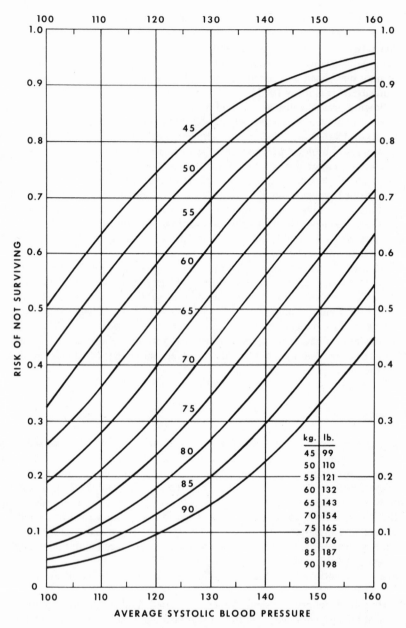

Figure 10-2. Relationship of Average Systolic Blood Pressure and Weight to the Risk of Not Surviving. (Weights in Kg are along the curves.) Source: Bartko, in S. Granick and R. Patterson, eds., *Human Aging II* (Washington, D.C.: Government Printing Office, 1971).

133

age of the subjects at the first study (r=−0.46), however, this cannot totally account for its high predictability of survival because the actuarial variable (which is directly related to age) was not a good discriminator.

Greater organization of behavior and intellectual ability (here measured by the mental status score) may be associated with greater survival because the better scoring men anticipated crises and actively planned effective responses which minimized any detrimental effect. This might be most easily identified with regard to medical illnesses where the high scoring men might be more alert to early signs of illness and get the needed care, thus avoiding death. In the emotional area, the higher scoring men might, for example, be able to avoid or minimize some depressions by well organized behavior. There is some evidence to suggest that depressions are associated with shorter survival (Roth and Kay 1956). Unfortunately, detailed data are not available from this study to test this hypothesis.

A second explanation of the association between certain psychological factors and survival may be that the psychological measures simply reflect the degree of arteriosclerosis present. The interaction of mental state, organization of behavior and survival discussed above suggest this is not an adequate explanation.

On the other hand, it seems likely that mental status, intelligence, morale, and organization of behavior may be related to the central nervous system's competence to respond appropriately in a behavioral *as well as* neuroendocrine way when under stress. Selye (1936, 1970) has shown that under stress, endocrine factors which are normally under control of the central nervous system can be crucial to survival in animals. He has also shown the role of the "stress hormones" in what he calls the "diseases of adaptation" which include hypertension, peptic ulcers and cardiac accidents. The relatively long lasting conditions of grief and depression may also influence the organism's neuro-endocrine responses and thus influence survival through similar mechanisms.

We do not know if a deliberate change in the level of organization of a person's behavior would have an influence on his survival. Similarly we do not know whether intellectual stimulation or "healthier" grieving for losses would improve responses to physiological stresses which threaten life. Interestingly, patients today are often given treatment on the assumption that such changes will prolong their lives.

Many other relationships between socioemotional states and increased risk of death are known and many of them are discussed in other chapters of this volume. Two which have a particular relation to our findings will be discussed here.

The first is a study by Rees and Lutkins (1967) which found an increased death rate among relatives (spouse, child, parent, or sibling) in the year following death of an index case. They interpreted this as evidence of an increase in mortality due to the psychological state of grief. Our study supports this finding in that people with greater psychosocial losses survived less frequently. In the Rees and Lutkins study one must assume that the psychological state was primary and that it affected survival. In other situations the causal chain may be unclear; for example, in the association of intelligence and survival, some third factor such as degree of arteriosclerosis may be affecting both intelligence and survival, thus leading to the association of the latter two.

The second study of interest is one on "Voodoo Death" by Cannon (1942). He reviewed reports by observers of primitive people that a curse placed on a man might lead to his death within a matter of hours to a few days. He felt that the evidence for such deaths was convincing and suggested a physiological mechanism. Cannon found that extreme fear similar to the feelings of a cursed native led to marked sympathetic nervous system stimulation and adrenal hormone secretion in animals. If the fear state was maintained more than a few hours, especially without water intake, cardiovascular collapse and death occurred. This is an appealing explanation of the mechanism by which a psychological state can lead to death.

Whether or not the explanation can serve in some modified form to explain increased death rates in long-standing mildly disturbed psychological states is an open question. However, Cannon suggested the applicability of these physiological principles to more gradual declines leading to death which are seen in our culture. He described how Australian aborigines totally withdraw social support and contact from a person who is presumed to be under the influence of black magic. The tribe's withdrawal makes the victim's social life completely collapse. Correspondingly, he makes no effort to live or to stay a part of the group. Before he dies the tribesmen come to him and perform a mourning ceremony. The ceremony has the purpose of cutting him off from the ordinary world and symbolically placing him in the world of the dead.

This description has some resemblance to behavior typical of the dying and the people around them in our culture. Often a dying person is socially isolated during a terminal illness and his family displays some mourning behavior in his presence. Normally, the patient is not thought of as dying to any degree *because* of the social circumstances surrounding his dying, since his physical disease is the recognized cause. However, the occurrence of death when primitive tribes carry out the rituals associated with death in the absence of primary physical disease at least raises the question as to how much social and emotional factors play in at least the timing of death for persons in our culture.

The results of the present study support the idea that social and psychological influences are associated with length of survival. In particular they point to those factors which determine the complexity of one's daily behavior. Also, even in very healthy men, aspects of central nervous system function appear to be very sensitive predictors of survival.

Our finding of the important role of cigarette smoking in survival agrees with other recent studies (Preston 1970; Grannis 1970). Preston concluded that smoking is a major factor limiting life expectancy in civilized countries. Grannis has gone so far as to suggest that the excess number of elderly females in the United States population may be entirely accounted for by the excess deaths among smokers, who have more frequently been males. He reports that the increased sex ratio among the aged has developed during the past seventy-five years, a period during which smoking among males became widespread. This suggests that to an important degree the high frequency of widowhood in old age in our society is traceable to cigarette smoking among men.

Palmore used a regression analysis to predict longevity (Chapter 18). Using data from the Duke University longitudinal aging study, he found actuarial prediction of years remaining to be the most significant variable. In the risk approach used in our research actuarial prediction was not among the best predictors. There was no significant difference between the actuarial prediction of age of death for the survivors and nonsurvivors. Hence it does not serve as a discriminator. Further, for our selected group of healthy men the actuarial or life expectancy tables were not strictly applicable since the tables cover a broad spectrum of aged men in terms of health, environmental conditions, etc.

There is also a fundamental difference in the kind of questions being asked in the two approaches. Our study sought to discover physical and psychological factors which maximally *differentiated* a group of aged healthy male survivors from a comparable group of nonsurvivors. Our risk approach asks not for the specific number of years remaining, but for the probability of an old man's surviving eleven years. Our results indicate that behavior and smoking ratings, among others, are good predictors of risk and that age is not. However, in a regression analysis such as Palmore has done, the question becomes: how many years remain? The man's actuarial prediction of years remaining then becomes overwhelmingly the best predictor.

Summary

1. Forty-seven very healthy initially community resident men who were intensively studied physiologically and psychologically have been followed-up after an eleven year interval. There were significant relationships between survival and specific variables in every major area of study except cerebral physiology.
2. The dependence of the eleven-year probability of nonsurvival on a set of 15 variables was investigated using statistical multivariate discriminant functions.
3. Two of the variables were as good discriminators as all of the variables taken together. They were: a social psychological variable which measured the degree of organization and complexity of a subject's typical daily behavior and the presence or absence of cigarette smoking. The two variables correctly classified about 80 percent of both survivors and nonsurvivors. Further, in terms of a risk analysis, the greater the subject's organization of behavior score the lower was his risk of not surviving. Smokers had a much higher risk of not surviving.
4. When the analysis was restricted to behavioral variables alone, organization of behavior and mental status test score were the two significant variables. Higher mental status scores were associated with a lower risk of not surviving.
5. With physical variables alone for risk prediction, average systolic blood

pressure and weight were the significant variables. Lower blood pressure, even though in the normal range and *greater* weight (also in the normal range) were associated with lower risk of not surviving.

6. How long healthy old men will survive is moderately predictable. Measurements of physical and behavioral variables within the normal range may be used as predictors. It appears that some social and psychological influences may be remote, but important factors in causal sequences leading to death.

7. A possible role of neuroendocrine factors in survival and their relationship to the behaviors measured in this study is discussed.

References

Bartko, J.J. and Patterson, R.D. Survival Among Healthy Old Men: A Multivariate Analysis. In Granick, S. and Patterson, R., *Human Aging II: An Eleven Year Biomedical and Behavioral Study*. U.S. Govt. Printing Office, Washington, D.C., 1971.

Birren, J.E. et al., eds. *Human Aging: A Biological and Behavioral Study*. Washington, D.C., U.S. Govt. Printing Office, 1963.

Butler, R.N. Aspects of Survival and Adaptation in Human Aging. *Amer. J. Psychiat.*, 123:10, April 1967.

Cannon, W.B. Voodoo death. *Amer. Anthrop.*, 44:169-181, 1942.

Fisher, R.A. The use of multiple measurements in taxonomic problems. *Annals of Eugenics*, 7:179-188, 1936.

Granick, S. and Patterson, R. *Human Aging II: An Eleven Year Biomedical and Behavioral Study*. U.S. Govt. Printing Office, Washington, D.C., 1971.

Grannis, G.F. Demographic perturbations secondary to cigarette smoking. *J. of Geront.*, 25:55-63, 1970.

Kety, S.S. and Schmidt, C.F. The Nitrous Oxide Method for the Quantitative Determination of Cerebral Blood Flow: Theory, Procedure and Normal Values. *J. Clin. Invest.*, 27:476, 1948.

Libow, L.S. Medical Factors in Survival and Mortality of the Relatively Healthy Elderly: 11 Year Study. In Granick, S. and Patterson, R. *Human Aging II: An Eleven Year Biomedical and Behavioral Study*. U.S. Govt. Printing Office, Washington, D.C., 1971.

Palmore, E.B. Physical, mental, and social factors in predicting longevity. *Geront.*, 9:103-108, 1969.

Preston, S.H. Older Male Mortality and Cigarette Smoking: A Demographic Analysis. Monograph; 1970. University of California.

Rees, W.D. and Lutkins, S.G. Mortality of Bereavement. *Brit. Med. J.*, 4:13-16, 1967.

Roth, M. and Kay, D.W.K. Affective Disorders Arising in the Senium II. *J. Ment. Sci.*, 102:141-150, 1956.

Selye, H. A syndrome produced by diverse nocuous agents. *Nature*, London, 138:32, 1936.

Selye, H. Stress and Aging, *J. Amer. Geriatrics Soc.*, 18:660-681, 1970.

Society of Actuaries. *Build and Blood Pressure Study, Vol. 1*, Table 112. Society of Actuaries, Chicago, Ill., 1959.

Yarrow, M.R., Blank, P., Quinn, O.W., Youmans, E.G. and Stein, J. Social Psychological Characteristics of Old Age. In Birren, et al. *Human Aging: A Biological and Behavioral Study*. Washington, D.C., U.S. Govt. Printing Office, 1963.

11 The Prediction of Death and Longevity in Longitudinal Research

KLAUS F. RIEGEL

Developmental trends, as traditionally analyzed, confound individual growth with sociocultural changes. In some cases and in the view of some observers (e.g., Ryder 1955), social changes might out-pace those of individuals. Subsequently, persons (for instance, old individuals) without changing much themselves might increasingly fail to cope successfully with the "changing times." In other cases and in the view of most developmental psychologists, changes occur primarily in the individuals. Often, persons (for instance, young individuals) might change so rapidly that they out-pace the "changing times." Thus potentially, they produce "progress," whereby, to them, the existing sociocultural conditions attain the appearance of outmoded relicts. The growing friction between the individuals' expectancies and approaches on the one hand, and the changes in cultural conditions within which they occur on the other, has become painfully clear to us in view of the social and political life of the present days.

By going beyond the traditional methods of cross-sectional and longitudinal comparisons, i.e., by applying complex developmental designs (Baltes 1968; Schaie 1965), it has become possible to disentangle the confounded factors of social and individual change. This success achieved in psychological gerontology (Riegel, Riegel and Meyer 1967b; Schaie and Strother 1968), having by no means penetrated the minds of other developmental psychologists (see, however, Hilton and Patrick 1969; Baltes, Baltes and Reinert 1970), is to be questioned by observations of selective survival and selective test participation. The first implies a lack of homogeneity of the population (Riegel, Riegel and Meyer 1967a) and the latter a lack of uniformity of the sampling process across age levels (Riegel, Riegel and Meyer 1968).

While the refinements in developmental designs thus do not help us in deriving unbiased estimates of population trends, the further suggestions of defining this population in more specific terms (Baltes, Schaie and Hardi 1971), for instance, in terms of the most important predictors of survival, longevity, or cooperation, appeared to have provided a reasonable solution. This suggestion also brought the research closer to psychological considerations (made it more "relevant") rather than tying it to abstract discussions of developmental research designs.

However, the generality of this solution must be again questioned. In

Klaus F. Riegel is Professor of Psychology, University of Michigan, Ann Arbor, Michigan.

particular, our analysis will describe a "terminal-drop" in performance and behavior occurring less than five years prior to the death of subjects. This observation, previously made by Kleemeier (1961, 1962), Jarvik and Falek (1963), and Lieberman (1965, 1966), has the potential implication that all observed changes, though hidden through selective survival and selective test resistance, might be attributed to the performance of persons who do not survive the five years following the time of test administration. If we were to exclude these "high risk" subjects from the analysis, little or no changes might be observed as in most longitudinal studies. While selective survival and selective test participation lead to "underestimate" the decline during later years, the observation of a "terminal-drop" implies an "overestimation" and, generally, the idea that our data might describe nothing but trends in mortality of the aging population, i.e., that the observed decline is due to nothing but the "terminal-drops" of the nonsurviving subjects whose number increases with age.

Methods and Procedures

This report is based upon a cross-sectional study of an aged population in Northern Germany in 1956 (stage A), a retest-study after five years (stage B), and two inquiries into the fate of the subjects from the original sample, the first in combination with the retest study (stage B), the second ten years after the original testing (stage C).

Subjects. The original sample at stage A consisted of 190 females and 190 males. These cases were drawn from a group of about 500 subjects tested, and were subdivided into five age levels, including 38 females and 38 males each. The five age levels are: 55 to 59, 60 to 64, 65 to 69, 70 to 74, and over 75 years (average age 79.0 years). Aside from controlling for age and sex, each age level was matched against census statistics on the following criteria: occupation or former occupation, source of income, marital status, refugees vs. non-refugees, and religious affiliation. The samples can be regarded as representative for the population of Northern Germany. Fuller descriptions are given by R.M. Riegel and Riegel (1959), Riegel, Riegel and Skiba (1962) and by Riegel (1967).

At the time of the second testing at stage B, all subjects had moved precisely into the next higher age levels. Of the 380 persons originally tested, 202 participated in the second testing; 62 had died during the intervening five years; 116 refused to be retested. The number of retested subjects decreases rather regularly with age, whereas the number of deceased subjects increases. No systematic differences in the number of retest-resisters have been observed between age levels.

At the time of the third inquiry at stage C, a total of 162 subjects had died. A total of 152 of the 202 retested subjects survived but only 66 of the 116 retest-resisters. In other words, of the latter group 43.1 percent did not survive the five years following their refusal to be retested; of the retested subjects only

24.7 percent did not survive. Thus, cooperation in retest-studies is a powerful predictor of survival. Since we did not keep record of the 10 or 15 percent of subjects who refused to cooperate at the very first testing at stage A, it is not possible to generalize our conclusion from the retest-resisters to the original test-resisters. Intuitively, such a generalization is most reasonable. Future investigators should be advised to record the names of all subjects approached in order to check on the survivorship of noncooperative subjects.

There is a slight increase with age in the number of non-survivors in the group of retested subjects, adding up to 50 across ages; correspondingly, the number of survivors declines, adding up to 152 across ages. The figures of the refusing subjects change more markedly across ages, adding up to 50 non-survivors and 66 survivors, respectively.

Materials. The following measures have been applied both in the original and the retest study:

(a) Three short forms of the Hamburg Wechsler Intelligence Test for Adults (Wechsler 1956) consisting of combinations of three and four subtests, respectively. The subtests have been combined in such a way as to allow for equally good estimates of the total, verbal and performance IQ's, and have been grouped as follows:

General Information	Comprehension	Similarities
Arithmetic	Digit Span	Coding
Object Assembly	Picture Completion	Picture Arrangement
	Block Design	

Subjects were randomly assigned to a particular combination. To a subsample of 128 subjects the complete test was administered (R.M. Riegel and Riegel 1959). The results to be reported are based on IQ scores.

(b) Five multiple-choice verbal achievement tests (Riegel 1959, 1967) consisting of twenty items each, as in the following (translated) examples:

Synonym test: GRANARY means the same, or almost the same as:
    STABLE, MARKET, *SILO*, CORNFIELD, HARVEST.
Antonym test: STRONG means the opposite of:
    SHY, *WEAK*, SMALL, LIGHT, SICK.
Selection test: A GRANARY always has:
    GRAIN, ELEVATOR, CELLAR, MICE, *ENTRANCE*.
Classification test: GRANARY belongs with:
    FIELD, *STABLE*, FARM, *BARN*, PLOUGH
(note, two coordinates to the stimulus have to be selected).
Analogy test: GRANARY is related to WHEAT, as STABLE is related to:
    FIELD, *COWS*, GRAIN, COTTAGE, FARMER.

Half of the items of the tests of antonyms, selections and classifications were given in a mixed combination; the others were presented (like the remaining two tests) in separate blocks. The results to be presented are given in raw scores, i.e., denote the number of items solved.

(c) Three attitude and one interest test (Riegel and Riegel 1960) in which statements had to be endorsed on five-point rating scales with labels ranging from correct (or like it much) to incorrect (or dislike it much). The attitude measures include scales on behavioral rigidity, dogmatism and attitude toward life.

The rigidity scale has been divided into two subsets of items on general rigidity and personal ridigity, respectively. The items of the former were given as general phrases, such as, "In whatever one does, the 'tried and true ways' are always the best"; those of the latter were given in the first person singular, such as, "I much prefer to eat a familiar dish than something which I do not know at all."

The dogmatism scale has been divided into three subsets of items. The first two were given in the first person singular and test expressions of anxiety, such as, "I have often observed that strangers were looking critically at me" or expressions of intolerance, such as, "In a heated discussion I, generally, become so absorbed in what I am going to say that I forget to listen to what the others are saying." The remaining items denote general dogmatism and are given as general phrases, such as, "It is better to be a dead hero than a live coward."

The scale on attitude toward life has been subdivided into two sets of statements. In the first, some expectancies about the future are expressed or the present is evaluated in terms of the past (pro- and retrospective), and in the second, subjects had to express their present feelings of acceptance, usefulness, and well-being (contemporaneous). A typical item for the former is, "For the next years I already have quite a few plans," and for the latter, "I often think that I am only in the way of younger people."

The interest scale lists 14 adult activities and has been subdivided noting whether these imply primarily receptive and noncompetitive activities, such as "listening to music," productive and emotional activities, such as "doing art work," or physical activities, such as "working in the household."

(d) The questionnaire on the social and living conditions (Riegel, Riegel and Skiba 1962) consists of 77 open-ended or multiple-choice items most of which have been grouped into clusters.

The first five clusters are asking about subjects' living conditions, i.e., their educational, financial, and health status (the six items on education have been applied at stage A only). The next four clusters, measuring the habits of aging subjects, are asking about various activities, and thus are counterparts to the interest scale mentioned above, in which subjects express their preferences but not their actual engagement. Three of the four clusters inquire about physical, social, and leisure time activities; the fourth checked activities, covers all of the three areas, and is composed of five checklists, including a total of 55 activities. Finally, two scales on life adjustment are related to the scale on attitude toward life mentioned above and either expressed the subject's happiness about his social and living arrangements or compared his present situations with those at younger years. Three indexes of deterioration in intellectual and social behavior have been derived from the data obtained and have been described previously (Riegel, Riegel and Skiba 1962). The first of these measures compares the expressed interests with activities actually performed; the second is a measure of happiness and satisfaction; the third compares social and living conditions of subject's past with those of the present. All remaining entries represent single items and are self-explanatory.

All tests and measures were pretested and scrutinized by item analyses. Details of these investigations are given in the publications quoted above (see also, Riegel and Riegel 1962).

Results and Discussions

For cross-sectional, longitudinal, and time-lag comparisons, our data will be analyzed in terms of mean scores and trends across age levels. In the first two of the following sections the information on the fate of our subjects at times B and C will be used to make specific comparisons between subgroups and age levels. The results reported here are derived from the five verbal tests. In a third section, multiple regression predictions of survival and longevity will be reported using all the available data.

Homogeneity of the Population and Uniformity of the Sampling Process. As shown in Part A of Figure 11-1, the overall means (A_T) for the five verbal tests obtained from the first cross-sectional study (stage A) indicate a slight decline between the two age groups. When the two samples are subdivided on the basis of the information available at the time of the second testing (stage B), differential trends become apparent. Subjects retested at stage B (A_1) have above average scores; contrary to the slight decline in the total group (A_T), there is a slight increase in scores with age. Retest-resisters (A_3) as well as non-survivors (A_2) perform below average. The differences in scores between the retest-resisters and the total group (but especially the retest group) is larger for subjects above than below 65 years of age. This result indicates a more successful prediction of retest-resistance (on the basis of the first testing) for the older than for the younger subjects. On the other hand, the differences in scores between subjects who did not survive the five-year period following the first testing and the total group (but especially the retest group) is larger for subjects below than above 65 years of age. As to be confirmed below, this result indicates a more successful prediction of survivorship (on the basis of the first testing) for the younger than for the older subjects.

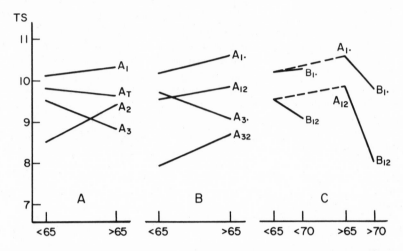

Figure 11-1. Average Scores on Five Verbal Tests for Two Age Levels, Various Subgroups and Two Times of Testing. (A = First Testing; B = Second Testing: 1st Subscripts = Fate of Ss at Stage B; 2nd Subscript = Fate of Ss at Stage C; T = All Ss; 1 = Retested Ss; 2 = Deceased Ss; 3 = Refusing Ss.)

As discussed previously (Riegel, Riegel and Meyer 1963, 1967a, 1968), our results allow for the following conclusions:

Because of the selective death (especially at the younger age level) of less able persons, the *population* from which consecutive age samples are drawn is *not homogeneous* but, increasingly with age, becomes positively biased. Subsequently, age trends reported in the literature underestimate the decline which would have resulted if all subjects had the same chances of survival and longevity, i.e., if the population would remain homogeneous. Furthermore, the age differences in the predictability of survival indicate that at the earlier ages death strikes subjects who are psychologically and sociologically distinctly different from the survivors, i.e., in general, less able. At the higher age levels (above 65 years) death strikes more randomly and the psychological and sociological differences between survivors and nonsurvivors are less marked.

Because of the selective retest-resistance (especially among the older subjects), the *sampling process* is *not uniform* across age levels. Over and above the effect of selective survival, increasing with age, there is a tendency among less able persons to refuse test-participation. Subsequently age trends reported in the literature, once more, underestimate the decline which would have resulted if all subjects at all age levels would remain equally willing to participate in the testing.

Terminal Drop in Performance. The information on the fate of our subjects obtained five or ten years after our first testing allows us to subdivide our original samples into the various subgroups shown in Part A and B of the figure. Furthermore, at stage B, a large proportion of subjects was retested. Thus our analyses can be supplemented by longitudinal comparisons. As shown in Part C of Figure 11-1, longitudinal records are available for the subgroup A_1 which can be further subdivided into those retested subjects who survived (A_1.) or did not survive (A_{12}) the five years following the retesting at stage B. The retest data obtained five years after the first testing will be denoted by B, yielding averages B_1. and B_{12} separately, for the two groups of younger or older subjects.

The retest scores of the younger surviving subjects (B_1.) fall closely upon the line derived from the original cross-sectional records of the same groups of young and old subjects (A_1.). Thus, the longitudinal comparison confirms the cross-sectional trend indicated by the upper dotted line in Part C of the figure and by the upper solid line in Part B. However, the longitudinal data for the older age group, extending five years beyond the cross-sectional comparison, drop off rather sharply. In order to provide an interpretation for this exceptional finding, we inspect, first, the longitudinal data of those retested subjects who did not survive the period following the second testing (B_{12}).

As shown in the lower section of Part C in the figure, the longitudinal means for both the younger and the older groups of retested subjects who do not survive until stage C (B_{12}) drop off rather sharply and, therefore, are at variance to the cross-sectional trend indicated by the dotted line in Part C and the solid line in Part B (i.e., A_{12}).

After carefully considering but failing to attribute these results to extraneous factors, the sharp drop in scores for the nonsurviving retestees strongly suggest that the changes in performance or behavior with age observed in cross-sectional studies are caused by sudden deteriorations, occurring during periods extending less than five years prior to the death of subjects. Little or no decline (if not continued improvements) seems to occur during periods more than five years prior to the death of a person.

Our longitudinal data thus confirm some previous research by Kleemeier (1961, 1962), Jarvik and Falek (1963) and Lieberman (1965, 1966), in which, through repeated testing, a sudden terminal drop in performance and behavior was observed. This terminal drop also suggests an interpretation for the change in performance of the older, surviving subjects of the retest group (see upper right section of Part A). These subjects, having by the time of the retesting attained an age of at least 70 years and at most of 93 years, might be so close to the "natural limit" of their life that the terminal drop is already occurring even though they are still cooperating in the testing. In support of this interpretation, it is noteworthy that their drop in performance is less marked than that of the nonsurviving older retestees (see lower right section of Part C). While our explanation seems quite reasonable, it requires an extension to over five years of the period during which such an terminal drop might occur.

Our conclusion derived from the observation of a terminal drop in performance and behavior can be formulated in a more staggering manner. At any time during the later periods of life, subjects who perform less well are likely to be closer to death than their more able age-mates. Differences in scores *within* age groups might thus be a function of survival probability; subjects scoring low have already experienced their terminal drop, those scoring high retain their abilities and have a good chance of survival. Differences in scores *between* age groups (diminished by selective survival and retest-resistance) might reflect the increasing number of persons with terminal drops; any observed decline in average scores might be attributed to those subjects likely to die; the performance and behavior of the long-term survivors (five years or more) remain essentially stable.

Multiple Correlations with Longevity. Our preceding interpretations have been limited to the results on the five verbal tests. This leaves us with the problem of relating the intelligence tests, the attitude and interest measures, as well as the array of items on the social conditions and possibilities, to one another and to the verbal scales mentioned. By directing our attention to the specific goal of predicting longevity and by using multiple correlation analysis, we take into consideration the intercorrelations of our variables and arrive at limited but systematic comparisons between them, namely in regard to their independent utility for our predictions.

Previously, multiple regression predictions of death (Riegel, Riegel and Meyer 1963, 1967a) and of retest-resistance (Riegel, Riegel and Meyer 1968) have been reported. Of these, we shall disregard the latter and extend the death predictions to cover the 10-year period from stage A to C of our investigation, as well as the second period from stage B to C. Both these extensions recapitulate and validate our previous predictions based upon the period from stage A to B. Finally, we introduce predictions, separate for males and females, on the number of years of expected survival, i.e., longevity. Whereas the death predictions are based on multiple-biserial correlations predicting either survival or death, the latter include the continuous variable of years and rely on Pearsonian coefficients. In the predictions of longevity, age is excluded and in all of the predictions sex is excluded as a variable since both these factors are expected to cover up the more interesting psychological and sociological variables. Since both age and sex are known to be good predictors of survival and longevity, their exclusion reduces the degree of our correlations.

Our predictions were made by successively reducing the probability of the F-levels at which variables would enter into the equations. The probability of the F-levels were set at 0.10, 0.25 and 0.50, respectively, but for each variable the F-level attained at the end of the procedures was also empirically determined. This was necessary because under the more lenient conditions, F-values for some of the variables already entered could have changed depending upon their correlations with the newly entering measures. Indeed, in some cases, high ranking predictor variables have been dropped altogether from the equations at a later stage in the analysis. Generally in a new field of investigation, it seems reasonable to lower the F-levels sufficiently and to go below the traditional levels of scrutiny in order to pick up unaccounted portions of the variance. Even though this will increase the likelihood of Type 2 errors, it seems appropriate to retain hypotheses initially, which after further research may turn out to be false, rather than to reject hypotheses too early that might turn out to be acceptable.

Table 11-1 shows the results of our analysis for the two age groups and the five types of predictions. Listed are the ranks under which the variables entered into the equations under the most stringent criterion of F = 0.10, and the empirically determined F-levels attained at the end of the procedure. At the bottom of the table is a listing of the number of variables entering into the equations at the three F-levels and the multiple correlations attained.

Looking at these last lines first, we notice that with very few exceptions, our predictions of both death and longevity are more successful for the younger than for the older subjects. Also for both age groups, the predictions of longevity are more successful than the all-or-none predictions of survival. For the younger subjects the longevity predictions, at the F-level of 0.50, reach the rather remarkable correlation of .91.

In delineating overall trends which determine the magnitude of the correlations, i.e., are consistent predictors of survival or longevity, we observe in the main body of the table that for the younger age group "subjective health" ratings enter consistently (4 out of 5 cases) and at the highest rank into the equations. For the older age group, this role is taken over by the ratings of "physical activities." In recognizing that several measures of intellectual performance (intelligence and verbal tests) are good predictors of survival and longevity for the older subjects (this has been discussed in the preceding sections) and that, in addition, the "time of rising," and "amount of free time" have a notable impact, we conclude that the chances for survival of older subjects are dependent upon (over and above good health) the opportunities and engagement in activities which, in turn, might guarantee a good maintenance of intellectual abilities.

Conclusions

The strong evidence for a terminal drop suggests that in a healthy population there may be no changes in performance and behavior during adulthood and aging. Since mortality increases with age, however, we observe an apparent decrement produced by the increasing number of persons exhibiting such a drop prior to their death.

This interpretation is congruent with and consolidates the discrepancies between cross-sectional and longitudinal findings. Cross-sectional results are confounded by selective death, selected test participation, and terminal drop, as well as by sociohistorical changes between the different cohorts tested. Although longitudinal results remain confounded in regard to the sociohistorical changes

Table 11-1

Multiple Regression Predictions of Death (D) and Longevity (L), for Data from the First (A) and Second Testing (B), over a Period of Five (5) or Ten (10) Years, for Females (F) and Males (M), and Below and Above 65 Years, Respectively.

Predictors	Below 65					Above 65				
	DA5	DA10	DB5	LAF	LAM	DA5	DA10	DB5	LAF	LAM
Performance Intelligence										
Antonyms		2 7.65	2 8.47						4 3.84	
Selections								3 8.70	3 8.14	
Classifications							2 4.15	1 18.89		
Analogies	4 7.18				4 8.74					
Mixed Tests										
Classification Time				5 12.20						
Mixed Time	7 4.90			4 21.47	7 6.34					
General Dogmatism	3 7.94		4 3.85			2 9.59				
Dogmatism Total		3 7.33								
Personal Rigidity				3 8.53			3 4.05			
Rigidity Total				10 4.09				4 7.57		
Pro-Retrospective										
Productive Preference	5 9.42									
Physical Preference				7 8.29						
Education 1					6 2.21					
Finances 1					3 8.21		4 3.30			5 3.27
Finances 2			5 2.77							
Health	1 12.61	1 12.48		1 7.58	1 5.04					3 9.39
Physical Activities						1 10.12	1 5.06	2 5.26	1 16.34	
Activities Total		5 3.34	3 5.53							
Checked Activities	6 5.67			6 17.18						

	1	2	3	4	5	6	7	8	9	10
Comparison Situations	4 4.39			2 11.77				5 3.11		
Deterioration 1	2 9.12									
Deterioration 2					2 0.56					
Deterioration 3					8 4.70					
Number of Siblings				8 6.94					2 6.94	
Number of Acquaintances					5 6.26				4 3.72	
Time Rising	1 7.54					3 3.55				
Free Time				9 5.33			5 2.79			2 9.01
Years Married				11 3.81						1 12.25
Number of Variables F.10	7	5	5	11	8	3	5	5	4	5
F.25	15	12	7	36	16	9	12	10	8	18
F.50	40	27	26	41	40	22	24	23	17	41
Correlations R.10	.57	.41	.50	.71	.65	.30	.34	.51	.49	.49
R.25	.60	.51	.53	.90	.74	.34	.37	.57	.54	.64
R.50	.68	.57	.63	.91	.85	.45	.45	.64	.59	.70

First figure indicates the rank at which variables enter into the regression equation. Second figure indicates the F-level attained at the end of the procedure. The number of variables entering into the equations at different strengths of the criterion and the corresponding multiple correlation coefficients are shown in the last six lines.

150

(affecting one cohort across the historical period during which the testing takes place), they allow the derivation of separate estimates of cross-sectional developmental differences between selected and, thus, "biased" subgroups (i.e., of nonsurviving subjects and retest-resisters) and longitudinal comparisons of the retestees. The latter, in particular, have consistently shown a high stability in performance and behavior or even increases with age for those retestees who survive, but marked drops for those not surviving additional years. Since the latter (being cooperative subjects) are most likely to enter into cross-sectional comparisons, they produce the notable decline in performance observed in all but a few of the cross-sectional studies.

This general interpretation, to be called "terminal drop—mortality model," does not consider the influence of selective survival, according to which the more able persons survive better than the less able. It assumes that death strikes persons in a random manner, whereas the chances of survival decrease systematically with age. On the other hand, the observations of selective survival and longevity call attention to the effectiveness of systematic factors. For the simplest extension of the "terminal drop—mortality model" we assume a connection between genetic factors of longevity and those performances and behaviors which served as predictors of survival in our multiple regression equations. In other words, this model proposes that there exist strains of individuals who perform at different levels and show variations in developmental trends as well as in longevity. All these behavioral signs co-vary and are genetically determined.

Our modified interpretation might be called the "genetic, terminal drop—mortality model," but this leaves any details of the genetic determinants and connections unexplained (see however, Strehler 1962). For the present purpose, it is of greater interest to consider another modification of our original interpretation which might be called the "mediated, terminal drop—mortality model."

Such a model assumes individual differences in performance and behavior without necessarily specifying whether these are primarily due to intrinsic or extrinsic factors. Certain persons cope less well with their environment, for instance, receive less education, lower income, worse nutrition, and little medical attention, etc. Subsequently, their chances for survival decrease and they drop out earlier than their more favored age-mates. Intuitively, it seems that such an interpretation allows for detailed explications of the determinants of survival and, most important, emphasizes the propedeutic and therapeutic possibilities of changing the course of development through social actions. It is for these reasons that we ought to pay special attention to such an interpretation.

References

Baltes, P.B. Longitudinal and cross-sectional sequences in the study of age and generation effects. *Human Development*, 1968, *11*, 145-171.

Baltes, P.B., Baltes, M.M., and Reinert, G. The effects of time of measurement in cognitive age-development of children: An application of cross-sequential sequences. *Human Development*, 1970 (in press).

Baltes, P.B., Schaie, K.W. and Hardi, A.H. Age and experimental mortality in a seven-year longitudinal study of cognitive behavior (unpublished manuscript), Department of Psychology, University of West Virginia, 1970.

Hilton, T.L. and Patrick, C. Cross-sectional versus longitudinal data: An empirical comparison of mean differences in academic growth. *Research Bulletin* 69-42, Educational Testing Service. Princeton, N.J., 1969.

Jarvik, L.F. and Falek, A. Intellectual stability and survival in the aged. *Journal of Gerontology*, 1963, *18*, 173-176.

Kleemeier, R.W. Intellectual changes in the senium or death and the IQ. Presidential Address, Division 20, Annual Convention of the American Psychological Association, New York, 1961.

Kleemeier, R.W. Intellectual changes in the senium. In: *Proceedings of the Social Statistics Section of the American Statistical Association*, Washington, D.C., 1962, pp. 290-295.

Lieberman, M.A. Psychological correlates of impending death; some preliminary observations. *Journal of Gerontology*, 1965, *20*, 181-190.

Lieberman, M.A. Observations of death and dying. *Gerontologist*, 1966, *6*, 70-72.

Riegel, K.F. A study on verbal achievements of older persons. *Journal of Gerontology*, 1959, *14*, 453-456.

Riegel, K.F. *Der spachliche Leistungstest SASKA*, Göttingen: Verlag Psychologie, 1967.

Riegel, K.F. and Riegel, R.M. A study on changes of attitudes and interests during later years of life. *Vita Humana*, 1960, *3*, 1977-2006.

Riegel, K.F. and Riegel, R.M. Analysis of differences in test performance and item difficulty between young and old adults. *Journal of Gerontology*, 1962, *17*, 97-105.

Riegel, K.F., Riegel, R.M. and Meyer, G. The prediction of intellectual development and death: A longitudinal analysis: In: *Proceedings 6th International Congress of Gerontology*, Copenhagen, Denmark, 1963, p. 194.

Riegel, K.F., Riegel, R.M. and Meyer, G. A study of the drop-out rates in longitudinal research on aging and the prediction of death. *Journal of Personality and Social Psychology*, 1967a, *4*, 343-348.

Riegel, K.F., Riegel, R.M. and Meyer, G. Socio-psychological factors of aging: A cohort-sequential analysis. *Human Development*, 1967b, *10*, 27-56.

Riegel, K.F., Riegel, R.M. and Meyer, G. The prediction of retest-resisters in longitudinal research on aging. *Journal of Gerontology*, 1968, *23*, 370-374.

Riegel, K.F., Riegel, R.M. and Skiba, G. Untersuchung der Lebensbedingungen, Gewohnheiten und Anpassung älterer Menschen in Norddeutschland. *Vita Humana*, 1962, *5*, 204-247.

Riegel, R.M. and Riegel, K.F. Standardisierung des Hamburg-Wechsler-Intelligenztests für Erwachsene (HAWIE) für die Altersstufen über 50 Jahre. *Diagnostica*, 1959, 5, 97-128.

Ryder, N.B. The cohort as a concept in the study of social changes. *American Sociological Review*, 1965, *30*, 843-861.

Schaie, K.W. A general model for the study of developmental problems. *Psychological Bulletin*, 1965, *64*, 92-108.

Schaie, K.W. and Strother, C.R. A Cross-sequential study of age changes in cognitive behavior. *Psychological Bulletin*, 1968, *70*, 671-680.

Strehler, B.L. *Time, cells and aging*. New York: Academic Press, 1962.

Wechsler, D. *Die Messung der Intelligenz Erwachsener*, Bern: Hüber, 1956.

12 Survival of Elderly Psychiatric Patients

PAUL E. BAER and
CHARLES M. GAITZ

There are now a number of corroborative studies which complement early findings by Kleemeier (1962) that changes in intellectual performance of the elderly are related to mortality, or conversely, to survival. In these studies, several different types of elderly populations have been examined, including noninstitutionalized normal (Riegel 1967, Jarvik and Falek 1963), institutionalized normal (Lieberman 1965), and institutionalized deteriorated individuals (Goldfarb 1966, 1969; Sanderson and Inglish 1961). However, in only two instances were nonintellectual physical status variables also assessed, in one with a normal (Riegel 1967) and in the other with a deteriorated sample (Goldfarb 1969). In each case, they were found significantly related to mortality, in conjunction with significant intellectual measures.

It is also of interest to note that a methodological difference between the various investigations appears to be associated with the type of population studied. The significant intellectual predictors for normal populations are typically found for change scores, while those for deteriorated populations are found for differences in absolute levels.

The present investigation was undertaken with an intermediate heterogeneous population obtained at psychiatric intake, restricted neither to normal nor to deteriorated persons. The measures were analyzed for differences in absolute levels. Included among the battery of measures were several indices of physical status. The intention was to test previously reported significant relationships between both intellectual and nonintellectual variables and survival, and to investigate the independence of these variables as predictors, particularly with respect to intellectual variables. Finally, the relationship of survival to disposition and institutionalization was explored.

Procedure

The 100 patients included in this study had been consecutively admitted to the Harris County Diagnostic Center, a receiving unit for psychiatrically disturbed

Paul E. Baer is Professor of Psychiatry, Baylor College of Medicine, Houston, Texas.

Charles M. Gaitz is Chief of the Gerontological Research Section, Texas Research Institute of Mental Science, Houston, Texas.

153

individuals. They were all at least age 60. These patients were studied as part of a demonstration project concerned with a multidisciplinary approach to the comprehensive care of older persons suspected of mental illness. All patients were evaluated within a day or two of initial hospitalization by a team consisting of psychiatrist, psychologist, nurse, social worker and internist, using a broad battery of procedures, the results of which were subsequently used to formulate diagnosis and disposition by team consensus. These initial evaluations were later stated in quantitative terms for follow-up assessments. Detailed follow-up was conducted at six and twelve months after intake. The results of the initial evaluation were also examined in relation to mortality within a 30-month follow-up period after the date of the initial evaluation.

Social histories obtained both from patients and informants yielded a variety of sociodemographic information. From the data concerning the patients' contact with social agencies and relevant professionals during the six-month period preceding intake, a visibility score was devised. In the present usage, visibility refers to active contact a patient has with agencies and professionals. The score consists of a summation of the variety of contacts made by the patient, or for the patient by his family, irrespective of the number of visits made to each of the agencies or professionals involved.

A complete battery of tests designed for assessment of impairment of cognitive and other functions in brain damage was administered to 60 of the patients during the initial evaluation. Of the remaining 40 patients, 24 others attempted to respond, but a scoreable record could not be obtained, and the failures were judged to imply impairment. The other patients refused the tests, had language problems or could not be induced to involve themselves in the tasks sufficiently to determine impairment. Fifteen measures were obtained; tapping rate, ratio of errors on the sensory component of the Reitan version of the Halstead-Wepman screening test for aphasia, WAIS vocabulary raw score, six scores from the subtests of the Wechsler memory scale, time to complete trail making A, time to complete trail making B, a rating for performance on the Weigl color form sorting test, time to complete a tactual performance test, ratio of errors on the screening test for aphasia except for number of errors on construction apraxia items, which were separately scored. Using data collected from other samples of hospitalized elderly patients with chronic brain syndrome, elderly schizophrenics and "normal" elderly individuals, a classification scheme for degree of cognitive impairment was devised. The four categories were: A, normal or minimally impaired; B, moderately impaired; C, severely impaired; and D, extremely impaired—record not satisfactorily scoreable. The classifications were made separately by two psychologists with virtually errorless reliability.

It was possible to obtain scoreable records for the Mental Status Schedule (MSS) (Spitzer et al. 1967) from 85 of the patients. The MSS consists of a series of 248 items in a structural interview and observational format. The patients' responses can be quantified on 16 factor-based scales, of which the first three are major summarized scales. They are labeled: feelings and concerns, confusion-retardation, delusions-hallucinations, inappropriate or bizarre appearance or behavior, belligerence-negativism, agitation-excitement, retardation-emotional withdrawal, speech disorganization, delusion-persecution-hallucination, grandiosity, depression-anxiety, suicide-self-mutilation, somatic concerns, social isolation, disorientation-memory, and denial of illness. An initial psychiatric diagnosis was also established, using clinical psychiatric impressions at intake. These diagnostic labels were subsequently checked by two psychiatrists working separately, disagreements were clarified, and the patients were classified into diagnostic groups, using the most recent psychiatric manual as a guide. For present purposes, only two classes of diagnoses were used, with or without organic brain syndrome, irrespective of other diagnosable problems.

Using the results of a physical examination conducted by an internist, and collateral information from hospitals, family and physicians, two raters, both physicians, independently classified each patient for the level of functional capacity. Information of a psychological or psychiatric nature was not used by the raters for this rating. The ratings were based on a scheme suggested by Zeman (1947). Rating A, the highest level of functional capacity, means that the patient is without obvious disability, and that there is no condition which interferes with ordinary activities. The next rating, B, means that the patient has some loss in functional capacity, but can be up and about in the community, i.e., can attend a clinic. The next rating, C, means that the patient is homebound, but can perform within the confines of his home, although there is considerable loss in functional capacity. The final rating, D, is reserved for patients whose functional capacity is severely reduced, and who are either bed-ridden or confined to a chair.

Each patient was rated by a nurse for the extent of need of nursing care in each of 14 nursing areas. A seven-point rating scale was used, ranging from no nursing care needed to critical need for nursing care. Ratings were collapsed into three sets: no or limited need for nursing care, moderate need, or severe need. A summary rating score was also obtained by summation of ratings over all 14 areas, which included: diet, fluids, feeding, bowel care, bladder care, toileting, skin care, oral care, grooming, rest, exercise, body movement, organization of environment, and medical regimen.

Finally, the patients were classified in accordance with the disposition which followed the initial evaluation and duration of any subsequent institutionalization. Five disposition classifications were used: (1) return to a noninstitutional setting, usually a family dwelling, (2) hospitalization in a local general hospital, (3) hospitalization in a local psychiatric hospital or ward, (4) hospitalization in a state psychiatric hospital, and (5) placement in a nursing home.

Predictors of Survival

Over a 30-month follow-up period after initial evaluation, 70 of the original 100 patients survived. In Table 12-1, several sociodemographic variables are shown in

Table 12-1
Survival and Sociodemographic Variables

Group	N	Sex*		Living Arrangements		Age		Education		Visibility	
		M	F	With spouse	Not with spouse	Years		Years		Years	
	N	N	N	N	N	$\overline{X}$	SD	$\overline{X}$	SD	$\overline{X}$	SD
Survivors	70	36	34	26	44	67.81	6.54	5.8	1.59	2.39	1.69
Non-Survivors	30	24	6	8	22	69.37	7.52	5.9	1.59	2.67	1.45

*χ^2 = 7.1, df=1, p < .01

relation to survival. Only sexual identity was significantly related to survival (χ^2 = 7.1, df = 1, p < .01), more male patients succumbing than females. Chronological age and the other variables were not significantly associated with survival. Another variable not shown in the table, whether or not the patient had a history of psychiatric hospitalization, was also not related.

Of the various measures obtained from the initial evaluations a number were significantly related to survival, more of them than would have been expected by chance from the total of measures considered. The index of cognitive impairment derived from the scores on the test battery was distributed differentially between the survival and nonsurvival groups. In the survival group the number of patients rated A was 20; B, 13; C, 12; and D, 10. In the nonsurvival group the ratings were: A, 3; B, 5; C, 7; and D, 14. (χ^2 = 11.8, df = 3, p < .01) Since 14 of the 29 nonsurviving patients for whom cognitive impairment ratings were available had D ratings, that is, they had incomplete protocols which could not be satisfactorily scored, the number of complete sets of cognitive test battery scores from the nonsurviving patients was limited to 15, in comparison to 45 from survivors. There were 15 test battery scores, but in none of the 15 comparisons did the mean score of one group significantly deviate from that of the other. Nevertheless, the differences between the mean scores of the surviving group and the nonsurviving group showed that on every one of the 15 measures the surviving group performed better or had fewer errors than the nonsurviving group.

The MSS was completed on 85 patients, of whom 62 were survivors. The mean scores on two scales differed significantly between the groups. For the scale, Confusion-Retardation, the mean score for the survivors was 56.42, SD = 18.36, and for the nonsurvivors it was 64.52, SD = 16.85. (t = 2.0, p < .05) On the scale Disorientation-Memory the mean score for the survivors was 62.44, SD = 23.39, and for the nonsurvivors it was 74.39, SD = 26.03. (t = 2.0, p < .05) The other 14 MSS scales did not yield significant differences between the two groups. Psychiatric diagnosis was examined for the presence or absence of organic brain syndrome (OBS) in relation to survival. The frequency of OBS patients in the survival group was 37 and in the nonsurvival group it was 24. The frequency of non-OBS patients in the survival group was 33, while in the nonsurvival group it was 6. (χ^2 = 4.6, df = 1, p < .05)

When ratings of functional capacity were examined, it was found that the distribution of these ratings was significantly related to survival. Among survivors, the number of patients rated A was 29; B, 23; C, 15; and D, 3. Among nonsurvivors, the number of patients rated A was 2; B, 7; C, 15; and D, 6. (χ^2 = 18.5, df = 3, p < .001) Among the nursing need care areas, only two of the 14 yielded a significant relationship with survival for the total 100 patients rated. Frequencies of the three levels of rating for need for bowel care among survivors were, respectively, 46, 13 and 11, while for nonsurvivors they were 13, 10 and 7. (χ^2 = 6.6, df = 2, p < .05) For bladder care the frequencies among survivors were 46, 13 and 11, while for nonsurvivors they were 11, 7 and 12. (χ^2 = 8.7, df = 2, p < .02) Moreover, for the survivors the mean summary nursing need score was 32.7, SD = 15.5, and for the nonsurvivors it was 40.6, SD = 18.2. (t = 2.1, p < .05)

Further analyses of the data were addressed to correlational evaluations of the measures which were significantly related to survival. These analyses were intended to be more exploratory than definitive, principally because cross-validation was not possible, and because of limitations in measurement characteristics and data distributions. The major goals were to obtain information regarding interrelations among measures related to survival, as well as some indication of the independence and relative power of them as predictors. The programs used routinely calculated product moment coefficients. For missing data the programs inserted mean values.

Table 12-2 shows the correlations of the measures significantly related to survival with actual survival, and the intercorrelations among them. One additional variable not previously shown related to survival was added, chronological age. The correlations of the measures cited above with survival and nonsurvival were either significant or approximated a significance level of .05. The highest correlation with survival was functional capacity (.45) and the second was cognitive impairment (.34). It is to be noted, however, that there were a large number of significant correlations among the predictors themselves. In Table 12-3, intercorrelations are shown for the predictor variables and the extent of survival: the number of months of survival following the initial evaluation. The sample consisted of the 30 patients who did not survive the 30-month follow-up period. In this instance only three of the measures, functional capacity, nursing need score, and bladder care rating, were significantly correlated with number of months of survival. Again, a large number of significant correlations within the set of predictor variables was found.

In a series of subsequent analyses, an attempt was made to isolate variables uniquely associated with survival by simplification of the intercorrelational pattern through factoring. It was difficult from the tabulation of intercorrelations to note whether some predictor variables for survival might not be

Table 12-2
Intercorrelations of Survival and Predictors of Survival for 100 Elderly Psychiatric Patients

Variable	Correlation Coefficients									
	2	3	4	5	6	7	8	9	10	11
1 Survival	.10	-.27*	.34*	.45*	.22*	.25*	.29*	.18	.19*	.25*
2 Age		-.02	.32*	.39*	.20*	.08	.23*	.20*	.19*	.41*
3 Sex			-.05	-.35*	-.17	-.16	-.18	.01	.00	-.06
4 Cognitive Impairment				.42*	.52*	.14	.29*	.67*	.64*	.67*
5 Functional Capacity					.55*	.37*	.53*	.18	.16	.44*
6 Nursing Needs						.60*	.74*	.35*	.35*	.41*
7 Bowel Care							.61*	.12	.13	.26*
8 Bladder Care								.15	.18	.27*
9 MSS Confusion–Retardation									.93*	.56*
10 MSS Disorganization–Memory										.58*
11 Chronic Brain Syndrome										—

*p ≤ .05

Table 12-3
Intercorrelations of Extent of Survival and Predictors of Extent of Survival for 30 Elderly Psychiatric Patients

Variable	Correlation Coefficients									
	2	3	4	5	6	7	8	9	10	11
1 Extent of Survival	-.10	-.03	-.17	-.30	-.39*	-.20	-.45*	.11	.02	-.07
2 Age		.11	.22	.19	-.03	-.25	.11	.10	.09	.33
3 Sex			-.13	-.20	-.10	.02	-.02	.06	.06	.04
4 Cognitive Impairment				.21	.45*	-.02	.22	.36	.40*	.54*
5 Functional Capacity					.41*	.41*	.43*	-.17	-.14	.41*
6 Nursing Needs						.69*	.80*	.09	.11	.25
7 Bowel Care							.73*	-.24	-.13	.08
8 Bladder Care								-.16	-.06	.21
9 MSS Confusion–Retardation									.92*	.50*
10 MSS Disorganization–Memory										.51*
11 Chronic Brain Syndrome										—

*p ≤ .05

primary or independent, but secondarily predictive through correlation with an independent predictor. Table 12-4 shows the results of a factor analysis of the significant predictor variables, age, and survival, rotated to a varimax solution, using the Data Text System, which was also used in subsequent analyses. Five factors were found beyond a limit of latent root = 1, or 10 percent of the communality. These five factors showed relatively little overlapping among the variables, and could be identified and rationalized with relative efficiency, using a cut-off point for factor loading of variables at .40. Physical status and cognitive variables loaded separately on two major factors, neither of which, however, included survival to an appreciable degree. Also, the survival variable did not load significantly on two additional factors, readily recognizable as concerned with chronological age and with sex. Finally, a survival factor appeared (#5) on which only one predictor variable also loaded (at .40), functional capacity. Several supplementary analyses were conducted, including a varimax solution (N = 73) on data limited to patients for whom scores on all measures were available, and a quartimax solution on all 100 patients. The factor structure obtained from these analyses corresponded very closely with that described above. In addition, the varimax solution for data from 100 patients was obtained with the survival variable excluded. A four-factor structure identical to the first four factors described above was obtained. Comparison of mean factor scores on all four factors between the group of surviving and the group of nonsurviving patients yielded no significant differences. Finally a fixed factor rotation was conducted

Table 12-4
Varimax Rotation of Factor Analysis of Survival and Correlates of Survival for 100 Elderly Psychiatric Patients

Variable	Rotated Factor Loadings					
	1	2	3	4	5	Communality
1 Survival	.15	−.15	−.12	.03	−.95	.96
2 Age	.14	−.06	.03	.92	.02	.87
3 Sex	.01	.11	.98	−.01	.12	.98
4 Cognitive Impairment	.75	−.19	.00	.30	−.26	.76
5 Functional Capacity	.11	−.47	−.33	.51	−.40	.76
6 Nursing Needs	.33	−.84	−.09	.14	−.02	.84
7 Bowel Care	.04	−.85	−.03	−.05	−.10	.74
8 Bladder Care	.07	−.86	−.07	.17	−.13	.80
9 MSS Confusion−Retardation	.95	−.07	.00	.01	−.01	.91
10 MSS Disorganization−Memory	.95	−.09	.00	−.01	−.01	.91
11 Chronic Brain Syndrome	.65	−.20	−.01	.45	−.15	.69

with the survival variable fixed for the first factor. Two variables loaded on the first factor in this procedure, functional capacity at .54 and cognitive impairment at .40. The loadings of all other variables were less than .30.

The data from the group of nonsurviving patients was treated similarly, with the variable, number of months of survival, replacing the survival variable. Other variables were the same as above. The results of a varimax rotation of these data are shown in Table 12-5. The survival variable was found isolated in one factor with no other variable loading substantially on it. These results must be considered cautiously because of the small number of patients, 30. Also, for 7 of these patients, MSS data were missing. Nevertheless, the factor structure of this small subsample is very similar to that obtained from the complete group of 100, except for alternation of the ordinal sequence of the first two factors. Inspection of a parallel analysis of the 70 surviving patients, for whom there was no survival variable, also yielded a similar factor structure.

The data were also submitted to stepwise multiple regression analyses. Table 12-6 summarizes the results for the 100 patients with survival and nonsurvival the target variable. After the first highly significant predictor variable, functional capacity, and its associated partial correlation with the other predictor variables have been accounted for, no additional predictor variable contributed substantially to the multiple correlation, although bowel care rating and cognitive impairment have the second and third largest F values. The results were similar when the data for the 73 patients without missing data were examined.

Table 12-5
Varimax Rotation of Factor Analysis of Extent of Survival and Correlates of Extent of Survival (N=30)

Variable	Rotated Factor Loadings					
	1	2	3	4	5	Communality
1 Extent of Survival	−.27	.04	−.10	−.01	.88	.85
2 Age	−.20	.06	.83	.16	−.20	.79
3 Sex	.01	.03	.06	.95	−.01	.91
4 Cognitive Impairment	.17	.59	.33	−.31	−.27	.65
5 Functional Capacity	.55	−.14	.59	−.32	.03	.76
6 Nursing Needs	.84	.23	.01	−.13	−.31	.87
7 Bowel Care	.94	−.14	−.13	.07	.06	.92
8 Bladder Care	.84	−.03	.14	.03	−.32	.84
9 MSS Confusion−Retardation	−.13	.94	−.02	.06	.07	.91
10 MSS Disorganization−Memory	−.05	.94	−.02	.08	.01	.90
11 Chronic Brain Syndrome	.26	.61	.60	−.02	.15	.82

Similarly, as shown in Table 12-7, for the nonsurviving patients with number of months of survival the target variable, only one variable, need for nursing care in the area of urinary incontinence, contributed significantly to the multiple regression. In such analyses, the major contribution to the regression and the first to be treated is the variable having the largest correlation. Also, F values cannot be tested because of the mix of continuous and discrete measures. On the whole, however, these results are consistent with those obtained by factoring.

Table 12-6
Stepwise Regression Analysis with Survival the Target Variable (N=100)

Variable	Step Number	Multiple Correlation	F
Functional Capacity	1	.45	24.56
Cognitive Impairment	2	.48	3.64
Sex	3	.50	2.39
Nursing Needs	4	.51	1.51
Bowel Care	5	.54	4.53
Bladder Care	6	.55	1.79
Age	7	.57	1.73
Chronic Brain Syndrome	8	.57	.19
MSS Disorganization—Memory	9	.57	.22
MSS Confusion—Retardation	10	.57	.50

Table 12-7
Stepwise Regression Analysis with Extent of Survival the Target Variable (N=30)

Variable	Step Number	Multiple Correlation	F
Bladder Care	1	.45	7.12
Bowel Care	2	.49	1.23
Functional Capacity	3	.51	.80
Chronic Brain Syndrome	4	.52	.45
Nursing Needs	5	.54	.45
Sex	6	.55	.50
Age	7	.55	.16
MSS Disorganization—Memory	8	.56	.10
MSS Confusion—Retardation	9	.59	1.09
Cognitive Impairment	10	.59	.12

Role of Institutionalization

For analysis of the role of institutionalization with respect to survival, the initial placements of the patients were classed into two categories. The first category contained patients who were not institutionalized, or who had brief periods of hospitalization in either a psychiatric or general hospital located in the community. Of the 54 patients in this category, 44 survived and 10 did not. The second class consisted of custodial types of placements involving long-term institutionalization in a nursing home, a home for the aged, or in a state psychiatric hospital. Of the 46 patients in this group, 26 survived and 20 did not. (x^2 = 5.7, df = 1, p < .05) Several measures were checked to explore further whether this association between placement and survival was a function of institutionalization or due to survival-associated characteristics of patients which may have determined the placements. It was found, for example, that the mean MSS score on confusion-retardation for noninstitutional placement survivors was 52.6 and for nonsurvivors 63.5 (t = 1.5), while for custodial placements the mean value for survivors was 63.5, and for nonsurvivors 65.1 (t = .27). Survivors compared across placements differed significantly (t = 2.3, p < .05), but nonsurvivors did not differ. The general tendency was to place more impaired persons into custodial settings. Nonsurvivors had scores suggesting impairment, irrespective of placement. Also, patients who survived in custodial settings had scores similar to those of the nonsurviving patients in these settings. Other indexes such as nursing needs, functional capacity, and cognitive impairment yielded corroborative results. In the case of functional capacity, a subsample of the least capable (rated C and D) patients was inspected to determine whether among them there would be differential survival in relation to placement. In the group of patients in noninstitutional placements, 10 survived and 9 did not, while in the group of custodially placed patients, 8 survived and 12 did not. Thus, survival was not significantly associated with placement, even among those whose indexes suggested the least likelihood of survival.

The number of months spent by surviving and nonsurviving patients in any one of four institutional settings during a one year follow-up period was also examined. It was necessary to prorate duration of institutionalization for those patients who did not survive the twelve-month period. Also, patients considered for institutionalization may have entered the institution after initial evaluation or at any time during the follow-up year. Among the survivors, 28 patients were in nursing homes an average of 9.0 months, 21 in a local mental hospital 2.1 months, 15 in a local general hospital 1.4 months, and 23 in a state psychiatric hospital 5.8 months. Among the nonsurvivors, 12 were in nursing homes 9.2 months, 3 in a local mental hospital 3.0 months, 10 in a local general hospital 3.6 months, and 14 in a state psychiatric hospital 8.4 months. The nonsurvivors had a significantly longer mean stay at a state psychiatric hospital than did the survivors. (t = 2.0, p < .05) Duration of institutionalization elsewhere did not differ significantly between the groups. Elaboration of this finding showed that the longer mean stay at the state hospital for nonsurvivors was entirely due to the effect of prorating the length of stay for patients who died so on after admission.

Discussion

The results of the present study substantiate previously published data that the likelihood of survival among elderly individuals is related to testa ble and observable characteristics. That these characteristics can be found in both intellectual and physical status domains was also confirmed. The fact that the present study utilized measures which differed in detail from those of the preceding studies while being similar in essence adds considerably to the reliability of these findings. Although the magnitudes of the correlations do not account for substantial portions of variance, they are nevertheless of de finitive signficance. An additional finding suggests that predictors may differ dep ending on the nature of the target variable, survival. In the present case, both intellectual and nonintellectual variables were significantly correlated with survival over the period of two and a half years. However when only nonsurviving individuals were considered and correlates of duration of survival were sought, it was found that only nonintellectual, physical status variables were significantly correlated with duration of survival. It is worth noting that the term prediction may be misleading since it is being used on a posthoc basis. In that connection it may also be noted that cross-validation is possible for survival per se, but is not readily possible for duration of survival in the sense in which it is used in the present context.

The correlates of survival and extent of survival were frequently and significantly correlated among themselves. Using factor analytic methods to simplify the pattern of intercorrelations, it was found that a stable factor structure could be determined. The factor structure consisted of a factor concerned with cognitive variables involving impairment, a factor concerned with physical status involving functional capacity and need for nursing care, a factor concerning sex, a factor concerning chronological age and to some extent cognitive impairment, and finally, a factor concerning survival, on which also a measure of physical status, functional capacity, loaded. When the survival variable was fixed for the first factor position, cognitive impairment as well as functional impairment loaded on the factor which contained the survival variable. When the intercorrelations were factored for the nonsurviving patients only, using extent of survival, the factor structure obtained was essentially similar to that described except that no other variable loaded substantially on the factor which contained extent of survival. What is notable about the factorial approach is not only that a strong survival factor including both survival and significant predictors could not be found, but that at the same time a factor structure was obtained which sensibly reflects important dimensions of aging. These dimensions are evidently better established, structurally more well defined, and more stable in their own right than they are in conjunction with survival, at least as far as the present sample is concerned. The intercorrelations among the predictors are more apparently important than the correlations between predictors and survival. These findings put the search for predictors of survival into perspective. They further stand as a reminder that while it is possible to find statistical predictors, these do not necessarily reflect processes involved in the predictive relationship. The factorial results suggest that the variance for prediction of survival which can be accounted for may be more readily explained on physical status than on cognitive grounds. These findings create an atmosphere of caution for acceptance of cognitive processes as indicative of survival, especially in the absence of parallel exploration of noncognitive processes.

The regression analyses generally support these impressions. When the largest correlation with survival (physical status) and its associated partial correlations with the other predictive variables were accounted for, no substantial increment in the multiple correlation was contributed by any other predictor variable. As far as survival is concerned, the physical status variables appear to take a primary position in importance over the cognitive variables. Despite the fact that they appear only in a secondary position, the cognitive or intellectual variables cannot be entirely discounted. In these analyses, when they do appear, they do so independently of nonintellectual variables. In the case of extent of survival, however, only a relatively specific physical status variable, that of urinary incontinence, is significantly predictive. This observation accords well with the data previously reported by Goldfarb (1969). In cases where the terminal state appears to be already in progress, this variable may be of particular importance. Nevertheless, prediction of extent of survival is less potent than predictors of survival.

The present analysis was based on differences in absolute measures related to survival. What appeared to have occurred was that these measures distinguished the patients who were in a preterminal state and similar to the patients described in other studies where the sample was institutionalized and deteriorated. The rest of the patients in the present sample, had there been sufficiently long follow-up, might have shown a relationship between change scores and survival, similar to that observed in studies where the subjects were normal elderly individuals. The relationship between absolute differences and change scores is of some importance, since change scores require differences between pairs of absolute levels. With the passage of time or declining competence, elderly individuals become progressively more susceptible to prediction of survival by using absolute levels only.

In view of the popular concern that facilities for institutionalization are apt to be incapable of caring for the elderly and thus may hasten their demise, the present findings are illuminating. They indicate that for the present sample, survival was not readily explained on the grounds of either placement in an institution or duration of institutionalization. They also make it clear that it is possible to obtain significant relationships between variables associated with institutionalization and survival but that these may be artifactual in nature. It is important to recognize that if placement in an institution is related to the

166

patient's survival, it may not be because of the institutionalization but because of the characteristics of the patient which have led to institutionalization.

References

Goldfarb, A.I., Fisch, M., and Gerber, I.E. Predictors of mortality in the institutionalized aged. *Diseases of the Nervous System*, 1966, *27*, 21-29.

Goldfarb, A.I. Predicting mortality in the institutionalized aged. *Archives of General Psychiatry*, 1969, *21*, 172-176.

Jarvik, L.F., and Falek, A. Intellectual stability and survival in the aged. *Journal of Gerontology*, 1963, *18*, 173-176.

Kleemeier, R.W., Intellectual change in the senium. In *Proceedings, Social Statistics Section, American Statistical Association*, 1962. pp. 290-295.

Lieberman, M.A. Psychological correlates of impending death. *Journal of Gerontology*, 1965, *20*, 181-190.

Riegel, K.F., Riegel, R.M., and Meyer, G. A Study of the dropout rates in longitudinal research in aging and the prediction of death. *Journal of Personality and Social Psychology*, 1967, *5*, 342-348.

Sanderson, R.E., and Inglis, J. Learning and mortality in elderly psychiatric patients. *Journal of Gerontology*, 1961, *16*, 375-376.

Spitzer, R.L., Fleiss, J.L., Endicott, J., and Cohen, J. Mental Status Schedule. *Archives of General Psychiatry*, 1967, *16*, 479-493.

Zeman, F.D. The functional capacity of the aged, its estimation and practical importance. *Journal of the Mt. Sinai Hospital*, 1947, *14*, 721-728.

13

Some Issues in Studying Psychological Predictors of Survival*

MORTON A. LIEBERMAN

Despite growing attention to psychological dimensions relating to survival in the aged (Jarvik and Falek 1963; Kleemeier 1961; Lieberman 1965; Lieberman and Coplan 1969; Riegel and Riegel 1970), a number of difficult problems remain because of the lack of theory by which new information can be integrated. Much of the information on psychological parameters related to survival has accrued fortuitously as a function of the attrition characterizing aged samples. Accordingly, it is not surprising that theoretical developments have lagged behind empirical developments. Such explanation, however, does little to reduce the frustration inherent in working without theoretical guidelines.

Data from several studies of adaptation and survival of the aged under stress may be illustrative of the problems still facing investigators.† In the absence of a cogent theoretical framework for looking at psychological characteristics relating to survival, several sources were explored in selecting variables for these studies. The research in the area of human stress of Irving Janis (1958) and others (Appley and Trumbull 1967; Funkenstein, King and Drolette 1957; Lazarus 1966) was instrumental in leading to an emphasis on psychological dimensions related to coping, as well as to thinking of adaptation in terms of strategies for dealing with anticipated threat, such as denial and processes of "psychological resolution."

The studies of psychological factors mitigating reaction to physical diseases, such as those of LeShan (1961) on cancer, or of Greenfield et al. (1959) on infectious diseases, while lacking a comprehensive framework, contained recurrent suggestions that various indices of emotional states were important predictors of ability to recover from physical illness. These ideas suggested the selection of a number of dimensions reflecting emotional states of the study population.

Perhaps the major influences on the choice of variables were empirical and theoretical inquiries directly related to aging. These influences were manifested in diverse forms ranging from the inclusion of variables such as cognitive

*Presented at the 23rd Meeting, Gerontological Society Meetings, Toronto, October 22, 1970: Symposium—Predictors of Survival.

†These investigations were supported wholly by PHS Research Grant No. HD-00364, NICHHD and by Research Career Development Award 5-K 3-H D 20-342.

Morton A. Lieberman is Associate Professor, Committee on Human Development and Department of Psychiatry, University of Chicago.

functioning, that have been associated with developmental decrements, to the inclusion of variables relating to functions such as reminiscence, which has been assigned critical importance by theorists such as Erikson (1959) and Butler (1963).

A series of 41 measures was developed to assess: cognitive functioning, energy output, physical level, level of mental health, emotional states, introspection, affective complexity, future-orientation, self-esteem, self-consistency, personality traits, interpersonal relations, coping mechanisms, reminiscence functions, and source of stress. Table 13-1 describes the 41 variables examined in this chapter.

The findings discussed in this chapter are based on studies of 180 aged men and women (average age, 78 years) followed for two years. The study population included 100 aged individuals in relatively good psychological and physical condition, awaiting entrance into three homes for the aged (Stressed Group) and two control samples (Nonstressed Group)—a matched community group who did not anticipate institutionalization, and a group who had lived in these institutions over three years and had retained a psychological status which would still have allowed them admission to the institutions. Thus the phenomena were not those involved in the usual attrition study, for a much lower survival rate had been anticipated at the outset for the Stressed Group (those awaiting entrance into the homes for the aged) than for the Nonstressed Group (the two control populations). Based on previous studies with similar populations (Lieberman 1961), it was expected that upon relocation, the mortality rate for the Stressed Group would be over twice that of the Nonstressed Group. The reported findings here are based upon a comparison of psychological factors associated with survival in both the Stressed and Nonstressed Groups.

Each group was measured at the onset of the study (Time I) and two years later (Time II). Survival was evaluated in a broader sense than that of simply staying alive. Information from tests and interviews was used to classify subjects into two groups: those who retained the same level of physical, mental, and behavioral functioning from Time I to Time II and those who evidenced appreciable deterioration or who were dead at Time II. Although rated independently, psychological, physical, and mental deterioration overlapped considerably in the second group (.9 average correlation), suggesting that these individuals had crossed over a "threshold level" of deterioration and had low chances of surviving much beyond the arbitrary two-year limit. When these survival criteria were applied to the Stress Group, 52 percent of subjects had the same level of functioning at Time I as at Time II, whereas 48 percent had died or seriously deteriorated by Time II. For the Nonstressed Group, 65 percent were intact and 35 percent had died or were deteriorated by Time II.

Results

To what extend and in what areas do psychological dimensions predict stable or deteriorated status? Findings are presented separately for the Stressed and

Nonstressed Groups, because many of the predictive psychological dimensions were different for these two samples, despite their being closely matched.[1]

The Stressed Group

Overall Power of Prediction. The overall power of psychological dimensions in predicting survivorship was determined by use of a linear discriminate analysis. A combination of 15 psychological indexes yielded a discriminate function that correctly classified 90 percent of the subjects into "survivors" and "nonsurvivors." This statistical procedure made clear that psychological parameters could be powerfully related to survival, although an accurate assessment of the true power of the discriminate function would require replication of the procedure on another sample. The single most powerful discriminate was the bipolar personality trait of passivity-aggressivity; differences on this trait correctly identified outcome status for 69 percent of the subjects.

Specific Predictors. Table 13-2 shows the means and p levels for the 41 measures. Low levels of cognitive functioning (#1), diminished output of energy (#2), and poor physical status (#3) were all significantly related to nonsurvival. Mental health (#4, 5) did not discriminate. Cognitive functioning was particularly powerful. (It should be noted that the sample selection procedures eliminated seriously cognitively-impaired individuals; the differences in level of cognitive functioning reflected here are not comparable to those reported in studies in which moderate to severe organic brain damage was involved (Goldfarb 1958)).

None of the measures (#6-14) of emotional states and emotional organization were predictive of survival. In the area of time-perspective and hope (#15-17), however, it was revealed that the degree to which an individual can extend himself into past and future time (#15, 17) was a powerful predictor of survival status—low scores on time extension and futurity were associated with deterioration. Level of self-esteem (#18) and self-image based on current (rather than past or fantasied) interpersonal world (#19) were positively related to survivorship.

Classifications of psychological functioning by personality traits (#20-26) yielded dimensions that were highly predictive of survivorship status. Of the four approaches (factored rating of interviews, Q-Sort Factors, dimensions based on self-description and a standardized test) only the standardized personality tests (Catell 16 PF) yielded no significant prediction of survival status. The central trait appeared to be passivity-aggressivity or a dominant-nondominant stance. Dominant-aggressive individuals had higher survival probabilities than did communion-oriented (Bakan 1966), passive-withdrawn individuals.

A number of approaches were used to determine and categorize reminiscence

---

[1] A series of comparisons on test measures of personality and cognitive function demonstrated the homogeneity of these samples (Lieberman, Prock, Tobin 1968).

Table 13-1

	Variable	Description
1	Cognitive Sign-combined score on Mental Status, Learning-retention, Visual organization, Perceptual adequacy, Time judgment and Perseveration	Weighted sum of scores on the Mental Status Questionnaire (Kahn, Pollack and Goldfarb 1961); Paired-word association learning test (Inglis 1959); Bender-Gestalt designs (Bender 1938); Pascal and Suttell Scoring (Pascal and Suttell 1951); Murray TAT Cards 1, 2, 6BM, 7BM, 10 and 17BM; Dana system (Dana 1955); Time judgments of 30 and 60 sec. intervals; Reitman Stick-Figure Test scored for perseveration (Reitman and Robertson 1950).
2	Energy	Word count (output) on three standardized situations, Murray TAT cards, Daily round questionnaire and sentence completion test (S.C.T.).
3	Physical Function	Self report on mobility, locomotion, level of needed care (National Opinion Research Center, 1962).
4 & 5	Mental Health	4) Ratings of interviewer using Block Q-Sort Technique (Block 1961); 5) rating of interviewer for Life Satisfaction (Neugarten, Havighurst, and Tobin 1961).
6 & 7	Anxiety	6) Rating of S.C.T. by Gottshalk method (Gottshalk 1961); 7) Catell 16PF (Form C).
8 & 9	Depression	Rating of S.C.T. by Gottshalk method for depression (Gottshalk 1961); rating of S.C.T. items for death, hopelessness, boredom.
10-12	Body Image	10) Body Preoccupation—20 S.C.T. items scored for number of introduced body references; 11) Negative body image projection on Reitman test (Reitman and Robertson 1950); 12) Body Image—Negative or positive qualities associated with three body items on the S.C.T.
13	Introspection	Adaptation affect interview of Gendlin's rating system for level and degree of introspection (Gendlin 1964; Gorney 1968).
14	Affective Complexity	Number of different emotional themes used in telling stories to five Murray TAT cards.
15-17	Hope	15) Time extension—degree to which person extends himself into both future and past; rating for amount of extension, explicitness and sense of prescience based on number of questionnaire items. 16) attitudes toward life

Table 13-1. *(cont.)*

Variable	Description
	(Srole) and 17) Futurity, attitudes toward future events, ratings in response to interview questions—"planning ahead, meaning of time, reflections on past and future."
18 Self-esteem	Number of positive self items selected from 48 self descriptions.
19 Self-consistency Maintenance	Adequacy of utilizing realistic evidence for maintaining self consistency (Rosner 1968).
20-26 Personality Traits	20 & 21) 48 Self-descriptive statements based on Leary scoring system (Leary 1957), 2 dimensions, Dominance and Love. 22-25) Factor analysis of Trait rating based on total interview; Authoritarian; Passive-Aggressive; Introspective; Friendly.* 26) Catell 16PF, Introversion-Extroversion scale.
27-33 Reminiscence	Ratings based on life history and a life evaluation questionnaire. 27) Life evaluation. 28) Life review—avoidance of past to complete resolution and acceptance of past. 29) Affect toward one's past. 30) Reminiscence activity—amount of time spent in such activity. 31-33) counts based on the content of recollections: 31) number of satisfaction, 32) number and intensity of deprivations; 33) ratio of adult to childhood memories (Falk 1969).
34-36 Coping with anticipated threat	34) Denial—Perceptual avoidance or distortion of Institutional TAT themes (Lieberman and Lakin 1963). 35) Anticipatory working—number of times S spontaneously introduces in the interview topic of institutionalization. 36) Expected Loss—Gain-Loss anticipations, rated from interview (Pincus 1968).
37-40 Relations with People	37) Number of actual roles S is currently engaged in. 38) 11 hypothetical situations requiring S to indicate availability of real persons that could be called upon. 39) Interviewer ratings on transaction with S. 40) Interpersonal Role Playing Task, scored for avoidance of relationships.
41 Accumulated Life Stress	Number of current crises events impinging on S.

*A factor analysis of the 100 Block Q-sort items produced, dimensions highly correlated with these factors.

Table 13-2
Comparisons–Survivor Status

		Variable	Stressed Sample[1] Means		Nonstressed Sample[2] Means	
			Intact	Not Intact	Intact	Not Intact
Functional Capacities	1	Cognitive Malfunction	.84	2.02***[3]	.77	1.39*
	2	Word Count	65.30	56.20*	63.80	58.20
	3	Self Care Inability	1.25	3.12***	1.53	2.06**
	4	Q-Sort Mental Health	.17	.17	Not available	
	5	Life Satisfaction	15.70	16.10	17.40	16.30
Affects	6	S.C.T. Anxiety	19.80	19.40	14.80	18.00*
	7	Catell Anxiety	26.30	27.30	27.20	25.40
	8	S.C.T. Depression	13.40	14.20	11.10	12.80
	9	S.C.T. Despair	1.80	1.90	1.50	2.10**
	10	Body Preoccupation	3.81	3.80	1.94	1.65
	11	Neg. Body Image	1.24	1.32	1.29	1.50*
	12	S.C.T. Body Image	1.88	1.87	1.88	1.50*
	13	Introspection	2.27	1.95	2.05	1.61**
	14	Affective Complex	4.02	4.47	5.23	5.31
Hope	15	Time Extension	19.90	16.40***	23.20	19.40**
	16	S Role	15.40	15.00	14.80	17.70***
	17	Futurity	6.60	5.50***	6.21	4.45***
Self	18	Self-esteem	20.40	18.60**	19.60	17.40
	19	Self Consist. Maint.	.42	−1.84**	3.70	−.23*
Personality Traits	20	S.S. Dominance	.02	−.37*	.32	.32
	21	S.S. Love	.06	.41*	−.03	.14
	22	Authoritarian	.16	−.17*	Not available	
	23	Passivity	−.46	.49***	.25	.23
	24	Introspective	.13	−.13	Not available	
	25	Friendly	−.05	.05	Not available	
	26	Introv. Extrov.	21.10	21.10	22.10	21.60
Reminiscence	27	Life Evaluation	3.33	3.10		
	28	Life Review	3.74	3.85		
	29	Affect	3.07	2.67		
	30	Rem. Activity	113.80	97.30*	Not available	
	31	Amount, Satis.	19.90	16.20		
	32	Amount, Depriv.	7.42	6.20*		
	33	Emphasis, Child.	.59	.63		
Coping	34	Denial	7.07	7.90**	Not appropriate	
	35	Working	1.96	1.22*	to	
	36	Anticipated Loss	10.10	9.00**	Nonstressed Group	
Interpersonal	37	Total Role	9.52	8.56	10.30	8.70
	38	Availability	4.16	4.13	Not available	
	39	Relations-Interview	11.20	11.20	10.36	8.81***
	40	Interpersonal Denial	.82	1.57**	.90	1.83**
	41	Accumulated-Stress	3.05	2.73	Not appropriate to Nonstressed Group	

[1]Statistical analysis: analysis of covariance, covariates were age, sex and type of environment at Time 1. Overall contribution of these covariates was found to be minor, affecting significance levels for 2 variables, 18 and 30, both of which become statistically significant only in covariance analysis.

[2]One tailed t test used.

[3]* p level ⩽.10, ** p level ⩽.05, *** p level ⩽.01.

variables (#27-33); the overall results were uniformly negative (at p of .05)—it seemed to make little difference for survival whether an individual was highly involved or relatively uninvolved in reminiscence activity, or whether there were many or few signs of restructuring, reworking, or life-reviewing.

Strategies of coping with anticipated threat (#34-36) were predictive of survival status. The probability of survival was significantly low for those who approached the anticipated threat by denial (#34), who did not go through internal psychological work regarding the impending threat (#35), and who perceived the situation as involving loss (#36). Most of the interpersonal variables (#37-39), number of roles, availability of help, and relations in interview, as well as level of environmental stress (#41) did not prove predictive of survival. The exception was the Interpersonal Role Playing task (#40) in which less denial predicted survival.

Generalized Prediction. Taken together, the 41 variables involved a number of alternative ways of looking at psychological functioning and yielded a surprisingly large number of survival predictors. Do these predictors as a group describe an underlying, more generalized predictor? Several attempts to examine this issue suggest that such an explanation does not fit the data. These 41 variables represent a set which had been highly refined from a larger group. Some were derived through factor analysis; others through combinations of scores. Of the 41 variables, 17 studied showed univariate statistical significance associated with survivorship. Intercorrelation among these 17 variables yielded a small proportion with correlations above .2 (76 percent under .2, 13 percent between .2 and .29, 10 percent between .3 and .39, and 2 percent > .4), suggesting that most did not represent overlapping or redundant constructs. (This "discovery of nonoverlapping variables" is partly artifactual, for considerable effort was spent originally in eliminating redundant variables.)

A more precise procedure for determining redundance was the use of multivariate statistics. A step-down analysis of variance was employed to determine whether the variables predictive of survival status through univariate statistics maintained statistical significance, when the effects of other variables were partialled out. Six variables were analyzed: cognitive malfunction (#1); self-care (#3); time extension (#15); self-consistency maintenance (#19); the passive-aggressive personality trait (#23); and psychological working on anticipated threat (#35). These variables represented a wide range of psychological functions and had yielded the highest level of statistical significance in discriminating outcome status. Six step-down analyses of variance were calculated by systematically rotating entrance of the six variables. Table 13-3 presents the results of this analysis. This analysis indicated that four variables—#1, 3, 15 and 23—maintained high levels of statistical significance in predicting survival status no matter what other variables were entered into the prediction equation; variables #19 and 35 were somewhat diminished.

The implication of these analyses is that it may be difficult to develop sound theory relating psychological characteristics to survival, since positive findings

Table 13-3
Step Down Analysis of Variance

Variables	1 Cognitive Malfunction		3 Self-Care Inability		15 Time Extension		19 Self-Consistency Maintenance		23 Passivity		35 Working	
	P	Step	P	Step	P	Step	P	Step	P	Step	P	Step
1. Cognitive Malfunction	.0003	1	.04	6	.06	5	.08	4	.03	3	.0008	2
3. Self-Care Inability	.006	2	.01	1	.05	6	.02	5	.02	4	.006	3
15. Time Extension	.07	3	.03	2	.009	1	.25	6	.16	5	.11	4
19. Self-Consistency Maintenance	.37	4	.08	3	.13	2	.04	1	.27	6	.40	5
23. Passivity	.01	5	.0004	4	.0002	3	.0001	2	.0001	1	.01	6
35. Working	.98	6	.76	5	.86	4	.60	3	.30	2	.09	1

appear to accrue from a number of ways of looking at psychological functioning. A number of relatively independent psychological variables, which as yet cannot be encompassed by more generalized predictors, appear related to survival in the present studies. Statistical manipulations—e.g., factor analysis—did not yield more productive abstractions.

All of the preceding analyses were based on mean differences. The 17 variables significant in discriminating survival status were re-analyzed to determine the sensitivity of each predictor variable in discriminating at both ends of its range. The scores on each variable were divided into thirds—high, medium, and low—chi squares were computed, relating each of the 17 variables to survival status (2 X 3 tables). Some variables discriminated only at their low range—e.g., poor cognitive functioning predicted deteriorated status, but good cognitive functioning was less able to discriminate between surviving and deteriorated groups. For example, poor self-care (#3), high denial of anticipated threat (#36) and the personality trait of love (#21) were predictors of deteriorated status, although high scores on these variables did not discriminate. Other variables were primarily sensitive at their high range: self-consistency maintenance (#19), the personality trait of dominance (#20), and psychological working on anticipated threat (#35) were associated with survival, whereas low scores did not discriminate as well.

Thus, the most sensitive predictors of survival were not simply the converse of the most sensitive predictors of nonsurvival. The development of a psychological theory of survival, therefore, may be further complicated by the need to account for these nonsymmetrical psychological relationships.

The Nonstressed Group

The two control samples more closely approximated other populations studied in attrition research, insofar as they were made up of people who were not undergoing events associated with accelerated morbidity and mortality. Procedures similar to those used for the experimental group were employed to define survivorship and nonsurvivorship. To minimize sample variance each of the control groups was treated separately. The community group had too few deteriorated cases to warrant analysis, so that these analyses are based on 34 persons who were long-term residents of homes for the aged. Table 13-2 gives the means and p levels.

Of the 41 variables, 18 were untested, either because data were not available or the measures were inappropriate for this sample. Measures used to assess coping with anticipated threat (#34-36) and accumulated stress (#41) were inappropriate; data were unavailable on the measures of reminiscence (#27-33) and several of the personality measures. On the variables where replication was possible, it can be seen from Table 13-2 that most of the variables which were predictive for the Stressed Group did not evidence a corresponding pattern in the Nonstressed Group. Cognitive function (#1) (although statistically significant) and the measure of energy output (#2) did not operate as powerful predictors of survival status; physical level (#3) proved to be equally predictive for the Stressed and Nonstressed Groups. Personality traits found to be significant predictors in the Stressed Group did not bear the same relation to survival for the Nonstressed Group; no significant personality trait differences were found to relate to survival.

The ability to utilize adequate information in maintaining a stable self-system (#19) and degree of hope (#15-17) were related to survivor status in both groups. Several areas of psychological function—affects, body imagery, and interpersonal relationships—which did not show predictive relationships to outcome in the Stressed Group showed relationships to survivor status in the Nonstressed Group: deteriorated status in the Nonstressed Group was predicted by low introspective capacity (#13), negative body image (#11, 12), high anxiety (#6), high despair (#9), and disturbed interpersonal functioning (#39). Those who did not survive appeared to be less warm, less spontaneous, and less motivated individuals, fitting with their bland, dysphoric affective life (#6, 9, 11, 12, and 13).

Discussion

In a highly homogeneous group of elderly persons large differences were determined in psychological parameters associated with survivorship. Life context was found to alter the kind of relationships obtained between psychological functions and survival status. The number of psychological variables found in the Stressed Group which served as predictors of subsequent status makes sense once the particular kind of stress on these individuals is considered—the basic issue for this group was the radical change in life-space; the common event for aged persons undergoing such change is the requirement to adapt to a new set of complexities. Many of the psychological functions that proved to be powerfully related to survival can be understood in such a context. The ability of aged people to adapt to radical environmental change is predicated on such capacities as cognitive level and energy output which are needed to master new learnings in the altered life-space. Other factors, such as methods used to cope with anticipated threat, are also consistent with a stress model of survivorship.

Another condition (differences in time periods) that may affect relationships found between psychological functions and survival is suggested by a previous study (Lieberman 1965). As noted earlier, survival was defined in the present studies in terms of a two-year period. Other investigators have related psychological functions to survival status using time periods ranging from several months to ten years. Given these differences in assessment time, it is reasonable to ask whether they may account for some of the diversity in findings on psychological factors associated with survival. The previous study, however, indicated that certain psychological variables became predictive only within a period relatively close to death. In that study, systematic psychological changes were noted in a sample of 30 aged persons, 6 to 9 months prior to death, whereas no psychological characteristics predicted survivorship beyond nine months.

In the context of the present volume, the most important feature of these findings may be their indication of the primitive level at which the psychology of survival remains. A diverse range of factors, including environmental context, assessment-time, and numerous psychological dimensions, has been added to others observed by many investigators to be powerfully related to survival in the aged. Still, salient hypotheses to explain the meaning of these relationships have yet to be advanced. The present work, along with that which has preceded it, leaves little doubt that further relationships can be established between psychological dimensions and survivorship. The relative ease with which they are returned, however, and the independence which has been demonstrated between particular predictors and differing samples, suggests that the road to understanding of the phenomenon under discussion may lie less in the direction of piling up positive findings and more in the direction of some integrative theoretical breakthrough.

References

Appley, M.H. and Trumbull, R. (eds.): *Psychological Stress*. New York, Appleton-Century-Crofts, 1967.

Bakan, D.: *The Duality of Human Existence*. Chicago, Rand McNally, 1966.

Bender, L.: *A visual motor gestalt test and its clinical use*. American Orthopsychiatry Association, Research Monograph, No. 3, 1938.

Block, J.: *The Q-sort Method in Personality Assessment and Psychiatric Research*. Springfield, Ill., Charles C. Thomas, 1961.

Butler, R.N.: The life review: an interpretation of reminiscence in the aged. *Psychiatric Journal for the Study of Interpersonal Processes*, 26: 65-76, February 1963.

Dana, R.H.: Clinical diagnosis and objective TAT scoring. *J. abnorm. soc. Psychol.*, 50: 19-25, 1955.

Erikson, E.H.: *Identity and the Life Cycle*. New York, International Universities Press, *1*, 1959.

Falk, J.M.: The organization of remembered life experience of older people: its relation to anticipated stress, to subsequent adaptation, and to age. An unpublished doctoral dissertation, The University of Chicago, Committee on Human Development, 1970.

Funkenstein, D.H., King, S.H. and Drolette, M.E.: *Mastery of Stress*. Cambridge, Mass., Harvard University Press, 1957.

Gendlin, E.T.: A theory of personality change.. In P. Worchel and D. Byrne (eds.), *Personality Change*. New York, John Wiley and Sons, pp. 100-148, 1964.

178

Goldfarb, A.: Report to the New York State Commission on Aging, 1958.

Gorney, J.: Experiencing and age: patterns of reminiscence among the elderly. Unpublished doctoral dissertation, The University of Chicago, Committee on Human Development, 1968.

Gottshalk, L.A., Springer, K.H. and Gleser, G.C.: Experiments with a method of assessing the variations in intensity of certain psychologic states occurring during the psychotherapeutic interview. In L.A. Gottshalk (ed.), *Comparative Psycholinguistic Analysis of Two Psychotherapeutic Interviews*. New York, International Universities, pp. 115-138, 1961.

Greenfield, N.A., Roessler, R. and Crosley, A.P.: Ego strength and length of recovery from infectious mononucleosis. *J. nerv. ment. Dis.*, 128: 125, 1959.

Inglis, J.: A paired-associate learning test for use with elderly psychiatric patients. *J. ment. Sci*, 105: 440-443, 1959.

Janis, I.L.: *Psychological Stress*. New York, John Wiley & Sons, 1958.

Jarvik, L.F. and Falek, A.: Intellectual stability and survival in the aged. *J. Gerontol.*, 18: 173-176, 1963.

Kahn, R.L., Pollack, M. and Goldfarb, A.I.: Factors related to individual differences in mental status of institutionalized aged. In P.H. Hoch and J. Zubin (eds.),*Psychopathology of Aging*. New York, Grune and Stratten, pp. 104-113, 1961.

Kleemeier, R.W.: Intellectual changes in the senium, or death and the I.Q. Presidential Address, Division 20, American Psychological Association, New York, September 1961.

Lazarus, R.S.: *Psychological Stress and the Coping Process*. New York, McGraw-Hill, 1966.

Leary, T.: *Interpersonal Diagnosis of Personality*. New York, Ronald Press, 1957.

LeShan, L.L.: A basic psychological orientation associated with malignant diseases. *Psychiat. Quart.*, 35: 314-330, 1961.

Lieberman, M.A.: The relationship of mortality rates to entering a home for the aged. *Geriatrics*, 16: 515-519, October 1961.

Lieberman, M.A. and Lakin, M.: On becoming an aged institutionalized individual. In W. Donahue, C. Tibbitts, and R. Williams (eds.) *Processes of Aging: Social and Psychological Perspectives*, I. New York, Atherton Press, Chapter 22, 1963.

Lieberman, M.A.: Observations on death and dying. *The Gerontologist*, 6: #2, 70-73, June 1966. Presented at Gerontological Society meetings, Los Angeles, November 1965.

Lieberman, M.A.: Psychological correlates of impending death: some preliminary observations. *J. Gerontol.*, 20: 182-190, 1965.

Lieberman, M.A., Prock, V.N. and Tobin, S.S.: The psychological effects of institutionalization. *J. Gerontol.*, 23: #3, July 1968.

Lieberman, M.A. and Coplan, A.S.: Distance from death as a variable in the study of aging. *Developmental Psychology*, 2: #1, 71-84, 1969.

National Opinion Research Center. Questionnaire for cross-national survey of the aged, April, 1962.

179

Neugarten, B.L., Havighurst, R.J. and Tobin, S.S.: The measurement of life satisfaction. *J. Gerontol.*, 16: 134-143, 1961.

Pascal, G.R. and Suttell, B.J.: *The Bender-Gestalt Test: Quantification and Validity for Adults*. New York, Grune and Stratton, 1951.

Pincus, A.: An exploratory study of the effect of differing institutional environments on the adjustment of residents in homes for the aged. Unpublished doctoral dissertation, University of Wisconsin, January 1968. The definition and measurement of the institutional environments for the aged, paper presented at the Gerontology Society, St. Petersburg, Florida, November 1967.

Reitman, F. and Robertson, J.P.: Reitman's pin-man test: a means of disclosing impaired conceptual thinking. *J. nerv. ment. Dis.*, 112: 498-510, 1950.

Riegel, K.F., and Riegel, R.M.: Development, drop and death. Paper presented at the 23rd meeting, Gerontology Society, Toronto, October 27, 1970.

Rosner, A.: Stress and the maintenance of self-concept in the aged. Unpublished doctoral dissertation, The University of Chicago, Committee on Human Development, 1968.

14 Dependency, Illness, and Survival Among Navajo Men

DAVID GUTMANN

Introduction

This paper explores the relationship between illness, survival, and the management of passive-receptive character traits in a sample composed mainly of
traditional Navajo men. While such relationships can also be studied in our own
culture, tradition-oriented and remote living groups, such as the Navajo, are
particularly suited to a study of the relationship between somatic and
psychological states. If such a relationship exists it can best be observed in men
who have less than we in the way of extrinsic, medical, and nutritional supports.
If these men survive, it is by their own resources; and if psychological parameters
are included among these resources, then their contributions should be most
evident in these populations.

The hypotheses which guided this study were developed from the results of
previous investigations in the comparative psychology of later life, first
undertaken among urban Americans and then replicated among middle-aged and
aging men of various traditional and preliterate groups. By way of introduction
to the body of this report, some pertinent findings from the earlier studies will
first be briefly reviewed.

Background of Comparative Studies

The original American research, from which the body of orienting hypotheses
was derived, considered projective test (TAT) data from "Middle-Majority"
Kansas City men aged 35 and over. Age-blind analysis of these materials
suggested the possibility of a developmental framework in later life, involving an
age-graded movement through successive ego-mastery positions. The instru-
mental-productive orientation (active mastery) involves instrumentality towards
the outer world and is mainly found among younger men (aged 35-54). This
stage is superceded by a more passive-receptive orientation (passive mastery) in
which the self rather than the world is revised to meet the requirements of
external authorities and providers. After age 65 this conformist mode is to some
degree replaced by magical mastery, which involves projective rather than

David Gutmann is Professor of Psychology, University of Michigan, Ann Arbor, Michigan.

instrumental revisions of the world and/or the self. In this stage, primitive defensive operations (projection and denial) tend to substitute for realistic and reformative activity, whether towards production or conformity (see Neugarten and Gutmann 1958; also Gutmann 1964).

In order to test the hypothesis that these age differences had some intrinsic, "developmental" basis, replication studies were carried out with samples of men, similar in their age composition to the American cohort, drawn from the Lowland and Highland Maya (Mexico), Navajo (Arizona) and Druze (Israel: Galilean highlands) societies.[1] In each case, subjects were given the TAT and were interviewed concerning their history, their present conditions of life, their definitions of pleasure, pain and remedy, and their dreams.

The data analysis is not complete, but thus far the results from the various studies support the American findings: the active-productive, passive-receptive and magical orientations distribute more predictably by age in adult male populations than they do by culture. As in Kansas City, among the Navajo, the Maya, and the Druze tribesmen, the younger men rely on and relish their own instrumentality and the products of their industry; moreover, they see themselves as a source of provision to others. By contrast, older men come to rely on the accommodating techniques whereby they influence external providers in their favor; and the oldest men, especially in time of trouble, manage reality projectively and rely on the less adaptive illusions of security and comfort. In sum, the "species" age shift in men as it emerges from these comparative studies is away from the position of one who actively provides security for others and towards the position of one whose sense of security is based on the good will of powerful providers[2] (see Gutmann, 1969).

---

[1]The overall program of cross-cultural studies has been supported by Career Development Award no. 5-K3-HD-6043-04, from the National Institutes of Child Health and Human Development. Field expenses for Indian studies in Mexico and in the American Southwest were covered by Faculty Research Grants nos. 1344 and 1412 from the Rackham School of Graduate Studies, the University of Michigan, and by grant no. MH 13031-01 from the National Institutes of Mental Health. Israeli Druze research was supported by grant no. M66-345 from the Foundation's Fund for Research in Psychiatry.

[2]The objection has been repeatedly raised that these results represent generational rather than developmental differences. Cultures are changing, so the argument goes, and different age cohorts, within societies, have been exposed to different socializing and child rearing practices. Thus, the "mastery" types X age group distributions could represent the outcomes of different forms of nurture, rather than positions along a developmental or "life cycle" continuum. This objection has been tested in a second field trip to the Navajo reservation, in the course of which I re-interviewed my original panel of informants, and re-administered those TAT cards which had significantly discriminated age groups at time.[1] Seventy-five time[2] records were thus obtained, and in the majority of cases the later profiles show shifts away from the time[1] profile, in the passive and/or magical direction. Though the predicted shift did not show up in all cases, it is mainly important medicine men or tribal leaders who either replicate or improve on the time[1] estimate of their mastery status. These results counter the objection that the differences in mastery style that obtain between age cohorts could reflect age group differences in child rearing, degree of acculturation, etc., rather than developmental differences within individuals.

Passive-Dependency, Orality and Aging:
Some Findings and Hypotheses

By contrast to the more autonomous posture maintained by younger men, I will characterize the older man's stance as one of oral-dependency. In this, my authority derives from aspects of the psychoanalytic theory of character and from empirical evidence, which will be presented later. Thus, on the theoretical side, psychoanalysts propose an intrinsic association between the passive-dependent ego-orientations that we have observed transculturally in older men, and the oral needs of the personality.[3] From this theory comes our prediction that the older man's concern with external donations of affection and support, with powerful external providers, and with magical defenses against threat, should be matched by a heightened interest in the production, the preparation, and especially the pleasurable consumption of food.

Accordingly, if old men are more accommodating and succorant than younger men, then their explicitly oral interests should also be higher than those of younger men. Furthermore, since the relationship between the psychosexual and the psychosocial vectors of personality is presumed to be intrinsic and invariant, then we would expect to find that the predicted relationship is transcultural in its distribution: in *any* society, a high degree of manifest orality should predict, on the individual level, to character traits and behaviors that register a high degree of passive-receptivity, in terms of local standards.

Empirical support for this prediction is provided by Simmons (1965) who collected ethnographic reports from over thirty diverse but preliterate societies, bearing on the roles and personal characteristics of their aged members. He devotes his first chapter, (titled "Assurance of Food") to making the point that, across cultures, the aged are particularly concerned with oral supply. He notes,

---

[3]Thus Fenichel (1945, p. 491) states, "Just as the essential connection between the anal-social conflicts and the anal-erotic drives have been doubted, so also have the relations between dependence and oral eroticism. But their connection is an essential one. The biological basis of all attitudes of dependence is the fact that man is a mammal, and that the human infant is born more helpless than other mammals and requires feeding and care by adults. Every human being has a dim recollection that there were once powerful or, as it must seem to him, omnipotent beings whose help, comfort and protection he must depend on in time of need. Later, the ego learns to use active means of mastering the world. But a passive-oral attitude as a residue of infancy is potentially present. Often enough the adult person gets into situations in which he is again as helpless as he was as a child; sometimes forces of nature are responsible, but more often social forces created by man. He then longs for just such omnipotent protection and comfort as were at his disposal in childhood. He regresses to orality. There are many social institutions that make use of this biologically predetermined longing. They promise the longed-for help if certain conditions are fulfilled. The conditions vary greatly in different cultures. But the formula, 'If you obey, you will be protected,' is one that all gods have in common with all earthly authorities. It is true that there are great differences between an almighty god, or a modern employer, and a mother who feeds her baby; but nevertheless it is the similarity among them that explains the psychological effectiveness of authority."

for example, that older men have typically used their prestige to ensure the choicest foods for themselves, by making them taboo for younger men.[4]

Scoring for Orality

In order to further check the hypothesis that oral interests, like passive and magical mastery, become more prominent in later life, the Navajo and Druze[5] data collected by the author were coded for the orality variable. All references to eating, food preparation, purchase, or production were assigned weights which reflected the intensity of oral need presumably expressed through them. Thus, mentions of food production or preparation received lower scores than mentions of food consumption; and mentions of food consumption by others received lower scores than mentions of food consumption by the respondent himself. In addition, a distinction was made between those oral references embedded in the body of the interview proper, and those found in the subject's projective protocol (TAT or dream reports).

The age, cultural, and regional distributions of the various orality sub-scales are reported in another paper (Gutmann 1970). Here, we will restrict ourselves

---

[4]While Simmons and I agree on the fact of senescent orality, we disagree on the interpretation. Where I see in these developments the tracings of universal psychological laws that for the most part operate outside of human consciousness, Simmons explains them as a direct consequence of human awareness, in this case, the awareness of mortality. Simmons' basic position is summed up in this statement (ibid., p. 20): "A dominant interest in old age is to live long, perhaps as long as possible. Therefore, food becomes a matter of increasing concern. Its provision in suitable form, on regular schedule, and in proper amounts depends more and more upon the efforts of those who are in a position to provide or withhold it. And, as life goes on, the problem of supplying and feeding the aged eventually reaches a stage at which they require the choicest morsels and the tenderest care."

[5]The theoretical basis of this exercise comes from western psychoanalysis; but the two cultures in which the assumptions concerning the increased orality of later life were tested are distinctly nonwestern in their cultural values and social forms. Furthermore, while the Navajo and the Druze groups are both composed of traditionally oriented agriculturalists, they are also strikingly unlike each other. The Navajo are herdsmen, migratory within fixed ranges, whose small bands, largely based on kinship, are scattered across the high desert plateau of northeastern Arizona. Their world is dynamic: what are for us neutral events are for them charged with personal, often magical significance. And the Navajo character mingles opposing traits: suspicion and humor, toughness and vulnerability, pragmatism and superstition, apathy and a delight in movement. By contrast, the Galilean Druze are sedentary agriculturalists, who live in organized villages. In their values and in their social forms they are similar to other Arabic speaking agriculturalists of the Levant; but while they worship Allah, they have a special religion, and they are accounted heretics in Islam. They have survived 800 years of consequent persecution through cultivation of industry, courage in battle, and political sophistication. Where the Navajo character is a blend of opposites, the Druze are almost rigidly self-consistent: their character combines piety, stubbornness, a valuing of rationality over emotion, and a reserve that takes the form of extreme politeness and formality. Despite these marked cultural differences, Navajo and Druze aged have a fairly secure and valued status.

to the *Syntonic Orality Score* (SOS) which is produced by the subject's references to his own ingestion of food or beverage, in the past or in the present, and by his mentions of pleasure in such consumption. Included in this score are references to food and beverage as a remedy against discontent. Examples of references scored for SOS are: "I feel better about these problems when I drink good coffee," (Druze) or, "My relatives bring me the food, sometimes they bring that great big roast rib" (Navajo). Oral references occurring in dreams or in the TAT record are not coded as SOS. Because raw SOS could be a function of interview length, which varied from respondent to respondent, it is expressed for computational purposes as a percentage of the respondent's Total Orality Score (TOS), a scale which sums *all* the respondent's references to nutriment, including those not having to do with his own pleasurable consumption of food and drink.

*Age and Regional Variations in
the Orality Score*

As a further step, the Navajo and Druze samples were divided into three matching regional subgroups: traditional-remote men (residents of conservative settlements, remote from population centers and main roads); traditional-proximal men (residents of conservative settlements, remote from population centers but close to main roads); and secular-urban men (residents of "modern" settlements, close to population centers). The SOS mean was then computed for each Age X Region X Culture cell, and the resulting distribution is plotted in Figure 14-1. This display indicates that syntonic orality clearly increases as a function of age for both the Druze and Navajo cultures and across the three settlement types. There is a regional effect in that for any age group, traditional remote men, whether Druze or Navajo, have the lowest SOS, while Druze and Navajo "urbanites" tend to have the highest SOS; but the age effect is clearly independent, both of culture and of settlement type within cultures.

*The Orality Scores in Relation to Other
Personality Measures*

This age effect in regard to syntonic orality was predicted from the prior findings concerning the age-grading of passive ego states, and thereby supports the hypothesis of a relationship between these variables. However, before we can use the SOS as a valid barometer of passivity, its predictive power vis à vis independent registers of this trait must also be demonstrated. Accordingly, partly in order to test the relationship between SOS and the deeper fantasies of our Navajo subjects, Krohn and Gutmann (1970) estimated the ego position— active, passive, or magical—represented through the formal and content aspects of dreams reported by the most traditional men. Krohn selected a sample of those dreams in which a mastery orientation was clearly represented through

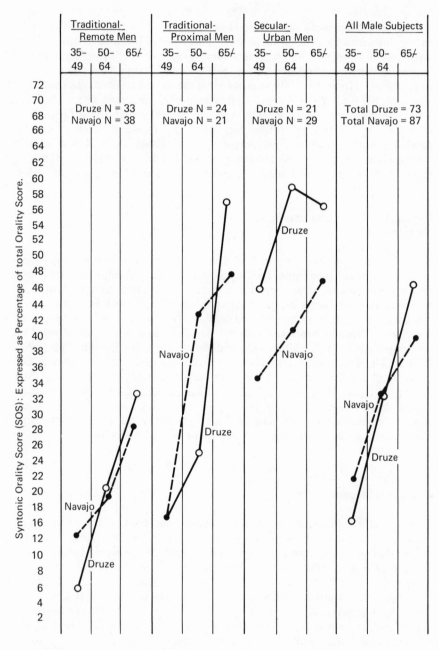

Figure 14-1. Comparison of Navajo and Druze Syntonic Orality Scores.

various expressions of that position. Thus, active mastery dreams were typically set outdoors and, regardless of dream content, the subject played a central and organizing role in the fantasied action. In passive mastery dreams the subject was either absent from the dream scene, or peripheral to it: characters other than himself are the main actors, and in the dream the subject is either inert or at the mercy of arbitrary force. Dreams classified as "magical" had all the passive characteristics, though the dream events tended to be highly improbable; and the subject believed that the dream events were portents of specific events in his waking life. Our prediction was that men with active mastery dreams would have syntonic orality scores below the median for the traditional Navajo group; and that men with passive or magical mastery dreams would have syntonic orality scores above that median. The results of the median test, shown in Table 14-1, indicates a significant association in the predicted direction: the subject's mastery style, as portrayed in his dream, predicts fairly well his level of syntonic orality.

Along similar lines, the TAT protocols of Navajo subjects are being analyzed for the central mastery tendency represented in component stories. The hypothesis states that subjects whose syntonic orality scores lie below the median would show a majority of active mastery stories in their TAT protocols, and that subjects with a preponderance of passive and/or magical mastery stories would have syntonic orality scores above the median. Thus far, a preliminary analysis, restricted to remote-traditional Navajo subjects, shows a significant association between respondent's mastery type, as represented in TAT content, and his degree of syntonic orality, as shown in Table 14-2.

The Orality Scores and Navajo Drinking Patterns

Finally, many Navajo drink heavily, sometimes enough so that the habit is noted in the medical records of the Public Health hospitals to which we had access.

Table 14-1
Distribution of Navajo Dreams: By Mastery Style and by Syntonic Orality Scores

Mastery Style of Dream	Subject's SOS *below* Median	Subject's SOS *above* Median
Active Mastery	17*	8
Passive or Magical Mastery	8	19

N=52

*Chi-square = 7.641, D.F. = 1, p <.01

Again, other investigators, especially Wolowitz (1968), have noted a significant relationship in American populations between alcoholism and oral receptivity, and it was accordingly proposed that a similar relationship would be discerned among the Navajo subjects as well. Accordingly, the Navajo sample was divided into three categories, whose criteria referred to various degrees of alcoholic intake. Category 1 grouped those men who reported no drinking and whose self-reports and medical records also contained no mention of drinking, nor of injuries sustained in brawling. Category 2 grouped those men who reported that they had given up drinking (usually after a conversion to Christianity or to Peyotism) and those men whose medical records mentioned injuries sustained in fights.[6] Category 3 included all those men who admitted, usually reluctantly, to chronic drinking and those men whose medical records mentioned alcoholic psychoses, or organic syndromes caused by heavy drinking.

Respondents were further sorted, depending on their SOS, into the first, second, or third tercile of the syntonic orality score distribution; and a chi square was calculated for the resulting SOS X Alcohol intake distribution. If we compare only the non-drinkers of all ages to the chronic drinkers of all ages, the resulting chi square is significant at the .10 level. However Table 14-3 indicates that the SOS discriminates drinking patterns in the case of men under 70 much more sharply than it does for men 70 and over. The percentage of possible, reformed, and chronic drinkers is much lower (19 percent) in the older cohort than it is for the younger men (57 percent). This finding suggests that the older men are a particularly abstinent group. The possibility that cultural factors specific to the over-70 group may in their case inhibit the hypothesized relationship between orality and alcoholic intake allows us to compute a chi square comparing only the younger non-drinkers and chronic drinkers. In this case, the chi square is at the .02 level.[7]

Table 14-2

Distribution of Navajo Remote Traditionals: By Projected Mastery Styles (From TAT) and by Syntonic Orality Scores

	Subject's SOS *below* Median	Subject's SOS *above* Median
Majority of respondent's TAT stories have active mastery theme and organization	12	5
Majority of respondent's TAT stories have Passive and/or Magical Mastery theme and organization	6	14

N=37

p < .05 by Fisher's Exact Probabilities test

[6]The logic being that the Navajo are typically restrained and pacific, except when intoxicated.

In sum, the SOS varies with age across two disparate cultures as predicted by theory; furthermore, it varies as predicted with passive fantasy content and with the degree of drinking behavior in Navajo subjects. Accordingly, we can have some faith that this score is a valid measure of passive tendencies in personality, such as might steer overt forms of behavior. We will now investigate the hypothesis that the SOS, considered as a barometer of passivity, is related to the health status of middle-aged and elderly Navajo subjects.

Passivity, Orality, and Health Status

The Autonomy of the Traditional Survivor

The hypothesis that passivity, as a personality dimension, might influence the health status of Navajo subjects was based on our interviews with Navajo men

Table 14-3
Distribution of Navajo Subjects by Drinking Patterns and by Syntonic Orality Scores

	Without Evidence of Drinking		History of Brawling or Reformed Drinker		Chronic Drinker	
SOS less than or equal to .08 (First Tercile)	Aged 35-69	18#	23*	8	9	3	3
	Aged 70+	5		1		0	
SOS less than or equal to .29 (Second Tercile)	Aged 35-69	9	20	9	9	9	9
	Aged 70+	11		0		0	
SOS equal to or above .30 (Third Tercile)	Aged 35-69	7	13	7	11	9	10
	Aged 70+	6		4		1	

* x^2 (of the "without evidence" and "Chronic" cell totals) = 5.027, DF=2, P < .10.

x^2 (for 35-69 years old cell totals in the "without evidence" and "Chronic" columns) = 8.358, DF=2, P < .02.

---

[7] These findings can be contested on the grounds that respondent mentions of drinking may have elevated their SOS, thereby bringing about an artificial association between SOS and drinking pattern. This is very unlikely: even confirmed Navajo drinkers customarily refer to their own or other's drinking practices in pejorative terms, as leading to imprisonment, fighting, or serious accidents. Such mentions do not meet the criteria for Syntonic Orality, and would instead be coded as "Oral Rejection" (a subscale that will be discussed in a future publication). Accordingly, the SOS, while it can co-vary with overt drinking behavior, is independent of verbal reports of such behavior.

aged 70 and over. Given the harsh conditions of Navajo life on the arid, remote Arizona deserts, we considered men living to this age as "survivors," whose longevity—in view of the relative absence of adequate nutrition, housing and medical care—presumably reflected their own physical and psychological resources. In our contacts with such men, my students and I have been impressed by the psychological and physical differences between this longevous cohort and those "normal" Navajo men in their late fifties and sixties, elderly but not old enough to merit the classification of "survivor." These differences are most marked in regard to the issue of passivity: the presurvival Navajo elder typically expresses the fantasy, cognitive and behavioral metaphors of passive mastery, but the survivor of seventy, eighty, or even ninety years of age is, particularly in his behavior and in his ideology, "counter-passive." While the survivor's dreams and TAT's give evidence of passive wishes, these do not find their way into his behavior or value systems. The essential difference between these cohorts seems to reside not in the sheer degree of passive wishes, but in their management. Where the presurvivor tends to indulge his passivity, to take it easy and to rely on others for his security, the survivor treats such temptation as a danger signal, even as a precursor of death, and his response is to swing into action; at such times instead of lying down he goes out to herd sheep, to plant corn, to cut wood, or to haul water.[8]

It seemed reasonable to assume that the surviving Navajo were not "normal" men who had undergone a massive character reformation towards counter-passivity after they reached age seventy. Rather, their life histories suggested that these had always been unusually vital men (by the standards of any culture) whose proportion increased in the highest age brackets owing to the greater mortality rates of "normal" Navajo. Accordingly, if mortality was highest among "normal" men, those who also gave free expression to passive mastery, it seemed reasonable that the longevity of the survivor cohort might in some manner be related to their counter-passivity. This line of reasoning led to the hypothesis tested in this study, namely, that the health status of middle-aged and elderly Navajo would be related to their management of passivity. If SOS is taken as an index of overt passivity, then low SOS should reflect a successful management of passivity and should coincide with reasonable health. By the same token, a high SOS should reflect inadequate management of passivity, and should coincide with poor health and premorbid conditions.

---

[8]The tendency towards active modes of coping with passive wishes in "survivor" populations appears to be characteristic of survivor populations in other cultures that I have studied. For example, among the Druze it is customary for older men to sign over their land to their sons, to give up physical labor, and to rely on the support provided by their sons or by the Israeli government in the form of Social Security. But the oldest "surviving" Druze tend to be "hold-outs" against this cultural pattern for easing them into dependence: either they refuse to give up their land, or if they do, they continue to interfere in their son's management of it. And when these men reject Social Security payments they draw their rationales from the "counter-passive" morality: they refuse to be supported by tax monies that "were not given willingly."

Re-Study of the Navajo Sample

This hypothesis was tested in the summer of 1970, through a re-study of the panel of Navajo subjects who had first been contacted in the summer of 1966. One hundred and thirteen men of the original sample were either seen at the re-study, or, where deaths had occurred, friends and kin-folk of the deceased were interviewed concerning the circumstances of death.[9] The interviews, whether with our original subjects or with their surviving kin, were focused mainly on health-related topics, with particular reference to the subject's health status during the four years since time 1. Those 5 TAT cards which had most significantly discriminated age cohorts at time 1 were also readministered on this occasion. Furthermore, in all but four cases we were able to inspect the usually detailed medical records kept by the USPHS Indian hospitals on the Navajo reservation.[10] The Navajo (as is the case with other American Indian tribes) have the use of Indian hospital services, without charge, and accordingly resort to them for minor as well as major complaints. As a result, the individual records are in most cases very detailed and cover an average span of ten years. With some help from USPHS resident physicians it was quite feasible in most cases to make a rough estimate of the subject's overall health from these records and from his self-report.

Drawing on the interview and medical data, the Navajo subjects were sorted into three major health status categories, which define a continuum from relative health to serious disease, as listed below.

Category I. This included all men whose interviews and medical records gave evidence of a continuing state of good health. That is, they were without chronic or crippling disease, and they had mainly complained, if at all, of upper respiratory and gastrointestinal infections, the latter being endemic on the reservation. In some cases there was a record of serious, acute infections, e.g., bronchopneumonia, but these were quickly overcome, apparently without damaging sequelae, and had not recurred. Older men grouped here sometimes complained that their "health is down" but in evidence they cited only vague "aches and pains" and "tired feelings" that accompanied physical exertion but were not troubling enough to keep them from their work. In a few cases these complaints were supported by medical evidence of mild osteoarthritis; but in the main the old men grouped here were not identifying a distinct syndrome but

---

[9]Two students, Mr. Jeffrey Urist of the University of Michigan, and Miss Sally Haimo of the University of Chicago, both helped with the interviewing. Also, three members of the Navajo tribe, Mr. Harvey Bilagodi, Mr. Charles Bracker, and Mr. Max Hanley, Sr., helped us locate our subjects, performed interpreting services, and Mr. Bilagodi carried out independent interviews. Such assistance was invaluable and is gratefully acknowledged.

[10]The author wishes to thank Dr. George Bock, Chief of the Indian Health Service of the Navajo Reservation, and Mr. Tony Lincoln, of the Navajo tribe, for granting me access to the medical records kept by the USPHS Indian hospitals on our Indian subjects.

were ruefully noting the usual physical symptoms of aging. It was not pain and fatigue that they minded so much as the loss of vigor and the attendant limitations on their mobility and productivity.

Category II. This was a residual category which grouped all men who had chronic but not fatal disease. They ranged from probable psychosomatic cripples and malingerers to men with cases of severe arthritis, glaucoma or T.B. that had been either arrested or controlled. Some of these men seem to have used their illness as an excuse to quit work and to get on welfare; others were clearly incapacitated by blindness or degenerative joint disease. But for all of them, illness—whether psychosomatic or organic—either was important, or had been at one point important in their lives.

Category III. This category included two subgroups—those men who had either died from or were still enduring a major illness (e.g., congestive heart failure) contracted before time 1; and those men who were apparently in good health at time 1 but who had since developed a potentially terminal illness (with death resulting in three instances). Thus, this category included all subjects whose deaths since time 1 are clearly traceable to illness and all those who suffered from potentially terminal conditions contracted before or after time 1.

The Covariance of SOS and Disease

The above groupings were made without knowledge of the individual subject's syntonic orality scores. These scores were computed from time 1 data by a research assistant who had no knowledge of the individual subject's time 2 health status. The median SOS was computed for all subjects in the time 2 sample, the hypothesis being that subjects with SOS below the median would be found mainly in Category I and that subjects with SOS above the median would be found mainly in Category III. Table 14-4 shows the SOS distribution relative to the median, the three health status categories, and subject's time 2 age. A highly significant association between SOS and health status obtains for subjects younger than 70, though SOS does not discriminate successfully between sickness and health for men aged seventy and over at time 2. In sum, the SOS shows a high degree of association with health status, in line with our prediction, for the "normal," presurvivor Navajo sample.

*Implications of the SOS-Health
Status Relationship*

The high degree of association between somatic status and a score that presumably registers the degree of psychological passivity does not allow us to assume that passivity as an independent variable precedes illness and death. For one thing, while orality may be the register of a psychic orientation, it is also a synonym for "hunger," which is, after all, a fairly common somatic condition. Thus, the orality of unhealthy Navajo may be only another physical symptom, the expression of somatic illness rather than the expression of some independent psychological "cause" of somatic illness.

But appetite is more likely to decline with illness than to be increased by it, and so the above objection to our finding does not hold up. However, a more sophisticated explanation of the association between orality and illness derives from psychoanalytic theory itself, which proposes that heightened oral need can be reactive to anxiety: the anxious person turns to oral gratification as a form of comfort and tension release. By this reasoning, unhealthy Navajo, frightened by the mortal implications of their illness, seek magical reassurance by reviving the passive-dependent relationships of the early, "oral" period of development, when food stood for maternal love and maternal protection against inner and outer dangers.[11] Again, in this quite plausible formulation, oral passivity does not precede the onset of serious illness, but is a side-effect, and illness is the independent event.

At least 10 and possibly 15 Navajo subjects who appeared healthy at time 1 had died or contracted a potentially terminal disease by time 2. The median distribution of their SOS scores against those of a matched sample from the consistently healthy Type I population shows the predicted trend towards higher SOS scores in the "recent onset" group, though not at a significant level. In any

Table 14-4
Median Distribution of Syntonic Orality Scores: by Health Status and by Age

		Health Status I (Healthy)		Health Status II (Moderate Chronic Illness)		Health Status III (Potentially Terminal Illness)	
SOS equal to or less than .18 (median)	Aged 35-54	10		8		2	
	Aged 55-69	12	24*	10	25	3	8
	Aged 70+	2		7		3	
SOS equal to or above .19 (median)	Aged 35-54	2		4		8	
	Aged 55-69	3	11	8	19	10	26
	Aged 70+	6		7		8	

*x^2 = 15.167 (of cell totals)
DF = 2
P < .001

[11] Should this be the case, one does not need to propose a heightened level of *appetite* in reaction to illness, but only a re-activation of orally-tinged *fantasies*, which is quite a different matter.

event, the number of men unexpectedly ill or dead since time 1 is too small for an adequate test of the hypothesis that passivity is the precursor of important illness, particularly since the "recent onset" sample is filled out with 5 doubtful cases.

Passivity as the Precursor of Disease:
Some Relevant Findings

At this point we can neither demonstrate nor finally refute the central hypothesis of this study, namely, that passive ego states, as represented by the SOS, predict important illness. However, while severe pathology can clearly put even the most autonomous individuals in a passive and dependent frame of mind, there are scattered findings from the Navajo data which support the idea that passivity as a personality dimension contributes significantly to the occurrence of chronic, disabling, or fatal disease. For example, we find that while a personality shift towards passivity may precede the actual onset of significant pathology, such shifts—as measured by the TAT—are not a likely sequel to such onset. In this regard, we measured the differences in mastery position reflected in the time 1 and time 2 TAT protocols of our Navajo subjects. Comparisons were limited to thematic material generated by those five cards which were used on both occasions, and which had significantly discriminated Navajo age groups at time 1. The results of this comparison show that the Type I men were more likely than the significantly ill Type III men to show a time 1-time 2 shift in the regressive direction towards passive and magical mastery. Indeed, 37 percent of the Type I men shifted in this manner, as against 23 percent of the Type III men; and only 26 percent of the Type I men held on to or improved their time 1 mastery position, as against 54 percent of the Type III men (see Table 14-5).

While these intertype differences are not statistically significant, they do support the contention that illness is not necessarily productive of passive orientations, and they leave open the possibility that increases in passivity may be prodromal to disease. Certainly, it is still a testable hypothesis that those

Table 14-5
Relationship Between Health Status and TAT Changes in Mastery Position

Health Status	No Change: or T1–T2 Shift Towards Active Mastery	Notable T1–T2 Shift, Towards Passive and Magical Mastery
Type I (N=35)	26%	37%
Type II (N=44)	33%	33%
Type III (N=34)	54%	23%

Type I men who showed a significant regressive shift by time 2 will prove to be overtly ill by time 3.

The regional variations in orality and in disease-proneness also support the hypothesis that passivity is prior to disease. Thus, as Table 14-6 indicates, we find that an inordinately high proportion (60 percent) of the healthiest men in our sample hail from the traditional-remote (Navajo mountain) region of the reservation, while the secular-urban sector contributes only 11 percent of the Type I population. These proportions are reversed for the significantly ill Type III group: 48 percent from the Tuba City area, and 23 percent from Navajo mountain. These striking regional differences in the distribution of significant disease are unexpected, the more so since supportive missionaries, welfare agencies and especially medical services are much more available in Tuba City, an Indian agency center, than on Navajo mountain.

The great majority of the chronically ill Tuba City men were already established residents of the region at the time that their disease revealed itself; they did not first become ill and then move to Tuba City in order to be close to a hospital. Accordingly, the finding that the frequency of Navajo illness increases in step with the availability of supportive agencies may be related to the special characteristics of the population which is attracted to those services prior to serious illness. In this regard, our interviews and observations strongly suggest that the Tuba City population, when contrasted with the Navajo mountain group, has a notably larger proportion of those passive-dependent types for whom we would predict the highest illness rates. As an administrative, trading, and road center, Tuba City has attracted many of the most vigorous and talented Navajo on the reservation; but it has also either attracted or generated a significant number of the more passive, dispirited types. Thus, it is in this secular urban population that we are most likely to find early retirees, dependent on welfare payments, on the provident missionaries, and on their wives' rug-weaving income. They are in marked contrast to those hardy remote-living Navajo who choose to maintain personal control over the sources of their security by following the traditional life-way of the semimigratory sheep-herder around

Table 14-6
Regional Representation in Navajo Health Status Categories

Regions	Type I (Healthy) (N=35)	Type II (Moderate Chronic Illness) (N=44)	Type III (Potentially Terminal Illness) (N=34)
Remote-Traditional	60%	41%	23%
Outlying Areas	29%	25%	29%
Secular-Urban	11%	34%	48%

Navajo mountain. Our impression that the more passive-dependent Navajo tend to collect around Tuba City is borne out by the regional differences in SOS, which, as shown by Figure 14-1, are strikingly higher, for any age cohort, in the Tuba City subsample than they are for the Navajo mountain subsample.

In sum, given its special endowment of medical facilities, there are no features peculiar to the Tuba City region which can explain the special susceptibility of its adult male inhabitants to disease. And there are no obvious features of the Tuba population which might account for their special vulnerability except for the high degree of passivity found among many of its members. In their case, passive-dependency seems to be a precondition rather than a side-effect of disease.[12]

The Somatic Consequences of Passivity: Some Speculations

Let it be clear that I am not suggesting some mystic "mind over matter" causation in somatic illness: I am not suggesting that passivity is a metaphor of death, nor that it involves a resignation which by itself brings on disease and actual death. The idea is attractive to psychologists: we like to believe that the psychic states which are the subjects of our interest are also the great independent variables of human existence. However, at least in regard to the Navajo, it is quite likely that passivity and disease are related in a fairly straightforward way, via those behaviors which express the passive attitude and which are *incidentally* deleterious to health. Take the matter of exercise, its antecedents and consequences. We have found that counter-passive Navajo survivors force themselves, by sheer effort of will, to herd sheep or to hoe corn. Their intent is to demonstrate their continued independence, but they incidentally keep their cardiovascular systems in tune and probably extend their lives. By the same token, the more overtly passive Navajo, who sends his grandchild out with the sheep, may think that he is conserving his energies, but he is more likely contributing to the deterioration of his arteries.

Probably more crucial is the relation between passivity, alcohol intake, and disease. Table 14-3 showed a significant relationship between SOS, considered as a measure of passive-dependency, and alcohol intake. Table 14-7 shows a strong positive relationship between organic disease and such intake: 47 percent of the Type III men drink to a significant degree, as against 23 percent of the healthy

---

[12]The possibility that a regression towards passive-dependency and primitive ego function precedes death has also been suggested by Lieberman (1965, 1969), who collected longitudinal psychological data from the population of an old age home. He reviewed the premorbid protocols of subjects whose sudden deaths had not been predicted by medical personnel; comparisons with earlier data from the same subjects and equivalent data from still surviving inmates showed a drastic shift towards dependent imagery and thought processes structured along magical mastery lines in the period prior to the unexpected death.

Type I men. Accordingly, if passivity indeed predisposes Navajo men to disease, the relationship is probably mediated, in a high proportion of cases, by alcohol: the passive-dependent man of high oral needs in a culture that sponsors drinking will be most likely to turn to alcohol as an anodyne against the anxiety and depression to which he is particularly prone; and this chronic reliance on alcohol could result in a heightened suceptibility to degenerative and infectious disease.

If there are other links between passivity and disease, they are masked in the Navajo case by the high incidence of heavy drinking that marks this group. If there is a relationship between passive-dependency and disease that works through agents other than alcohol, it can only be revealed through studies undertaken in societies which maintain strong cultural sanctions against drinking. The Druze are such a society, and most of our Druze subjects live by traditional religious precepts which forbid drinking. If our projected time 2 study of the Druze reveals the same degree of association between SOS and health status that we found among the Navajo, then we can more seriously consider the possibility that there is an intrinsic relationship between passive-dependency and morbid somatic conditions that has species-wide distribution.

Table 14-7
The Relation Between Alcoholism and Health Status

	Type I (Healthy) (N=35)	Type II (Moderate Chronic Illness) (N=44)	Type III (Potentially Terminal Illness) (N=34)
Percentage of Men With History of Heavy and/or Chronic Drinking	23%	29%	47%

References

Fenichel, O. *The Psychoanalytic Theory of Neurosis*. New York: Norton, 1945.
Gutmann, D. "An Exploration of Ego Configurations in Middle and Later Life." In B. Neugarten, (ed.) *Personality in Middle and Later Life*. New York: Atherton, 1964.
Gutmann, D. "The Country of Old Men: Cross-Cultural Studies in the Psychology of Later Life." *Occasional Papers in Gerontology*, Institute of Gerontology, The University of Michigan—Wayne State University, April, 1969.
Gutmann, D., "The Hunger of Old Men," (1970), In press: *Trans-Action.*
Krohn, A. and Gutmann, D. "Changes in Mastery Style with Age: A Study of Navajo Dreams." In press: *Psychiatry*, Aug. 1971.
Lieberman, M. "Psychological Correlates of Impending Death: Some Preliminary Observations." *Journal of Gerontology*, vol. 20, No. 2, April, 1965.
Lieberman, M., and Coplan, A. "Distance from Death as a Variable in the Study of Aging." *Developmental Psychology*, vol. 2, No. 1, 1969.

Neugarten, B., and Gutmann, D. "Age-Sex Roles and Personality in Middle Age: A Thematic Apperception Study." *Psychological Monographs*, No. 470, 1958.

Simmons, L. *The Role of the Aged in Primitive Society*. New Haven: Yale University Press, 1945.

Wolowitz, H., and Berker, M. "Alcoholism and Oral Passivity." *Quarterly Journal of Studies on Alcohol*. vol. 29, No. 3, Sept. 1968.

15

Cognitive Declines as Predictors of Mortality in Twin Pairs: A Twenty-Year Longitudinal Study of Aging*

LISSY F. JARVIK and
JUNE E. BLUM

Over a decade has passed since the suggestion was first made that decline in intellectual functioning might serve as an indicator of morbidity and mortality (Jarvik et al. 1957; Kleemeier 1962). Specifically, decrements on three subtests measuring cognitive performance (vocabulary, similarities and digit symbol substitution), when incorporated into a formula for "Critical Loss," distinguished subjects on the basis of five-year survival (Jarvik 1962). Since then, the association between mental impairment and mortality, originally described in twins, has been confirmed for single-born elderly subjects by a variety of investigators (Birren 1964; Granick and Birren 1969; Palmore 1969; Riegel 1969). Using medical evaluation, mental status examination and behavioral ratings rather than standard psychological test scores, Goldfarb (1969) also found a positive relationship between mental functioning (chronic brain syndrome) and subsequent mortality in a group of institutionalized elderly.

While progress has been made in describing this psychobiological relationship, it has only been as a result of current studies (Jacobs et al. 1969; Pfeiffer, 1970; Wang et al. 1970; Eisdorfer 1970) that relevant biological information is beginning to accumulate. For example, Wang and colleagues recently reported that a decrease in cerebral blood flow (usually indicative of cerebrovascular disease) was associated with a decline in cognitive functioning (Chapter 8).

Since cerebrovascular, like cardiovascular, disorders may have a significant

*The research from which the latest findings were derived was supported in part by Grant HD 01615, National Institute of Child Health and Human Development, National Institutes of Health. Grateful acknowledgement is made of the assistance of F. Goldstein in the most recent follow-up, J. Allen, E. Knell and M. Reiter in psychological testing, Dr. J. Fleiss in providing valuable statistical advice, and particularly our twin subjects who enabled us to pursue this study. Based in part on a paper presented at the annual meeting of the American Psychological Association, Washington, D.C., September 1969. Lissy F. Jarvik, M.D. is Psychiatrist, Department of Medical Genetics, New York State Psychiatric Institute and Associate Professor of Clinical Psychiatry, College of Physicians and Surgeons, Columbia University. This paper was completed while the senior author was on leave, holding appointments in the Department of Psychiatry, University of California at Los Angeles and in the Veterans Administration Center for Psychosocial Medicine at Brentwood. June E. Blum is Senior Clinical Psychologist, Department of Medical Genetics, New York State Psychiatric Institute and Research Associate in Psychiatry, College of Physicians and Surgeons, Columbia University.

199

genetic component (McKusick 1965), information on the comparative mortality of aged monozygotic twin partners, concordant and discordant for intellectual decline, is of value. Such data have not been published as yet and it is the purpose of the present report to fill this gap.

Subjects

The subjects of this study were 52 survivors of a group of 268 senescent twins, tested initially at age 60 and older. They were chosen from 1,603 index twins, residents of New York State and closely adjacent areas (Kallmann and Sander 1949), in accordance with the following criteria:

a) Twin partners of the same sex (to facilitate intrapair comparisons in view of the well-known sex difference in survival);
b) Both twins in good health and residing in the community rather than in institutions (to obtain base-line data);
c) Both twins literate, English-speaking (to avoid linguistic bias) and white (there were only a few non-whites in the original sample).

A complete description of the 268 twins (134 pairs) selected in 1946-1949 having been given elsewhere (Blum 1969), the pertinent features for this report may be summarized as follows: In accordance with statistical expectation based on sex differences in life span, there was an excess of female over male pairs; the proportion of females in the twin sample was even higher than that in the corresponding New York State population (1940 United States Census). This discrepancy may be attributed to the large representation of monozygotic female pairs concordant for survival which constituted the largest subgroup (Jarvik et al. 1960). The educational level for the twins was comparable to that of the New York State population in that 29 percent of the former and 27 percent of the latter went beyond elementary school (1940 United States Census). While similar to the general population of New York State in sex ratio and educational background, the majority of our twins resided in rural and small urban communities. The marked under-representation of metropolitan residents (40 percent of the twins vs. 80 percent of New York State population) derives, in part, from the sampling technique, which depended upon voluntary reporting and thus favored stable close-knit communities. In addition, the exclusion of foreign-born persons with language differences further reduced urban representation.

Psychological tests were administered three times to 78 of the 268 subjects, twice between 1946-1949 (initial test-retest round) and once between 1955 and 1957 (third testing). Among the 78, there were 62 who had taken the three critical subtests (vocabulary, similarities, and digit symbol substitution) on all three occasions. The latter 62 included 26 intact twin pairs (52 twin subjects), and it is to them that the present analysis has been restricted. These 26 twin pairs, in mean age, at initial testing closely approximated the entire group of 78 (67.6 vs. 67.5 years).

In comparison with the original sample of 134 twin pairs, these 26 pairs included an even higher proportion of monozygotic female pairs (53.8 percent vs. 37.3 percent) and a correspondingly lower proportion of dizygotic females (7.7 percent vs. 19.4 percent). These proportions are due to the following contributing factors: The average age of the total original sample was 69.7 years and a requirement for inclusion in the present study was survival of *both* twin partners long enough to be tested three times (usually seven additional years). Because of the longer life expectancy of females, compared to males, and the higher concordance for survival of monozygotic, compared to dizygotic twins, it is monozygotic female pairs who had the highest chance of surviving intact, and therefore of participating in the present study.

The educational level of the 26 intact pairs was higher than that of the original group of 134 pairs (60 percent vs. 29 percent with at least some secondary education) and higher also than that of the total 78 retested subjects, of whom 44 percent went beyond elementary school. In view of the high correlation between educational achievement and intellectual ability (Birren and Morrison 1961; and Granick and Friedman 1967) on the one hand, and intellectual functioning and survival on the other, it is not surprising that the group most highly selected for survival also showed the largest percentage of subjects with better than primary education.

Intellectual performance at initial testing followed a similar progression, the 52 surviving twins showing the higher mean scores on nearly all subtests (Table 15-1). Likewise, Granick and Birren (1969) found survivors in their longitudinal study to have functioned at a consistently higher level on initial testing than nonsurvivors on both verbal and performance tests. Riegel (1969 and Chapter 11) also reported nonsurvivors to be less intelligent (particularly on verbal tests) than survivors, whereas Palmore (1969 and Chapter 18) observed a high correlation between WAIS performance scores and longevity approximately 13 years after initial testing.

Methods

The tests used throughout this longitudinal study of senescence (Kallmann and Jarvik 1959) included five subtests (similarities, digits forward, digits backward, block design, and digit symbol substitution) from the Wechsler-Bellevue test (Wechsler 1944), Vocabulary List 1 of the Stanford-Binet test (Terman 1916), and a tapping test to measure simple speed involving eye-hand coordination (Feingold 1950).

From previous analyses, three tests of cognitive functioning (vocabulary, similarities, and digit symbol substitution) emerged as predictors of subsequent survival. A formula for "critical loss" evolved (Jarvik and Falek 1963) upon observation that decrease in Vocabulary—defined as a score on the third testing

Table 15-1
Comparative Mean Raw Scores on First Testing (1946-1949)

Test	Original Group Tested 1946-49 268 twin subjects (134 intact pairs)	Subgroup Tested Three Times 1946-55 78 twin subjects (34 intact pairs)	Intact Pairs With Critical Loss Scores 52 twin subjects (26 intact pairs)
Vocabulary	28.4	29.4	29.9
Similarities	9.2	9.9	10.1
Digit Symbol Substitution	28.4	31.0	30.9
Digits Forward	5.8	6.1	6.4
Digits Backward	4.1	4.5	4.5
Tapping	66.6	70.8	72.3
Block Design	13.5	14.5	14.9
Mean Age (in years) at first test	69.7	67.5	67.6

which was lower than that on either of the first two testings—was associated with five-year mortality (a concept borrowed from clinical medicine). In addition to a diminishing Vocabulary score, persons who died within five years of their third testing had also shown a more rapid rate of decline on two other tests (similarities and digit symbol substitution) than had subjects who survived their last testing by five years.

The annual rate of decline (ARD) was computed by subtracting the score of the third test round (T_T) from the higher of the first two scores (T_H) and dividing the result by the product of T_H and the number of years intervening between the tests (Y);

$$\frac{\text{ARD}}{\text{(in percent)}} = \frac{T_H - T_T}{T_H \times Y} \times 100.$$

Using this formula, an annual rate of decline of ten percent or more on similarities distinguished decedents from survivors, as did an annual rate of decline of at least two percent on digit symbol substitution. Based on the above observations, the concept of critical loss was formulated to include two or all three of the following: (1) any decline on vocabulary, (2) an annual rate of decline of at least ten percent on similarities and (3) an annual rate of decline of at least two percent on digit symbol substitution (Jarvik 1962).

At first sight, multiple regression analysis with mortality as the dependent variable and the three loss measures as the independent variables would appear to be the most reasonable method of analyzing the data. It was decided not to employ this technique because the measures of loss utilized did not seem to satisfy the assumptions of linearity and equal variability required for regression analysis.

Results and Discussion

Previous Findings

As mentioned above, an interim analysis of longitudinal test results (Jarvik and Falek 1963) revealed the positive relationship between five-year mortality and critical loss. However, at that time 31 of the 78 subjects tested three times could not be included in the analysis because five years had not elapsed since their third testing and, consequently, their five-year status was still unknown. In 1967, it was established that 60 of the 78 subjects had survived their third testing by five years. These 60 included 14 survivors who did not take each of the three critical tests on all three occasions and, therefore, had to be eliminated from the analysis as did two of the 18 decedents. There remained 62 subjects (46 survivors and 16 decedents) for whom critical loss could be determined. Only four of the 46 survivors, but 11 of the 16 who died within five years of their last testing showed a critical loss. As previously reported (Blum, Clark, and Jarvik 1968) the differences between the groups, survivors and decedents, was statistically significant (chi square 7.9, p < 0.01).

Present Findings

The past analyses were concerned with longitudinal changes in a given individual. The present analysis takes advantage of the unique composition of the sample, i.e., twin pairs.

In 16 of the 26 intact pairs, both members were five-year survivors; in nine pairs only one of the twin partners survived five years, and in the 26th pair both twins died within five years of their last testing (Table 15-2).

With regard to five-year survival, members of monozygotic twin pairs, whether male or female, did not show higher concordance in mortality than dizygotic twin partners. The lack of difference between the zygosity groups is probably due to the small number of subjects, particularly dizygotic twins, inasmuch as significantly smaller intrapair differences in longevity between monozygotic than between dizygotic co-twins have been demonstrated even for age groups beyond 70 (Jarvik et al. 1960).

It may also be seen from Table 15-2 that monozygotic twins showed higher concordance for critical loss than did dizygotic twins (13 out of 21, or 62

Table 15-2
Critical Loss[a] and Five-Year Survival According to Zygosity and Sex

Critical Loss	Both 5-Year Survivors Monozygotic m	Both 5-Year Survivors f[c]	Both 5-Year Survivors Dizygotic m	Both 5-Year Survivors f	One 5-Year Survivor Monozygotic m	One 5-Year Survivor f	One 5-Year Survivor Dizygotic m	One 5-Year Survivor f	Both Died Within 5 Years Monozygotic m	Both Died Within 5 Years f	Both Died Within 5 Years Dizygotic m	Both Died Within 5 Years f	Total
Neither Partner	3	7	1	1	–	3	–	–	–	–	–	–	15
One Partner[b]	1	1[e]	1[d]	1[d]	2[d]	3[d]	1[d]	–	1[e]	–	–	–	11
Total	4	8	2	2	2	6	1	–	1	–	–	–	26

[a]See text for definition

[b]In no pair did both partners show a Critical Loss

[c]m—male   f—female

[d]Partner with Critical Loss now dead, co-twin still alive

[e]Both twins now deceased, partner with Critical Loss died first

percent vs. 2 out of 5, or 40 percent). Even though this difference is statistically not significant, the trend is in accordance with expectation.

In the 11 pairs discordant for critical loss, the partner with the critical loss always succumbed earlier to death (10 pairs) or to illness (one pair, both partners still alive). In the pair of twins who were still alive in 1967 at age 84.6 years, the twin with the critical loss was diagnosed as having severe organic brain syndrome on an arteriosclerotic basis while his co-twin was in vigorous health. The previously postulated relationship between critical loss and mortality is thus reinforced.

The terminal illnesses were cardiovascular (6 cases) or cerebrovascular disease (one case), diabetic coma (one case), pulmonary embolus following a hip fracture (one case) and metastatic carcinoma (one case). In view of the high frequency of arteriosclerotic disease, the decline in those specific psychological functions constituting critical loss may reflect subclinical cerebral dysfunction. In fact, Wang and colleagues (1970) noted an association between a decrease in cerebral blood flow and a decline in intellectual functioning.

Roth and colleagues (1969) reported a high correlation between degenerative cerebral changes (quantitatively assessed post-mortem) and psychometric scores. Furthermore, the amount of histopathological change was highly correlated with length of survival.

Even as early as 1962, Kleemeier (p. 293) suggested that the shape of the curve of intellectual ability in the senium (65 years and over) implies ". . . that factors related to the death of the individual cause a decline in intellectual performance. . . . It therefore appears that we have here strong evidence for the existence of a factor, which might be called terminal drop, or decline, which adversely affects intellectual performance and is related to impending death of the aged person."

A case history exemplifying the relationship between intellectual decrement and early death is that of the monozygotic twin sisters "A" and "L" (Fig. 15-1), who remained single and lived together their entire lives with the exception of a six-year period during their early twenties when their jobs as monotypists took them to different cities. At their first testing, there were remarkably few differences between the twins. However, at the time of their third testing, A showed a critical loss (combination of all three tests) while the scores of L had remained unchanged on vocabulary as well as on similarities, and had actually increased on digit symbol substitution. A died within three years of her third testing. L, on the contrary, was still a vital, active person when last seen at age 81. The crucial factor eventually differentiating their life histories was the onset of myocarditis (possibly rheumatic) when A was in her late fifties.

While the reason for the occurrence of critical loss and earlier mortality remains elusive, two factors can be excluded here: The twins being monozygotic, *neither genetic variability nor differences in chronological age* can be held responsible for the observed *discordance* in intellectual decline and mortality.

Elimination of age as a factor contributing to critical loss is in accordance with our previous results (Jarvik 1962) and those of others who failed to detect a significant influence of chronological age in the relationship between psychological test scores and survival (Birren 1964; Lieberman 1966; and Goldfarb 1969). Palmore (1969), too, recently suggested that there were factors more important for longevity than chronological age, at least between the ages of 60-69 years, and concluded that maintenance of mental abilities was one of them.

The twin pair described above was one of 11 pairs characterized by discordance for critical loss, eight monozygotic and three dizygotic (Table 15-2). Like monozygotic twin partners of younger ages, as well as the larger original sample (Jarvik et al. 1957), the eight monozygotic pairs discordant for critical loss did not show statistically significant intrapair differences in mean scores at any time (Table 15-3).

Yet, at their third testing, approximately seven and one-half years later, the twin partners with the critical loss exhibited statistically significant declines ($p < 0.05$), not only on the three tests constituting critical loss, but on the other four as well. Even though the co-twins without critical loss also declined on all subtests, their loss was significant only on two speeded tasks (tapping and block design). This finding lends support to the hypothesis that *decline on speeded psychomotor tasks represents a normal concomitant of aging, while decrements in cognitive functioning are pathognomonic of cerebral disease* (Jarvik 1967; Birren 1968).

Of the eight co-twins *without* critical loss, three were still alive in 1967, while the remaining five died, on the average 5.6 years after their third test. Aside

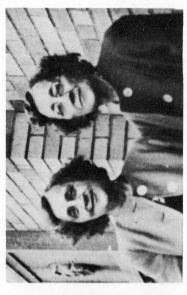
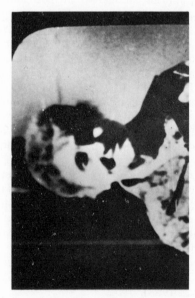

Figure 15-1. The "A&L" Twins ("L" on Left) in Their Teens and at Age 60. Survivor "L" at 80. (Photos courtesy Department of Medical Genetics, New York State Psychiatric Institute.)

Table 15-3
Mean Scores of Monozygotic Twins (Eight Pairs) Discordant for Critical Loss[a]

Tests	First Test-Retest Round Critical Loss		Third Testing Critical Loss	
	Without	With	Without	With
Vocabulary[b]	33.3	33.9	31.8	30.6*
Similarities[b]	12.1	10.9	10.9	8.1*
Digit Symbol Substitution[b]	33.9	34.0	30.9	25.4*
Digits Forward	6.8	7.0	6.3	6.3*
Digits Backward	4.9	5.3	3.8	4.4*
Tapping	77.1	81.6	61.0*	61.7*
Block Design	19.7	17.6	15.0*	13.6*
Mean Age (in years)	67.0		74.7	

[a]See text for definition
[b]Three Critical Loss Tests
*First vs. third testing $p < 0.05$

from a single survivor, the subjects with critical loss died, on the average, 3.1 years after the third testing, again confirming the association of cognitive decline and imminence of death.

One might question the necessity for the computation of critical loss when it is becoming increasingly apparent that higher mean scores generally discriminate survivors from nonsurvivors (Blum et al. 1968; Riegel 1969; Granick and Birren 1969, and Table 15-1, present paper). The advantage of the former is that, unlike group means involving raw scores, critical loss is useful in individual predictions, identifying high risk persons.

So far, the discussion has been concerned with the eight monozygotic pairs discordant for critical loss (Table 15-3). Among the remaining 13 monozygotic pairs (neither partner exhibited a critical loss) were six in which one partner survived long enough to be retested in 1967 while the other did not. In contrast to the critical loss group, where the deceased twin died after a mean interval of three years, here the mean interval between third testing and death was nearly 10 years (9.8 years). Comparing the test scores of the six surviving monozygotic partners with those of their deceased co-twins (Table 15-4), no significant intrapair differences were noted. The only significant within-group declines occurred between first and third testing on digit symbol substitution and

Table 15-4

Mean Scores of Monozygotic Twins (Six Pairs) Discordant for Survival to 1967 (Neither Critical Loss[a])

| | First Test-Retest Round | | Third Testing | | 1967 Testing |
	Alive	Dead	Alive	Dead	Alive
Vocabulary[b]	32.5	31.2	32.0	31.7	31.3
Similarities[b]	13.7	12.7	13.0	10.7	10.5**
Digit Symbol Substitution[b]	37.0	35.3	31.7*	31.4*	20.3**
Digits Forward	6.8	6.7	6.8	6.5	6.2
Digits Backward	5.2	5.2	4.6	4.8	4.2
Tapping	71.7	77.8	58.8*	65.7	46.7**
Block Design	18.5	17.3	17.5	17.0	12.2**
Mean Age (in years)	65.2		73.5		84.9

[a]See text for definition
[b]Three Critical Loss tests
*First vs. third testing $p < 0.05$
**Third vs. 1967 testing $p < 0.05$

tapping. Inasmuch as it was the survivors who decreased significantly on both tests, these declines are of no help in predicting mortality. Once again, *decline on speeded tasks is seen to accompany advancing age rather than to suggest underlying pathology*.

Further inspection of Table 15-4 indicates that in 1967, more than eleven years after their third testing, the scores of the six surviving co-twins did show significant declines on the majority of the tests—including two of the three critical loss tests. But by then, the surviving co-twins (tested in 1967) were in their ninth decade, and consequently had a reduced life expectancy. The imminence of death thus became a factor for the majority of them.

However, this was not true for those twin partners who had evidenced a critical loss and, like one of the W twins, died soom thereafter. When the W twins were tested for the third time, at the age of 70.5 years, they were both vigorous men, who, because of their good health, refused to consult a physician until CW's sudden and fatal diabetic coma two years later. Had the meaning of CW's cognitive decline been known at the time of his third testing, he might have been convinced to undergo a thorough medical examination. Rather than dying at the age of 73, it is possible that, like his monozygotic twin brother, he might have enjoyed another eight years of life.

Conclusions

Results of a twenty-year longitudinal study of intellectual changes during senescence demonstrate the usefulness of the critical loss formula in predicting mortality. The formula, based on specified rates of decline on three tests of cognitive functioning (vocabulary, similarities, and digit symbol substitution) distinguished survivors from decedents even when variability due to both genotype and chronological age was eliminated. The discriminatory ability of critical loss was demonstrated in spite of the limited number of twin pairs available for comparison, only 26 pairs having survived intact. In only eleven of these did at least one of the partners show a critical loss (in the remaining 15 pairs neither partner had a critical loss; there was not a single pair with both partners showing a critical loss). In ten of these eleven discordant pairs the partner with the critical loss was the first to die; in the eleventh pair the partner with the critical loss, though still alive at last report, showed marked physical and mental deterioration while his co-twin had remained in good health. *Critical loss thus emerged as a powerful predictor of morbidity and mortality for the given individuals.*

In contrast to the pathology suggested by the cognitive declines measured as critical loss, *decreasing scores on speeded motor tasks* appear to be normal concomitants of aging and *not indicative of impending mortality.*

The above results suggest that tests measuring cognitive functioning may have diagnostic value far beyond that presently assigned to them. Since more than a third of the monozygotic pairs (8 out of 21) were discordant for critical loss, it should be feasible to collect a series of such discordant pairs of identical genotypes. They would constitute an ideal group for controlled trials of dietary and other therapeutic regimens.

Eventually, the relationship between rate of cognitive decline and morbidity, if validated by prospectively designed studies on large representative samples, may find applicability in terms of prophylaxis and possible reversal of early morbid changes.

References

Birren, J.E.: Neural basis of personal adjustment in aging. In P. From Hansen, (ed.), *Age with a future*. Copenhagen: Munksgaard, 1964, pp. 48-59.

Birren, J.E.: Psychological aspects of aging. *Gerontologist*, 1968, *1*, 16-20.

Birren, J.E. and Morrison, D.F.: Analysis of the WAIS subtests in relation to age and education. *J. Geront.*, 1961, *16*, 363-369.

Blum, J.E.: Psychological changes between the seventh and ninth decades of life. Doctoral dissertation, St. John's University, 1969.

Blum, J.E., Clark, E.C., and Jarvik, L.F.: Longitudinal changes with advancing age: report of follow-up study. Paper read at American Psychological Association, San Francisco, September, 1968.

Eisdorfer, C.: The body and the mind. Paper read at American Psychological Association, Miami, September, 1970.

Feingold, L.: A psychometric study of senescent twins. Unpublished doctoral dissertation, Columbia University, 1950.

Goldfarb, A.I.: Predicting mortality in the institutionalized aged. *Arch. Gen. Psychiat.*, 1969, *21*, 172-176.

Granick, S. and Birren, J.E.: Cognitive functioning of survivors versus non-survivors: 12 year follow-up of healthy aged. Proceedings of the Eighth International Congress of Gerontology, Washington, August, 1969, Vol. II, Abstract #240, p. 67.

Granick, S. and Friedman, A.S.: The effect of education on the decline of psychometric test performance with age. *J. Geront.*, 1967, *22*, 191-195.

Jacobs, E.A., Winter, P.M., Alvis, H.J. and Small, S.M.: Hyperoxygenation effect on cognitive functioning in the aged. *New Eng. J. Med.*, 1969, *281*, 753-757.

Jarvik, L.F.: Biological differences in intellectual functioning. *Vita Hum.*, 1962, *5*, 195-203.

Jarvik, L.F.: Survival and psychological aspects of aging in man. *Symp. Soc. Exper. Biol.*, 1967, *21*, 463-482.

Jarvik, L.F. and Falek, A.: Intellectual stability and survival in the aged. *J. Geront.*, 1963, *18*, 173-176.

Jarvik, L.F., Falek, A., Kallmann, F.J., and Lorge I.: Survival trends in a senescent twin population. *Amer. J. Hum. Genet.*, 1960, *12*, 170-179.

Jarvik, L.F., Kallmann, F.J., Falek, A. and Klaber, M.M.: Changing intellectual functions in senescent twins. *Acta Genet. Statis. Med.*, 1957, *7*, 421-430.

Kallmann, F.J. and Jarvik, L.F.: Individual differences in constitution and genetic background. In J.E. Birren, (ed.), *Handbook of Aging and the Individual*. Chicago: Univ. of Chicago Press, 1959, pp. 216-263.

Kallmann, F.J. and Sander, G.: Twin studies on senescence. *Amer. J. Psychiat.*, 1949, *106*, 29-36.

Kleemeier, R.W.: Intellectual change in the senium. Proceedings of the Social Statistics Section of the American Statistical Association, 1962, pp. 290-295.

Lieberman, M.A.: Observations on death and dying. *Gerontologist*, 1966, *6*, 70-72.

McKusick, V.A.: Coronary artery disease. In Neel, J.V., Shaw M. and Schull, W.J. (eds.) *Genetics and the Epidemiology of Chronic Diseases*. Washington, D.C., U.S. Dept. H.E.W. (U.S. Print. Off., Pub. N. Service Pub. #1163), 1965, pp. 133-143.

Palmore, E.B.: Physical, mental, and social factors in predicting longevity. *Gerontologist*, 1969, *9*, 103-108.

Pfeiffer, E.: Survival in old age: physical, psychological and social correlates of longevity. *J. Amer. Geriatrics Soc.*, 1970, *18*, 273-285.

Riegel, K.F.: Research designs in the study of aging and the prediction of retest-resistance and death. Paper read at Eighth International Congress of Gerontology, Washington, 1969.

Roth, M., Tomlinson, B., and Blessed, G.: Quantitative measures of psychological impairment and cerebral damage (at post-mortem) in normal and demented elderly subjects with a note on the significance of threshold effects.

Proceedings of the Eighth International Congress of Gerontology, Washington, August, 1969, Vol. II, Abstract #180, p. 49.

Terman, L.M.: *The Measurement of Intelligence*. Boston: Houghton-Mifflin, 1916.

Wang, S.W., Obrist, W.D., and Busse, E.W.: Neurophysiological correlates of the intellectual function of elderly persons living in the community. *Amer. J.` Psychiat.*, 1970, *126*, 1205-1212.

Wechsler, D.: *The Measurement of Adult Intelligence*. Baltimore. Williams and Wilkins, 1944.

Part IV
Social Predictors

Some of the previous chapters have already reported the importance of several predictors with a social component such as organization of behavior (Chapter 10) and activity (Chapters 11 and 14). Thomas Garrity adds evidence that a measure of behavior in the hospital, based on observations of patient's attitudes and interactions, is a strong predictor of survival six months after hospital discharge. Eric Pfeiffer found that long-term survivors in the Duke Longitudinal Study, compared to short-term survivors, are characterized by greater education, financial status, higher occupation, and being married, as well as having better health and higher intelligence. With a multiple regression analysis of the factors related to the Longevity Quotient (which controls for the effects of age), Erdman Palmore found that the four strongest factors related to longevity among the Duke study participants were work satisfaction, happiness ratings, physical functioning, and avoiding tobacco. He concludes that the most important ways to increase longevity are maintaining a useful and satisfying role in society and maintaining a positive view of life.

Robert Kastenbaum discusses the concepts of hope, hopelessness, dread, the will-to-live, and the caring environment; and presents some preliminary evidence that they may be related to survival and longevity.

Finally, Richard Kalish discusses the social problems as well as the opportunities which will be presented by the addition of at least ten more years of life expectancy by 1990.

16 A Behavioral Predictor of Survival among Heart Attack Patients*

THOMAS F. GARRITY and
ROBERT F. KLEIN

Introduction

A number of studies have shown that the physical dimension of cardiac rehabilitation can be predicted by certain physical antecedent variables. Croog et al. (1968) recorded a number of studies which showed an association between the severity of attack and the physical outcome of the recovery process. It makes good sense that the physical condition of the patient at the time of the attack is related to the later physical condition of the patient.

What is not so intuitively obvious is that the behavioral response of the patient to the attack might be related to the long-term physical outcome. There has been a good bit of evidence that social and psychological factors play a role in the emergence of illness (Holmes et al. 1957; Hinkle and Wolff 1957; Jacobs et al. 1968). Behavioral factors have also been known to have an effect on the physical recovery of patients from various illnesses (Janis 1958; Sussman et al. 1964; Klein et al. 1968).

The study reported in the following pages is an attempt to relate behavioral characteristics of the heart-attack patient during hospitalization to his physical condition six months after hospital discharge. The general hypothesis is that patients exhibiting behavioral disturbance and poor adaptation during the acute phase of hospitalization will experience negative physical outcome within six months of hospital discharge. This relationship is expected to hold even when the effect of the patient's physical condition during hospitalization is controlled.

Study Patients

All patients entering the coronary care unit of a large teaching hospital over a six-month period were considered for the study. We were interested only in

*This research was supported by contract TH 43-67-1440, National Heart Institute, and is an expansion of a paper read at the Southern Sociological Society meetings, Atlanta, Georgia, in April, 1970. The authors wish to acknowledge the editorial assistance of Mrs. Joanne Baseheart.

Thomas F. Garrity is Instructor, Department of Behavioral Science, College of Medicine, University of Kentucky, Lexington, Kentucky.

Robert F. Klein, is Associate Professor, School of Medicine, University of Rochester, Rochester, N.Y.

patients with heart attacks diagnosed by the usual criteria of clinical history and electrocardiographic and/or enzyme changes. Forty-eight patients were eventually included.

Table 16-1 shows the breakdown of the group with respect to sex, race, age, and hospital economic status. The diversity of social characteristics represented in this group makes it somewhat less desirable for testing this this hypothesis than a socially homogeneous group. However, the effect of these social variables will be examined later in the discussion of behavioral patterns.

Behavioral Observations: The Independent Variable

Observations of the patient's behavior were made during the acute phase of the heart attack, i.e., during the first five days following hospitalization for the attack.

Observations were recorded on a check list (Table 16-2) similar to that reported by Bunney and Hamburg (1963); however, the items were modified to reflect types of behavior typical of patients in a coronary care facility. In constructing the checklist, items requiring a great deal of inference on the part of the observer were minimized.

The checklist consisted of 18 items descriptive of behavioral disturbance, such as anxiety, hostility, depression, etc. (Items 1-18), and 3 items descriptive of positive behavior such as calmness, cheerfulness, etc. (Items 19-21). Each item was scored from 0 to 4 depending upon the intensity of the particular trait. It

Table 16-1
Selected Social Characteristics of the Study Patients

	Men	Women
Total	32	16
Race		
Caucasian	24	9
Negro	8	7
Age		
40-49	2	1
50-59	12	4
60-69	13	4
70-79	4	5
80 plus	1	2
Hospital Economic Status		
Charity patient	19	11
Private patient	13	5

Table 16-2
Checklist for Behavior Rating Used by Nursing Personnel

Date   Shift   Patient
Rater   History #

Please indicate to what extent each of the following items was present in the patient during *this shift*. Check the appropriate place on each scale.

		Absent	Slightly	Moderately	Much	Extremely
1.	anxiety	——	——	——	——	——
2.	restless	——	——	——	——	——
3.	tense	——	——	——	——	——
4.	seems afraid of some-thing	——	——	——	——	——
5.	becomes upset easily	——	——	——	——	——
6.	seeks reassurance from personnel	——	——	——	——	——
7.	hostility	——	——	——	——	——
8.	unfriendly to others	——	——	——	——	——
9.	impolite to others	——	——	——	——	——
10.	complains	——	——	——	——	——
11.	objects to some routine procedures	——	——	——	——	——
12.	angry	——	——	——	——	——
13.	depression	——	——	——	——	——
14.	seems to feel rejected	——	——	——	——	——
15.	sad appearance	——	——	——	——	——
16.	withdrawn	——	——	——	——	——
17.	quiet	——	——	——	——	——
18.	talks of gloomy things	——	——	——	——	——
19.	calm	——	——	——	——	——
20.	cheerful	——	——	——	——	——
21.	friendly	——	——	——	——	——

should be noted that at least eight of the items (6-11, 18, and 21) recorded interactional or social behaviors.

The intraclass correlations were calculated to assess the interrater reliability of each item. The reliability of each of the 21 items on the checklist exceeded the .01 level of agreement. The reliability of the 18-item behavioral disturbance score was far better than chance when used under two conditions. The intraclass correlation was .64 when the raters saw a film stimulus and .42 when the observers rated patients in the hospital setting. Approximately the same levels of agreement were found on the measures of positive behavior.

Assignment of observers (members of the patient care staff) to patients and shifts depended entirely on the vicissitudes of work scheduling and were made by the head nurse of the unit. There is no evidence that assignment of observers to patients was biased in a fashion that would affect this research. All observers were trained through regular meetings in which specific patients were discussed in terms of the checklist.

Observations began with the patient's admission and continued during the five days of the study. Observations for each patient were recorded on checklists by two independent observers at the end of the 7 A.M.-3 P.M. shift and at the end of the 3 P.M.-11 P.M. shift.

The scores for the individual items on the checklist were grouped by addition into a measure of behavioral disturbance (Items 1-18) and a measure of positive behavior (19-21). (As might be expected, behavioral disturbance and positive behavior are negatively correlated.) These two measures were graphed over the five-day observation period. The graphs were then used to sort the patients into two groups which were called the nonadaptor and the adaptor groups. The group names are simply labels which are descriptive of manifest behavior and are not meant to characterize any deeper levels of psychological adjustment.

Graphs sorted into the nonadaptor group showed either great behavioral disturbance and little positive behavior over the five days of observation, or increasing behavioral disturbance and decreasing positive behavior. Graphs sorted into the adaptor group showed either little behavioral disturbance and great positive behavior over the five-day period, or decreasing behavioral disturbance and increasing positive behavior.

Two investigators, one acquainted with each of the patients, and the other not acquainted with them, independently sorted the graphs according to the above criteria. There was disagreement on only 10 percent of the graphs and this occurred because these graphs lacked clear behavioral trends. The differences were resolved by jointly reviewing and reclassifying the disputed cases, adhering as closely as possible to the original criteria.

Two groups of 24 patients emerged. The groups did not differ significantly in sex, race, socioeconomic characteristics, or in the amount or type of sedatives and tranquilizers administered during the observation period. There is a slight, though nonsignificant, tendency for the nonadaptors to be older. It should be noted that the occurrence of equal number of patients in the two groups happened by chance rather than design.

The Physical Outcome: The Dependent Variable

Six months after hospital discharge, questionnaires were mailed to the patients to assess mortality and the physical status of survivors. The questionnaire consisted of a symptoms checklist and the Cantril Self-anchoring Ladder (Cantril 1965). From the symptoms checklist was derived the New York Functional Heart Classification (Friedberg 1949) as well as the Psychophysiological Disability Index (Langner 1962). The former is an index of heart-related symptomotology and the latter provides a measure of general somatic preoccupation and functional disability. The Cantril Self-anchoring Ladder was used to learn the patient's assessment of his present level of health.

Findings

The follow-up at six months post-discharge showed that 12 patients of the original 48 had died during the intervening period. It was found that 10 of the 12 dead were nonadaptors; 2 were adaptors. In other words, 41 percent of the nonadaptors died within six months of discharge as compared with only 8 percent of the adaptors. In the nonadaptors group, 8 deaths were directly heart-caused and 2 were of uncertain cause. The 2 deaths in the adaptor group were due to heart attacks.

The clinical impressions of the attending physicians were examined for evidence that the differential mortality rates of the two groups were due to differing overall levels of health in the two groups. No such evidence could be found: the two groups displayed nearly equal distributions of diabetes, hypertension, lung disease, renal malfunction, and alcoholism. By this measure the nonadaptors and adaptors have similar health profiles.

Several further questions need to be answered. First, can the mortality difference between the two groups be explained by the differential severity of the attacks of the two groups? Second, can the difference be explained by the history of heart trouble experienced by the two groups? And finally, are the behavioral pattern, severity of attack, and prior history independent of each other, and if so, which seem to be the better predictors of mortality?

The most parsimonious way of dealing with these multivariate questions is by the technique of multiple regression. From this perspective we have a single dependent variable which is to be predicted by three independent variables. The dependent variable is the outcome, that is, death or life. The first predictor is the behavioral pattern during the acute hospitalization, nonadaptor or adaptor. The second is the severity of the attack measured by the presence or absence of heart failure. The third predictor is presence or absence of previous heart trouble. Multiple regression enables us to assess the effect of each independent variable on the dependent variable when the influence of the others is controlled. The usefulness of applying regression to "dummy" or dichotomous variables has been discussed by Suits (1957).

Table 16-3 shows the correlation matrix of the four variables. All three of the predictors are found to relate significantly to mortality. Among the predictors, the behavioral dimension does not relate to severity, but it does relate significantly to the presence of prior heart trouble. Severity and prior heart trouble are not significantly related. The fact that these four variables come into play at distinct points in time helps to suggest a tentative processual explanation of what is happening. The temporal priority of previous heart trouble makes it a more likely determinant of behavioral response than vice versa; and the temporal proximity of behavioral response and death suggests that behavioral response is a more likely determinant of death than would be previous heart trouble. This postulation also seems probable since there is no relationship between previous heart trouble and severity of the attack. Severity, on the other hand, relates to mortality quite independently of behavioral pattern and past history. Expressed more simply, severity and behavioral pattern each affect mortality independently. Prior heart trouble affects mortality, but only through the agency of behavioral response. This tentative model is borne out by the regression equation in Table 16-4 which shows severity and behavioral response to have independent predictive power for mortality. The effect of prior heart trouble becomes nonsignificant after the first two have been included in the equation.

By suggesting that the presence of prior heart trouble may cause adverse behavioral response after an attack, we have raised a question which is too complex to be adequately explored by our data. However, we can point to a study by Rosen and Bibring (1966) which partially agrees with our observations. They have shown that blue-collar workers tend to display far more negative affect after the second attack than after the first. The implication is that a first attack is easily denied; the second makes that defense unviable. Our patients who were experiencing attack number two or three may be more threatened than the first timers, and hence, more upset.

Table 16-3
A Correlation Matrix of the Three Independent Variables (Behavioral Adjustment, Severity, Prior Heart Trouble) and One Dependent Variable (Mortality) (n=48)

	Severity	Prior Heart Trouble	Mortality
Behavioral adjustment	−.0419	.2581*	.3849**
Severity		−.1626	.3152*
Prior heart trouble			.2484*

*significant at .05
**significant at .01

Table 16-4
The Beta Weights, Standard Errors of the Betas, and the F-Values of the Three Independent Variables Derived from Their Multiple Regression on the Dependent Variable of Mortality

Independent Variables	Beta	S.E. Beta	F
Severity	.36	.12	8.18**
Behavioral adjustment	.34	.13	6.94*
Prior heart trouble	.21	.13	2.75

(with 1.44 degrees of freedom)

*significant at .05
**significant at .01

With regard to other possible predictors of outcome, the survivors of the nonadaptor and adaptor groups showed no difference in their physical status. The Langner PPDI, the New York Heart Classification, and the Cantril Ladder all show no important differences.

Discussion

Our study supports others in finding that severity of illness is a predictor of physical outcome. The general hypothesis of this study that patients exhibiting behavioral disturbance and poor adaptation during the acute phase of hospitalization will experience negative physical outcome within six months of hospital discharge is also supported.

The empirical relationship demonstrated in this study is not easily explained. An adequate explanation would have to show how the manifest behavior was transformed into the physical. If we assume that manifest behavioral disturbance indicates underlying psychic stress (a relationship requiring validation), we are led into psychosomatic theory for an explanation. One of the basic tenets of psychosomatic theory is that psychic stress works a harmful effect on the physiology of the organism.

One variation of the psychosomatic theory proposed by W.B. Cannon (1942) argues that the cognition of a threat sets off an overstimulation of the sympathicoadrenal system, leading to the breakdown of normal structure and function in the body. The behavioral manifestation is one of acute anxiety and fear. Richter (1957) modifies the Cannon notion. He suggests a reaction of hopelessness and depression rather than fear and anxiety. In this notion, bodily functions are seen to dwindle away through parasympathetic overactivation.

The psychosomatic models of Cannon and Richter offer a very promising interdisciplinary perspective from which to view the findings of this study. Heart attack is a most threatening event. Even when the acute phase of the illness is successfully passed, there remains the threat that it could happen again, ultimately bringing death with it. It is clear that some patients defend themselves successfully in both adaptive and maladaptive ways (Hackett and Weisman 1964). Others are not able to handle the threat very efficiently in either the short or long run. It seems possible that the nonadaptors in the present study were showing signs of difficulty in dealing with the threats involved in having had a heart attack, and possibly went out of the hospital never really having come to terms with the threat of still another attack and the possibility of sudden death. Since early signs of negative adaptation seem to portend long-term problems for the patient, treatment intervention should perhaps include counseling to promote more promising defenses.

Evidence has been presented that there is a relationship between short-term behavioral and long-term physical adaptation after heart attack. However, we do not know why some heart patients adapt poorly and others well. It has been conjectured that prior experience with heart illness may play some role; there is

222

also some evidence that Nonadaptors are habitually more disturbed (Lebovits et al. 1967; Bruhn et al. 1969). Other social, psychological, and physical factors surely affect the patient's coping ability as well. All of these matters need consideration in future work.

References

Bruhn, J.G., et al. "A psychological study of survivors and non-survivors of myocardial infarction," *Psychosomatic Medicine*, 31, 1969.

Bunney, W.B., and Hamburg, D.A. "Methods for reliable longitudinal observations of behavior," *Archives of General Psychiatry*, 9, 1963.

Cannon, W.B. "Voodoo Death," *American Anthropologist*, 44, 1942.

Cantril, H. *The Pattern of Human Concern*. New Brunswick: Rutgers, 1965.

Croog, S.H., et al. "The heart patient and the recovery process: a review of the directions of research on social and psychological factors," *Social Science and Medicine*, 2, 1968.

Friedberg, C. *Diseases of the Heart*. Philadelphia: Saunders, 1949.

Hackett, T.P., and Weisman, A.D. "Reactions to the imminence of death," in G.H. Grosser, et al. (eds.), *The Threat of Impending Disaster*. Cambridge: M.I.T. Press, 1964.

Hinkle, L.E., Jr., and Wolff, H.G. "Health and the social environment: experimental investigations," in A.H. Leighton, et al. (eds.), *Explorations in Social Psychiatry*. New York: Basic Books, 1957.

Holmes, T., et al. "Psychosocial and psychophysiologic studies of tuberculosis," *Psychosomatic Medicine*, 19, 1957.

Jacobs, M.A., et al. "The relationship of life change, maladaptive aggression, and upper respiratory infection in male college students." Paper read at meetings of American Psychosomatic Society, Boston, Mass., March, 1968.

Janis, I.L. *Psychological Stress*. New York: Wiley, 1958.

Klein, R.F., et al. "Transfer from a coronary care unit," *Archives of Internal Medicine*, 122, 1968.

Langner, T.S. "A twenty-two item screening score of psychiatric symptoms indicating impairment," *Journal of Health and Human Behavior*, 3, 1962.

Lebovits, B.Z., et al. "Prospective and retrospective psychological studies of coronary heart disease," *Psychosomatic Medicine*, 29, 1967.

Richter, C.P. "On the phenomenon of sudden death in animals and man," *Psychosomatic Medicine*, 19, 1957.

Rosen, J.L., and Bibring, G.L. "Psychological reactions of male patients to a heart attack," *Psychosomatic Medicine*, 28, 1966.

Suits, D.B. "Use of dummy variables in regression equations," *Journal American Statistical Association*, 52, 1957.

Sussman, M.B., et al. *Rehabilitation and Tuberculosis*. Cleveland Western Reserve University, 1964.

17 Physical, Psychological, and Social Correlates of Survival in Old Age*

ERIC PFEIFFER

Purpose of the Study

Goldfarb has found four characteristics associated with mortality among institutionalized elderly persons: a) psychiatrically determined chronic brain syndrome of severe degree; b) high proportion of errors in a brief mental status exam; c) diminished capacity for self-care and mobility; and d) incontinence (Chapter 7). Quint and Cody, on the other hand, found that prominent men over 45 listed in *Who's Who* had a mortality which was 30 percent below that of white males of like age in the general population (1968). In a similar vein, statisticians of the Metropolitan Life Insurance Company have reported that death rates from heart disease, one of the major causes of death in old age, was substantially lower among Standard Ordinary policyholders than among Industrial policyholders (1967). Standard Ordinary policyholders are drawn chiefly from urban middle and well-to-do classes engaged in the professions, in business, trade, and clerical occupations. Industrial policyholders are mainly members of wage-earning families in the lower income brackets.

The present study seeks to discover physical, psychological, and social factors which differentiate short-term from long-term survivors among elderly persons *living in the community*. Simultaneously, this study becomes a comparison between elite and nonelite groups of aged individuals. The study is an outgrowth of the larger interdisciplinary research on age-related changes, begun at the Duke University Center for the Study of Aging and Human Development in 1954 and still in progress. An overall description of the larger study is found elsewhere (Palmore, 1970).

Sample and Methods

In a previous longitudinal study which focused on sexual behavior in old age and which utilized a sample of some 260 community volunteers, a subgroup of 39

*This study was supported by Public Health Service Grant HD-00668 from the National Institute of Child Health and Human Development. Computer programming for this study was carried out by Mrs. Nancy Watson. Raafat S. Mishriky, gave valuable statistical advice. Revised and reprinted by permission from the *Journal of the American Geriatrics Society*, 8:4:273-285, 1970.
Eric Pfeiffer, M.D. is Associate Professor of Psychiatry, Department of Psychiatry and Center for the Study of Aging and Human Development, Duke University, Durham, N.C.

individuals (20 men and 19 women) was identified who showed the following characteristics: they had given codeable responses to interview questions about their sexual activity and sexual interest, on each of four separate examinations over a period of ten years (Pfeiffer 1969). When these subjects were studied more closely, it became apparent that they represented a kind of physical, psychological, and social elite, in comparison with the entire panel of subjects from which they had been drawn. In addition, these 39 subjects, whose average age was 67 at the start of the study, by virtue of surviving for at least ten more years, also represented a longevous elite. This observation became the starting point for the present study.

In this study we wished to compare this relatively long-lived elite with a group of subjects, drawn from the same panel and matched for age and sex, who represented the opposite extreme with respect to longevity. For this purpose we first selected the 39 subjects (20 men and 19 women) who had been the earliest to die following entry into the study. This procedure caused problems, since the average age at the start of the study in the group thus chosen was significantly greater for both the men and for the women than for the corresponding longevous groups. Since none of the persons in the longevous group had reached age eighty at the time of the start of the study, we therefore chose the 20 men and 19 women below age 80 who were the first to die. Using this procedure, the average age of the longevous males was 68 years and of the short-term surviving males was 71 years, a difference which was no longer statistically significant. However, we still had statistically significant age differences between the two groups of women. In order to include women of more comparable age, we eliminated the two youngest women among the longevous group and the two oldest women in the short-lived group, thus reducing the number of women in each group from 19 to 17. The average age of these two groups was 66 for the longevous women, and 68 for the women with short-term survival, a difference no longer statistically significant.

To assure comparability, only data collected during the first examination were utilized in this study. For while all of the subjects in the longevous groups were studied on four difference occasions, the majority of the short-lived subjects were studied only once.

Throughout the study, long-lived women are compared only with short-lived women, and long-lived men with short-lived men. It is well known that sex has a major determining influence on life expectancy as well as on a number of the other factors which were examined. Thus, analyses were carried out on the following groups:

17 long-lived women
17 short-lived women

20 long-lived men
20 short-lived men

The average interval from entry into the study to the time of death was 2.42 years for the short-lived men, 5.5 for the short-lived women. All of the long-lived men and women remained alive for at least 10 years following entry into the study, and all but one of those selected into the long-lived group are still alive at the time of this writing (July 1969).

The tests of significance used in this study were: the *t*-test, when comparisons among means were involved; the Kendall rank correlation coefficient, when ordinal distributions were compared; and the Chi-square test, when nominal distributions were compared. In the multiple regression analysis, the F-test was used to determine significance levels.

Health Factors

Attention is focused first on health factors. To facilitate comparison with results reported in a recent paper by Ryser and Sheldon (1969), data with respect to self-assessment of health status are presented first.

Subjects were asked: "How would you rate your health at the present time?" (Self-Health Rating) Responses were classified into three categories, as follows:

> excellent
> 1. excellent for my age
> good
>
> good for my age
> 2. fair
> fair for my age
>
> 3. poor
> very poor

Results for the four groups are presented in Table 17-1.

Subjects were also asked: "How concerned do you feel about your health troubles?" (Self-Health Concern) Responses were classified into three categories, as follows:

> 1. not concerned
> 2. moderately concerned
> 3. very concerned

Results are presented in Table 17-2.

Subjects were also asked: "How many days did you spend in bed last year because of not feeling well?" (Days in Bed) Responses were classified into three categories, as follows:

1. no days in bed
2. a few days in bed
3. 2 to 4 weeks in bed, up to "all the time"

Results are presented in Table 17-3.

Subjects were also asked: "How much do your health troubles stand in the way of your doing the things you most want to do?" (Degree of Limitation) Responses were classified into three categories:

Table 17-1
Self Health Rating

	Long-Lived		Short-Lived		
	N	%	N	%	P
1.	12	71%	7	41%	Women
2.	5	29%	6	35%	<.01
3.	0	0%	4	24%	
	17	100%	17	100%	
1.	14	70%	5	25%	Men
2.	5	25%	9	45%	<.001
3.	1	5%	6	30%	
	20	100%	20	100%	

Table 17-2
Self Health Concern

	Long-Lived		Short-Lived		
	N	%	N	%	P
1.	11	65%	9	56%	Women
2.	5	29%	6	38%	n.s.
3.	1	6%	1	6%	
	17	100%	16	100%	
1.	10	54%	7	37%	Men
2.	6	35%	9	47%	<.05
3.	1	11%	3	16%	
	17	100%	19	100%	

1. no limitation
2. some limitation (mild to moderate)
3. a great deal of limitation (severe)

Results are presented in Table 17-4.

As can be seen from these four tables, the majority of long-lived and short-lived women saw themselves in relatively good health, admitting to little or

Table 17-3
Days In Bed

	Long-Lived N	Long-Lived %	Short-Lived N	Short-Lived %	P
1.	8	50%	9	54%	Women
2.	6	38%	4	23%	n.s.
3.	2	12%	4	23%	
	16	100%	17	100%	
1.	16	80%	10	59%	Men
2.	3	15%	4	23%	<.05
3.	1	5%	3	18%	
	20	100%	17	100%	

Table 17-4
Degree of Limitation

	Long-Lived N	Long-Lived %	Short-Lived N	Short-Lived %	P
1.	4	33%	3	37%	Women
2.	7	58%	3	37%	n.s.
3.	1	9%	2	25%	
	12	100%	8	100%	
1.	7	50%	2	14%	Men
2.	6	43%	8	57%	<.001
3.	1	7%	4	29%	
	14	100%	14	100%	

no limitation in their functioning. This finding is in agreement with those of Ryser and Sheldon (1969), and of Shanas and her associates (1968). The Self-Health Rating was the only measure which differentiated the two groups of women.

While the majority of long-lived men also saw themselves in relatively good health, the same was not true for the short-lived men. On three out of the four health measures used, the short-lived men rated their health as significantly poorer than did the long-lived men. Heyman and Jeffers had previously found similar relations of health to survival (1963).

The self-assessments of health status presented thus far are relatively static measures, requiring subjects to rate themselves *only at one point in time*. These measures are not very successful in differentiating short-lived from long-lived women, and are only moderately successful in differentiating similar groups of men. We therefore wondered whether a measure which required the subjects to make a *longitudinal* assessment of their health might be a more sensitive indicator of remaining life expectancy. This was in fact the case. The subjects were asked: "Is your health better or worse now than it was when you were 55 years of age?" (Self Rating of Health Change) The responses were classified as follows:

1. better
2. the same
3. worse

The results of this analysis are presented in Table 17-5. The majority of persons who have only a short number of years left perceive their health as having declined since age 55, while only a few of the long-lived persons do so, a difference which is statistically significant at the .01 level for the women and the .001 level for the men.

Table 17-5
Self Rating of Health Change

	Long-Lived		Short-Lived		
	N	%	N	%	P
1.	8	47%	1	6%	Women
2.	3	18%	7	41%	<.01
3.	6	35%	9	53%	
	17	100%	17	100%	
1.	6	30%	0	0%	Men
2.	9	45%	4	20%	<.001
3.	5	25%	16	80%	
	20	100%	20	100%	

We also had available on each subject an "objective" health measure, the "physical functional rating." This rating was based on the physical examination and on the examining physician's assessment of pathology and disability. Physical functional ratings were classified as follows:

1. no pathology
   pathology; no disability
   disability, mild 0-20%

2. disability, moderate 20-50%
   disability, severe 50-80%
   total 80-100%

The results are presented in Table 17-6. As can be seen, this "objective" measure is not associated with survival in the groups of women and has a relatively low but significant association with survival in the groups of men.

It is of interest that the various health measures seem to have greater predictive value for the men than for the women. This may be related to the fact that the short-lived men on average were significantly nearer death than were the short-lived women at the time these measures were taken (2.42 vs. 5.50 years).

Intelligence Test Scores

Mean intelligence test scores for the long-term survivors were significantly greater than for short-term survivors. This was true for the verbal, performance, and full-scale weighted scores of the Wechsler Adult Intelligence Scale (WAIS). This finding is thus in agreement with those of Jarvik and Falek (1963) and of Riegel, Riegel, and Meyer (1967). (Table 17-7.)

Table 17-6
Physical Function Rating

	Long-Lived N	Long-Lived %	Short-Lived N	Short-Lived %	P
1.	10	59%	10	59%	Women
2.	7	41%	7	41%	n.s.
	17	100%	17	100%	
1.	12	63%	8	40%	Men
2.	7	37%	12	60%	<.05
	19	100%	20	100%	

Education

The mean number of years of education was greater for the long-term survivors than for the short-term survivors. The difference was statistically significant among the women and approached significance among the men. (Table 17-8.)

Social Factors

In order to obtain a subjective indication of the subjects' economic situation, they were asked: "How would you describe your present financial position in life?" (Financial Self-Rating). Responses were categories as follows:

1. wealthy
   well-to-do

2. comfortable

3. enough to get along
   can't make ends meet

As can be seen from Table 17-9 there was no significant difference in financial self-assessment between the two groups of women, but there was a very

Table 17-7
Intelligence Test Scores

	Means	Long-Lived	Short-Lived	t	p
	Verbal	66.58	46.17	2.96	<.01
Women	Performance	35.70	24.47	2.65	<.02
	Full-Scale	102.29	70.64	2.95	<.01
	Verbal	63.85	48.30	2.58	<.02
Men	Performance	31.35	21.26	2.65	<.02
	Full-Scale	95.20	70.42	2.59	<.02

Table 17-8
Years of Education

	Long-Lived	Short-Lived	t	P
Women	12.23	8.41	2.18	<.05
Men	11.65	7.60	1.94	N.S.

significant difference in financial self-assessment between the two groups of men, with 80 percent of the short-lived men ranking themselves at the lower end of the continuum.

Subjects were also asked: "Are you in a better or a worse position financially now than you were at age 55?" (Financial Self-Evaluation Change) Responses were categorized as follows:

1. better now
2. about the same
3. worse now

Results are presented in Table 17-10. The two groups of women did not differ from each other in this analysis, but the two groups of men differed

Table 17-9
Financial Self-Evaluation

	Long-Lived N	Long-Lived %	Short-Lived N	Short-Lived %	P
1.	1	6%	0	0%	Women
2.	9	53%	10	59%	n.s.
3.	7	41%	7	41%	
	17	100%	17	100%	
1.	0	0%	0	0%	Men
2.	14	70%	4	20%	<.001
3.	6	30%	16	80%	
	20	100%	20	100%	

Table 17-10
Financial Self-Evaluation Change

	Long-Lived N	Long-Lived %	Short-Lived N	Short-Lived %	P
1.	9	53%	9	56%	Women
2.	1	6%	3	19%	n.s.
3.	7	41%	4	25%	
	17	100%	16	100%	
1.	9	45%	5	25%	Men
2.	5	25%	3	15%	<.01
3.	6	30%	12	60%	
	20	100%	20	100%	

significantly, with the short-lived group of men showing significantly greater worsening of their financial status since age 55.

Occupation

As a rough but relatively objective indicator of socioeconomic status, subjects were categorized according to whether their principal occupation (or their husband's principal occupation, in the case of married or formerly married women) had been manual or nonmanual. Significantly fewer long-lived women were found in the manual category. The difference between the groups of men was in the same direction, but barely missed attaining statistically significance (Table 17-11).

Marital Status

Among the short-lived women the proportion of those not married was significantly greater than in the long-lived group. Among the two groups of men the trend was in the same direction but did not attain statistical significance. The results are presented in Table 17-12.

Other Factors

The racial distribution of the two long-lived groups did not differ significantly from that of the short-lived groups. The several groups were also compared, using a series of attitude and activity measurements. Only a few of these measurements were able to differentiate significantly short-term from long-term survivors, and the relatively meager average results are not included in this chapter. (See Chapter 18 for analysis of these factors.)

Table 17-11
Occupation

| | Long-Lived | | Short-Lived | | |
	N	%	N	%	P
Nonmanual	13	76%	5	29%	Women
Manual	4	24%	12	71%	<.01
	17	100%	17	100%	
Nonmanual	14	70%	8	40%	Men
Manual	6	30%	12	60%	n.s.
	20	100%	20	100%	

Longevity Index and Longevity Quotient

Palmore, working with data from the Duke longitudinal study, has recently developed two new concepts which are of interest in connection with the present study: the longevity index and the longevity quotient (Chapter 18). The *Longevity Index* is defined as follows: the number of years from the time of entry into the study to death, for those subjects who have already died; or, the number of years from the point of entry into the study up to the present, plus the expected remaining years, based on current life expectancy tables, for subjects still alive. For the four groups in the present study the means of the longevity indices were as follows:

long-lived women	19.30 years
short-lived women	5.50 years
long-lived men	17.22 years
short-lived men	2.42 years

The *Longevity Quotient* is defined as follows: the Longevity Index divided by the number of years the subject was expected to remain alive at the time of entry into the study. Thus, it is a measure of whether a subject lived a longer or a shorter time than would have been actuarially expected at the time of entry into the study. Thus, a longevity quotient of greater than 1.00 is indicative of longer than expected survival, a value of less than 1.00 is indicative of shorter than expected survival. The mean longevity quotients for the four groups were as follows:

long-lived women	1.32
short-lived women	0.44
long-lived men	1.56
short-lived men	0.24

Table 17-12
Marital Status

	Long-Lived N	%	Short-Lived N	%	
Married	12	71%	5	29%	Women
Nonmarried	5	29%	12	71%	$<.05$
	17	100%	17	100%	
Married	19	95%	15	75%	Men
Nonmarried	1	5%	5	25%	n.s.
	20	100%	20	100%	

These findings merely confirm that polar groups were indeed chosen in constituting the sample.

Multiple Regression Analysis

Having found a number of variables which significantly differentiated short-term from long-term survivors, we were of course interested in determining which of the variables contributed most to the variance observed and which did so independently. To accomplish this, a multiple stepwise regression analysis was carried out, using the Longevity Index (defined above) as the dependent variable. The findings are presented in Table 17-13.

For the women in this study, full-scale weighted WAIS score, perception of health change, marital status, physical functional rating, and change in financial status, in that order, contributed most significantly to the variance in longevity,

Table 17-13
Multiple Stepwise Regression Analysis of Selected Variables With Longevity Index

Women Variable	Zero Order Corr.	Multiple R.	Cummul Var.	Add. Var.
Full scale wgt. WAIS score	0.42	0.42	0.18	0.18
Self health change	0.40	0.52	0.27	0.09
Marital status	0.39	0.56	0.31	0.04
Physical function rating	−0.31	0.59	0.35	0.04
Financial status change	−0.02	0.60	0.36	0.02
Performance wgt. WAIS score	0.41	0.61	0.37	0.01
Self health rating	0.24	0.61	0.37	0.00
Financial status	0.23	0.62	0.38	0.01
Socioeconomic status	−0.33	0.62	0.38	0.01
Men				
Financial status	0.53	0.53	0.28	0.28
Self health change	0.51	0.61	0.37	0.09
Physical function rating	−0.46	0.66	0.44	0.07
Financial status change	0.21	0.70	0.49	0.05
Marital status	0.33	0.72	0.52	0.03
Verbal wgt. WAIS score	0.34	0.73	0.53	0.01
Socioeconomic status	−0.17	0.76	0.58	0.05
Self health rating	0.44	0.76	0.58	0.00
Performance wgt. WAIS score	0.36	0.76	0.58	0.00

and together these five factors accounted for 36 percent of the total variance observed.

For the men in the study, the findings were similar though by no means identical. Financial status, perception of health change, physical functional rating, change in financial status, and marital status, in that order, contributed most significantly to the variance in longevity, and together these five factors accounted for 52 percent of the total variance observed.

A number of other factors (performance weighted WAIS score and occupational status for the women, and self-health rating and verbal and performance weighted WAIS scores for the men) were also significantly correlated with longevity but did not make a significant *independent* contribution to the total variance in longevity.

Conclusions

The present study, utilizing subgroups of a panel of community volunteers, has presented evidence to suggest that group characteristics of long-term survivors differ sharply from those of short-term survivors in old age. It further suggests that there is no single factor which determines longevity but rather a constellation of biological, psychological, and social factors, amounting to what may best be described as *elite status*. Persons with high intelligence, sound financial status, well-maintained health, and intact marriages, may be expected to live significantly longer than their less intelligent and poorer brothers and sisters whose health is also declining and whose marriages are no longer intact. It is lamentable that many of the factors which we have identified as contributing to longevity are not readily subject to individual, social, or political manipulation, with the possible exception of financial factors. It is hoped that investigations in other parts of the country and with differing populations of elderly people may be able to determine whether the hypotheses put forward here apply to elderly persons generally. It would also be interesting to know if these factors are similarly important in influencing survival at other stages of the life cycle.

References

Heyman, D. and Jeffers, F.: Effect of time lapse on consistency of self-health and medical evaluations of elderly persons. *J. of Gerontology*, 18:2:160-164, 1963.

Jarvik, L., and Falek, A.: Intellectual stability and survival in the aged. *J. Geront.* 18:173-176, 1963.

Metropolitan Life Insurance Company: Cardiac mortality and socioeconomic status. *Statistical Bulletin*, June 1967.

Palmore, E.: Physical, mental, and social factors in predicting longevity. *Gerontologist*, 9:103-108, 1969.

Palmore, E. (ed.): *Normal Aging*. Durham, North Carolina, Duke University Press, 1970.

Pfeiffer, E.: The natural history of sexual behavior in a biologically advantaged group of aged individuals. *J. Geront.* 24:193-198, 1969.

Quint, J., and Cody, B.: Preeminence and mortality: longevity of prominent men. Paper given before the Annual Meeting of the American Public Health Association, November 13, 1968. A summary was also published in *Statistical Bulletin* of the Metropolitan Life Insurance Company, January 1968, pp. 2-5.

Riegel, K. and Riegel, R., and Meyer, G.: A study of dropout rates in longitudinal research on aging and the prediction of death. *Journal Personality and Social Psychology* 5:342-348, 1967.

Ryser, C. and Sheldon, A.: Retirement and health. *J. Amer. Geriat. Soc.* 17:180-190, 1969.

Shanas, E. et al.: *Old People in Three Industrial Societies*. New York, Atherton, 1968, pp. 49-70.

18 The Relative Importance of Social Factors in Predicting Longevity*

Erdman Palmore

Actuaries predict how many years a person will live simply on the basis of his age, sex, and race. These predictions are summarized in standard life expectancy tables and are widely used by life insurance companies, government agencies, and others to establish premium rates, annuity payments, benefit levels, etc. But the other chapters in this book have demonstrated that there are many factors other than age, sex, and race which are related to longevity. If we were able to give a person a complete series of physical, mental, and social examinations and if we knew how these examinations are correlated with longevity, we should be able to improve the accuracy of longevity predictions by adjusting for individual differences in these variables. Data from the Duke Longitudinal Study of Aging now allow us to test this hypothesis. We can also examine the relative importance of social factors in predicting longevity and how their importance varies by age, sex, and race. We can even construct prediction equations based on the most important factors and these equations can be used to predict, with a specified standard error, the number of years remaining for persons who are similar to persons in the longitudinal study.

Methods

Volunteers (268) in a longitudinal, interdisciplinary study of aging were examined the first time during 1955-1959. They were given a two-day series of physical, psychiatric, and psychological examinations, laboratory tests, and social history interviews (Busse 1969). At that time they ranged in age from 60 to 94 with a median age of 70. All were ambulatory, noninstitutionalized residents of central North Carolina. They did not constitute a random sample but their sex, racial, and occupational distribution approximated that of the area. The average panelist was somewhat above the average area resident in many respects, as reflected by the fact that the average panelist lived or is expected to

*This chapter is based on two articles: "Physical, Mental, and Social Factors in Predicting Longevity," *Gerontologist*, *9* (Summer, 1969), 103-108 and "Predicting Longevity: A Follow-up Controlling for Age," *Gerontologist*, *9* (Winter, 1969), 247-250. Research supported in part by NICHD Grant HD-00668.

live about one year more than would be predicted from this actuarial life expectancy at the time of initial testing.

Two measures of longevity are used in this analysis: the Longevity Index (LI) and the Longevity Quotient (LQ). The LI is simply the number of years a panelist lived after initial testing or, for a living person, an estimate of the number of years he will have lived after the initial testing. This estimate of years remaining for those living is made by adding the present number of years since the initial testing to the estimated number of years now remaining according to actuarial life expectancy tables. In order to know exactly how many years each person will live after initial testing we would have to wait another 20 or more years until all participants have died. In the meantime this estimate can be used for purposes of analysis because it will probably not be off by more than a few years for most persons, and in a sample of this size many of the errors tend to cancel each other out. If one were to analyze only those who have already died, he would have a one-sided picture because his sample would include only those on the lower end of the longevity distribution, i.e. the sicker and less able persons. The pattern of correlations for the panelists who died is similar to that of the total, but is generally lower because of reduced variance.

The Longevity Quotient is the LI divided by the actuarially expected number of years remaining at initial examination based on each person's age, sex, and race. Since the LQ is basically the observed years remaining, divided by the expected years remaining, it is analogous to an intelligence quotient (observed score divided by expected score for the age group). Thus, an LQ of 1.0 means that the person lived exactly as long as expected, an LQ greater than 1.0 means that he lived more than expected, and an LQ of less than 1.0 means that he lived less than expected. For example, if a man lived 15 years after examination and had an actuarial expectancy of only 10 years, his LQ would be 1.5.

The LQ controls or standardizes for the effects of age differences at initial examination while the LI does not. There are two main advantages to the LQ: (1) The LQ improves the homogeneity of variance at different age levels. The variance of the simple LI was smaller among those of older age because they had proportionately fewer years remaining on the average. Frequency distributions of the LQ, on the other hand, show fairly similar curves and means for younger and older subjects. (2) The LQ removes the effect of age from the independent variable side of the regression equations and allows us to focus attention on those independent variables in which we are most interested: health, attitudes, activities, etc. We already know that actuarial life expectancy based on age is strongly related to the number of years remaining. The analysis needed is to determine the relative importance of the physical, mental, and social factors on longevity *once the age related life expectancy has been allowed for*.

We will first examine the zero-order correlations of 39 items with the LI and LQ and then discuss the results of multiple regression analysis using the five strongest predictors of longevity: work satisfaction, happiness rating, physical functioning, use of tobacco, and intelligence. These five predictors were constructed as follows:

1. *Work Satisfaction* This is part of an attitude questionnaire designed to measure a person's satisfaction with various areas of life (Burgess 1949). The work satisfaction scale awards one point for agreement with each of three positive statements (I am happy only when I have definite work to do; I am satisfied with the work I now do; I do better work now than ever before) and one point for disagreement with each of three negative statements (I can no longer do any kind of useful work; I have no work to look forward to; I get badly flustered when I have to hurry with my work). Thus the score could range from 0 to 6 with a mean of 3.7 and a standard deviation of 1.2. If a person asked what was meant by "work," it was defined to include any useful activity such as housework, gardening, etc.

2. *Happiness Rating* This is a 10 point scale used by the interviewing social worker to evaluate the person's overall happiness. It ranged from 0 for "unhappy, discontented, worried, fearful, frustrated" to 9 for "very happy, exultant, great contentment." It had a mean of 3.6 and a standard deviation of 1.6.

3. *Physical Functioning Rating* This is a score given by the examining physician for the level of physical functioning in everyday activities on the basis of the medical history, the physical and neurological examinations, audiogram, chest x-ray, electroencephalogram, electrocardiogram, and laboratory studies of the blood and urine. For the present analysis the scores were reversed so that they range from 1 (total disability) to 6 (no pathology), with a mean of 4.4 and standard deviation of 1.2.

4. *Use of Tobacco* This score was based on responses to the question, "How often do you use tobacco?" The scores ranged from 0 for never used, through slight and moderate use, to a score of 4 for heavy use (11 cigarettes or more per day, cigar and/or pipe 5 or more per day, constant use of snuff or chewing tobacco). The mean was 1.6 and the standard deviation was 1.6. Few of the women used any tobacco.

5. *Intelligence* This is the performance IQ score of the Wechsler Adult Intelligence Scale (Wechsler 1955). It is made up of tests on digit symbols, picture completions, block designs, picture arrangement, and object assembly. The mean score for our panelists was 94 with a standard deviation of 19.

Results

Zero-order Correlations. From among the hundreds of measures taken during the two-day examinations, we selected 39 items to test for correlations with the LI and LQ (Table 18-1). Although many of the zero-order correlations with LI and LQ were similar, there were substantial differences in the correlations of some independent variables with LI as compared to the correlations with LQ. One marked difference is that the correlation of the physical functioning rating dropped from .43 with the LI to .21 with the LQ. We believe this reduction in correlation occurs because the LQ controls for age, which in turn has a negative

Table 18-1
Correlations of 39 Items with Longevity

Independent Variables	N	r with Longevity Index	r with Longevity Quotient
Health			
Physical functioning rating	261	.43	.21
Cardio-vascular disease	187	−.29	−.22
Cholesterol	139	.19	.14
Self health rating	268	.13	.23
Tobacco use	263	−.09	−.19
Hypochondria	265	−.02	−.07
Obesity and emanciation	262	−.01	−.04
Intelligencee (WAIS)			
Performance weighted score	259	.31	.21
Full scale weighted	259	.26	.20
Verbal weighted score	268	.22	.14
Performance IQ	258	.14	.22
Full scale IQ	258	.13	.20
Verbal IQ	268	.11	.19
Activities			
Total activity	263	.23	.15
Leisure activities	263	.23	.15
Economic activities	255	.18	.09
Health activities	262	.11	.20
Family and friends contact	259	.07	.01
Religious activities	263	.02	.02
Attitudes			
Total attitudes	263	.15	.26
Work satisfaction	266	.19	.26
Health evaluation	266	.19	.20
Usefulness	266	.16	.20
Religious attitude	266	.11	.02
Happiness	265	.10	.19
Economic security	266	.07	.10
Attitudes toward family	264	.04	.06
Attitudes toward friends	266	.00	.10
Adjustment Ratings			
Secondary group contacts	252	.24	.21
Primary group contacts	251	.14	.02
Nongroup activities	252	.12	.19
Emotional security	252	.05	.09
Prestige feelings	252	.04	.17
Master rating	253	.03	.21
Happiness rating	252	.01	.25
Socio-economic Status			
Education	268	.13	.18
Occupation	267	.09	.07
Parents' Age at Death			
Father's	230	.03	.03
Mother's	228	−.11	−.04

association with both health and longevity. On the other hand, the correlations of the self-health rating and of tobacco use are substantially increased, apparently because the LQ eliminates the complicating effects of age at entrance to the study. The greater influence of tobacco use is particularly strong among the men aged 60 through 69 (Table 18-2).

Among the intelligence scores the correlations of the simple weighted scores are reduced and the correlations of the IQ scores are increased, because the IQ scores are similar to the LQ in controlling for age (Table 18-1). Most of the activity measures show lower correlations with the LQ, again because the negative association of activities and age has been eliminated. The attitude measures, on the other hand, are generally increased in the LQ, indicating that one's attitudes are better predictors of how long one is likely to live *relative to his life expectancy* than they are of the absolute number of years left to live.

The adjustment ratings performed by the interviewers do not show consistent differences, but the last two items (the Master Rating and the Happiness Rating) show a dramatic increase from almost no association with the Longevity Index to a correlation of .21 and .25 respectively with the LQ. This may indicate that the interviewers, in giving adjustment ratings, were using flexible standards relative to the age of the subject, rather than absolute standards. Thus their "age-adjusted" standards would be more closely related to an age-adjusted longevity measure.

Of our two measures of socioeconomic status, the correlation for education is increased from .13 to .18 with the LQ. This higher correlation reflects somewhat better the known relationship of higher socioeconomic status with greater life expectancy. Thus, controlling for age through the LQ generally had the effect of increasing the importance of such social factors as socioeconomic status and adjustment.

The last two items, father's and mother's age at death, show almost no correlation with either the LI or the LQ. This is contrary to the widespread theory that longevity tends to run in families and is inherited genetically. Chebotarev recently reported a similar lack of inherited longevity in a large scale survey in the USSR (1969). This of course underlines the importance of environmental factors in determining longevity.

Multiple Regressions. When the five strongest independent variables (work satisfaction, happiness rating, physical functioning, tobacco use, and performance IQ) are combined in a step-wise multiple regression, work satisfaction is the best overall predictor of the LQ and accounts for about half of the final cumulative variance explained (Table 18-2). This work satisfaction score represents a person's reaction to his general usefulness and ability to perform a meaningful social role.

The second most important factor, the overall happiness rating given by the interviewer, is somewhat similar in reflecting a person's general satisfaction with his life situation. It is significant that the first two most important factors (for the total group) are these social-psychological dimensions rather than some measure of health or of mental abilities.

242

Table 18-2
Step-wise Regressions of Strongest Predictors with Longevity Quotient by Age, Sex, and Race

Predictors	Zero-Order Correlation (r)	Cumulative Variance (r^2)	%Final Cumulative Variance
Total Panel N=233			
Work satisfaction	.29	.081**	47
Happiness rating	.26	.135**	80
Physical functioning	.21	.161**	95
Tobacco	−.21	.170*	100
Total Multiple r with 4 predictors	.41		
Men aged 60-69 N=47			
Work satisfaction	.38	.144**	68
Tobacco	−.37	.212*	100
Total multiple r with 2 predictors	.46		
Men aged 70+ N=60			
Physical functioning	.38	.144**	60
Work satisfaction	.35	.205**	86
Happiness rating	.17	.239**	100
Total multiple r with 3 predictors	.49		
Women aged 60-69 N=66			
Happiness rating	.34	.113**	39
Physical functioning	.32	.197**	67
Work satisfaction	.30	.266**	91
Tobacco	−.32	.292*	100
Total multiple r with 4 predictors	.54		
Women Aged 70+ N=60			
Happiness rating	.27	.076**	69
Work satisfaction	.16	.110	100
Total multiple r with 2 predictors	.33		
Whites N = 153			
Work satisfaction	.27	.072**	52
Happiness rating	.23	.119**	86
Physical functioning	.19	.138*	100
Total multiple r with 3 predictors	.37		
Blacks N=80			
Intelligence (Performance IQ)	.49	.239**	90
Tobacco	.32	.264*	100
Total multiple r with 2 predictors	.51		

*Additional variance significant at .05.
**Additional variance significant at .01.

Multiple regressions shown only for first two variables or through the last variable which yields an increment in variance explained significant at the .05 level, whichever is greater.

The physical functioning rating given by the examining physician is the third most important factor, while tobacco use is the last factor which contributes a significant increment in variance explained (for the total group). The total multiple correlation using these four predictors is .41. This can be increased to .64 if the LI is used as the dependent variable.

The step-wise regressions for specific age, sex, and racial groups show some interesting variations (Table 18-2). Work satisfaction is more important among men than women, and is most important for the men in their 60's. This reflects the greater importance of the work role for men in general, and especially for men under 70. The prediction equations (Table 18-3) show that for the men in their 60's, work satisfaction could theoretically make a difference of up to nine years in longevity.

The happiness rating was more important among women than among men, and was especially important for the women in their 60's. Among these women the happiness rating could theoretically make a difference of up to 15 years.

Tobacco use is a particularly strong (negative) predictor of longevity among the younger men and among the blacks. The greater importance of tobacco in these two groups probably reflects their greater use of tobacco. The prediction equations show that tobacco use could theoretically make a difference of up to five years in longevity among men in their 60's.

It is also noteworthy that the physical functioning rating was most important for the older men. Apparently health factors become more important than social-attitudinal ones among men in this older group. Also, health was second in importance among women in their 60's, for whom it could make as much as 13 years difference. Earlier analysis had shown health measures to be strongly related to survival in this panel (Heyman and Jeffers 1963).

Table 18-3
Prediction Equations for Longevity Index

Group		Standard Error
Total	$Y = 12.7 + 0.87\chi_E + 1.07\chi_P + .71\chi_W + .06\chi_I$	5.2
Men 60-69	$Y = 13.0 + 1.30\chi_E + 1.71\chi_W$	6.1
Men 70+	$Y = \ 9.0 + 1.33\chi_E + 0.20\chi_I$	4.6
Women 60-69	$Y = 16.8 + 1.24\chi_E + 2.02\chi_P$	5.6
Women 70+	$Y = 11.7 + 0.86\chi_E + 0.09\chi_I$	4.3
Whites	$Y = 13.0 + 0.95\chi_E + 1.03\chi_W + .08\chi_I$	5.2
Negroes	$Y = 12.2 + 0.75\chi_E + 2.32\chi_P$	5.3

Note — Y = Predicted Longevity: years remaining after initial testing
χ = $x - \bar{x}$
E = Life expectancy at Time 1
P = Physical functioning
W = Work satisfaction
I = Intelligence (Performance)

It is somewhat surprising to see that intelligence is the most important predictor for blacks, because intelligence was not among the significant predictors in any of the other groups. The correlation of intelligence with LQ (.49) in this group is higher than any other single correlation in any other group. There were some unusually low intelligence scores among the blacks and these were strongly related to early deaths.

Prediction Equation. The LI was used to construct prediction equations because it is more easily translated into the predicted number of years remaining. As one would expect from the differences in the step-wise regressions, the LI prediction equations vary for different age, sex, and race groups in terms of the relative effects of the various factors on the regression slope of the LI (Table 18-3). The first or constant term in the equation, which is simply the mean LI for the group, varies from a high of over 16 for the younger women to a low of 9 for the older men. This demonstrates the generally true principle that being younger and female is associated with living longer.

The second term shows the factor to be applied to a person's life expectancy deviation from the average life expectancy for this group. This factor is lowest for blacks, which shows that life expectancy has less effect in predicting longevity among blacks than among the other groups.

The third term for the total group, for the younger women, and for blacks, shows the factor for the person's deviation from average physical functioning. Among the younger women and blacks, this factor is twice that of the total group, which reveals again the relatively great importance of general health for these groups.

The fourth term for the total group (and the third term for the younger men and whites) shows the factor to be used for a person's deviation from average work satisfaction. This factor is highest for the younger men, which again demonstrates the importance of work satisfaction in this group.

The last term for the total group, for the older men and women, and for whites, shows the factor to be applied to a person's deviation from average performance intelligence. This factor is much higher among the older men than any other group.

The standard error of estimates derived from these equations ranges from 4.3 for the older women to 6.1 for the younger men. This means that if the LI is normally distributed in a specified group, the chances are two out of three that the actual number of years remaining for a person in that group will be within plus or minus 1 standard error of his predicted longevity. For example, the average woman over 70 would have a predicted longevity of 11.7 years remaining and the chances would be two out of three that she would actually live between 7.4 and 16 more years. For the total group, the use of work satisfaction, physical functioning, and intelligence scores improved the accuracy of the predictions by one-third over the use of simple life expectancy tables.

Perhaps a case illustration will clarify how this prediction equation can improve on the actuarial life expectancy prediction. Case 8075 was a white male aged 81 at the initial study in 1955. His actuarial life expectancy at that time was 5.6 more years. But his health was average (PFR = 20% or less limitation), his work satisfaction was the highest possible, and his performance intelligence was high. Substituting his weighted deviations from the average in the prediction equation for the total group we get: Y = 12.7 −5.1 −.4 + 1.6 + .7 which equals a predicted longevity of 9.5 more years. Case 8075 actually lived 11.6 more years, even more than predicted by the equation. But it is clear that the actuarial life expectancy (5.6) was only half his actual remaining years (11.6) and the predicted longevity (9.5) was much closer, even though it too fell short.

Discussion

Generalizations based on a sample of 268 volunteers from central North Carolina should, of course, be made only with extreme caution. Also the measures of longevity used for this study are only best estimates for those who are still living, based on the number of years lived since initial testing plus their present life expectancy.

Our predictions might be improved by using Delta scores (differences between the scores at two points in time) rather than the absolute scores at one point in time. Thus, for example, it may be that a decline in physical functioning is more closely related to shortened longevity than is the absolute level at initial testing. This will be tested in future work. Also, various long transformations of the longevity measure were tested, but showed no improvement in distribution or correlations.

Finally, it should be remembered that correlation does not prove causality. However, if we keep all these qualifications in mind, it may be useful to speculate about the meaning and practical implications of these findings. The substantial improvement in predicting longevity which results from adjusting for work satisfaction, physical functioning, and intelligence suggests that life insurance companies and others concerned with longevity might substantially improve the accuracy of their estimates by using not only complete physical examinations but also tests of intelligence and work satisfaction (or a similar rating of social adjustment) to adjust their life expectancy scores.

The meaning of the high association between physical functioning and longevity seems obvious: a healthy and well-functioning person has a better chance of surviving the stress and trauma of aging longer than a sick and weak person. The meaning of the association between intelligence and longevity is less clear. Are the more intelligent better able to adapt to the problems of aging and take better care of their health because they are smarter? Or is their higher intelligence just a sign that they are aging slower in general? Or is intelligence mainly an indicator of higher socioeconomic status with its usual advantages in comfort and medical care? This, however, is unlikely because of the low correlations of socioeconomic measures with longevity.

Similarly, are the associations of work satisfaction and happiness with longevity spurious ones simply due to their associations with health? This too is unlikely because there are significant associations left even after physical functioning is statistically controlled in multiple regression. Does it mean that older persons who stay active in useful roles are better able to maintain high morale and functioning, which in turn increases their longevity? The latter interpretation is consistent with other evidence linking greater activity with greater satisfaction and adjustment (Jeffers and Nichols 1969; Havens 1968; Maddox 1964; Palmore 1968). Furthermore, other studies of longevity in the U.S., Germany, France, Netherlands, and Russia come to similar conclusions (Jarvik 1963; Riegel 1967; Clement 1969; Beek 1969; and Chebotarev 1969). The use of the LQ shows that when age is controlled, the sociopsychological factors of work satisfaction and happiness become even more important predictors of longevity than are health factors.

Summary

A longitudinal study of 268 volunteers aged 60 to 94 at initial testing showed that (a) work satisfaction, (b) happiness rating, (c) physical functioning, and (d) tobacco use are the four strongest predictors of longevity when age is controlled by the use of a Longevity Quotient. The two most important factors are closely related to social role and adjustment. Work satisfaction was strongest among men in their 60's, happiness was strongest among women, tobacco use was stronger among the younger men and among blacks, while physical functioning was the important factor among the older men. These findings suggest that, in general, the most important ways to increase longevity are: 1) to maintain a useful and satisfying role in society, 2) to maintain a positive view of life, 3) to maintain good physical functioning, and 4) to avoid smoking.

References

Beek, A., and R.J. van Zonneveld: Longitudinal surveys of the health condition of old people. Proceedings of the 8th International Congress of Gerontology, Washington, D.C., 1969, Vol. 2:60.

Burgess, E.W., Caban, R.S., Havighurst, R.J., and Goldhamer, H.: *Your Activities and Attitudes*. Chicago: Science Research Associates, 1949.

Busse, E.W.: A physiological, psychological and sociological study of aging. In E.B. Palmore (ed.), *Normal Aging*. Durham, N.C.: Duke University Press, 1970.

Chebotarev, E.F.: Longevity and the role of its investigation in the elucidation of aging process. Proceedings of the 8th International Congress of Gerontology, Washington, D.C., 1968, Vol. 1:382-385.

Clement, R.: Du pronostic de mort *à partir de diverses mesures. Proceedings of the 8th International Congress of Gerontology*, Washington, D.C., 1969, Vol. 2:62.

Havens, B.J.: An investigation of activity patterns and adjustment in an aging population. *Gerontologist*, 8:201-206, 1968.

Heyman, D., and Jeffers, F.: Effect of time lapse on consistency of self-health and medical evaluations of elderly persons. *Journal of Gerontology*, 18:2:160-164, 1963.

Jarvik, L.F., and Falek, A.: Intellectual ability and survival in the aged. *Journal of Gerontology*, 1963, 18:173-176.

Jeffers, F. and Nichols, C.: The relationship of activities and attitudes to physical well-being in older people. *Journal of Gerontology*, 16:1:67-70, 1961.

Maddox, G.L.: A longitudinal, multidisciplinary study of human aging. *Proceedings of the Social Statistics*. Washington, D.C., American Statistical Association, 1962.

Maddox, G.L.: Disengagement theory: A critical evaluation. *Gerontologist*, 4:80-83, 1964.

Palmore, E.B.: The effects of aging on activities and attitudes. *Gerontologist*, 8:259-263, 1968.

Public Health Service: *State Life Tables: 1959-1961*. Vol. 2, No. 27-51, HEW, Washington, D.C.: U.S. Government Printing Office, 1966.

Riegel, K.F., Riegel, R.M., and Meyer, G.: A study of the dropout rates in longitudinal research on aging and the prediction of death. *Journal of Personality and Social Psychology*, 5:342-348, 1967.

Wechsler, D.: *Manual for the Wechsler Adult Intelligence Scale*. New York: The Psychological Corporation, 1955.

19 Hope, Survival, and the Caring Environment

ROBERT KASTENBAUM and
BEATRICE S. KASTENBAUM

This chapter represents an invitation to look over some of the psychosocial phenomena which affect human longevity but which tend to be sidelined when major prediction efforts are made. What we have to offer will not be mistaken for an elegant treatment of a neatly delimited subject-matter. Our concern is with those shifting, complex, interrelated, hard-to-pin-down processes that we all glimpse in our private lives even if we judge them unsuitable for the materials of a science.

Hope, survival, and the caring environment have been selected as organizing concepts. Survival does not require special comment at this point, but will be touched upon later. We begin with introductory comments on the concepts of hope and the caring environment.

Hope

Definitions of hope vary. It is probable, however, that most of us would recognize these facets as attributes of hope: (a) a psychic or phenomenologic state (b) pointed toward futurity (c) with a predominantly positive affective glow. Except for those who eschew all mentalistic formulations, it might also be agreed that hope has implications for the individual's present self-organization and for his future actions. We will leave these consensual points undisturbed. Hope, in the general sense outlined above, is an important part of man's phenomenologic life. We do not mean to equate the two—there is more in our minds than the dynamics of hope. But through concentrating upon hope we will be able to keep the individual in focus as we follow him into the complex swirl of factors whose outcome is both survival and death.

Although accepting the consensual definition, we must move to greater differentiation and specificity. This can be done most economically by a series of brief position statements:

Robert Kastenbaum is Professor of Psychology and Director of Center for Psychological Studies of Dying, Death and Lethal Behavior, Wayne State University, Detroit, Michigan.

Beatrice S. Kastenbaum is at the Michigan Cancer Foundation and Center for Psychological Studies of Dying, Death and Lethal Behavior.

249

(1) Hope and expectation are not synonymous. One has a certain level of expectation for particular contingencies. The future is scanned on a probabilistic basis, e.g., I wish it would not rain tomorrow. The individual may keep the probabilistic and axiologic views of futurity rigidly separated in his mind, mix them confusedly, or submerge one or the other (Kastenbaum 1963). Thus, it is possible for a person to restrict himself to probabilistic forecasts without permitting himself to express either hope or hopelessness.

(2) Nevertheless, hope does have a probabilistic implication. One hopes only if the hoped-for state has a subjective probability greater than zero and less than 100 percent. The element of uncertainty or suspense is always present in what we (accurately) call hope, whether it be present in an unobtrusive or dominant way. Hopelessness is the view that the desired state has a zero probability of occurrence.

(3) Dread is a hope-related concept. It may be regarded as hope viewed from the wrong end of the telescope. The hoped-for event has a probability of not occurring, or the event with hope is dedicated to averting is seen as having a certain probability of taking place. Hopelessness is something in contrast; it is clearly different from the perception that an unwelcome event may occur or a welcome event not occur. Dread and hopelessness differ in that the former state focuses on the possibility of future adversity, while the latter assumes that nothing can be done to avert "what is to be"—there is no point in even thinking about the future.

(4) The lack of certainty in perceived futurity which is characteristic of both hope and dread places the individual in a vulnerable position. He is in a position to be influenced, affected, perhaps destroyed. He cannot see himself as wholly self-contained and invincible. Hoping is chancy. Perhaps there is always pressure being exerted against the vulnerability-inducing effects of hope. Under certain environmental conditions there may be a strong tendency to submerge hope, end the suspense, and thereby attain at least the illusion of invulnerability.

(5) The ability of the individual to hope (and dread) should be distinguished from particular hopes and dreads. One may replace a particular hope with a certainty (either positively or negatively-valued). One may lose interest in a previous hope. An upsetting turn of events may deprive one of his most significant or superordinate hope, yet not wipe out all his hopes or destroy his capacity to develop hopes anew. Another person, facing the same calamity, may suffer a paralysis or loss in his basic ability to organize the future in terms of preferences and desires.

Later we will shift focus from hope per se to another concept: will-to-live (WtL). The WtL concept draws much of its nourishment from hope. We will be concerned with both concepts throughout this paper, but with WtL stepping to the fore because it seems more directly related to behavioral outcomes. First, however, we should acknowledge the environment.

The Caring Environment

In the most general way possible we wish to suggest that environments be assessed in terms of their caring or life-protective valencies. The size of the environmental unit can vary according to our best judgment of what a particular problem demands. The environment may be an operating room, an industrial complex, etc.

"Caringness" can be assessed in accordance with multiple criteria. One might compare, for example, the environment's self-perception of its caringness with objective descriptions and outcome measures. It would also be natural to distinguish between environments established with the explicit purpose of protecting life and those environments which have other primary functions. Is a hospital really more "caring" than, say, a place of work or education? We would not have to restrict ourselves to environments defined wholly in spatial terms, nor would we have to overlook the possible usefulness of identifying sets of environments nesting within each other, possibly exerting differential caringness at various levels of environmental structure.

We have been a little casual in this discussion because the task of detailing an approach to the caring environment is too extensive to be undertaken here. We hope some of the main outlines have come across in this brief introduction.

We now begin our more intensive exploration with a discussion of WtL.

Will-to-Live

Is it *despite* or *because* of limited research attention that the will-to-live concept has retained viability? Would sophisticated investigation puncture the notion that there really is such a phenomenon—or reveal WtL to be an indispensable consideration in any thoroughgoing approach to human behavior? These questions cannot be answered at present. However, we will argue in favor of the provisional use of the WtL concept based upon the following observations:

(1) It is valuable to include in our scientific vocabulary at least one expression which acknowledges the organism's orientation toward its own continued survival. Other assumptions or hypotheses can be introduced *ad libitum*. But the mere existence of the WtL concept serves the function of drawing together many scattered observations that could prove to have something significant in common. At this minimum level, one would not have to accept any particular propositions about WtL other than the proposition that it is a potentially useful term, one that would be more perilous to exclude than to admit for serious consideration.
(2) One could substitute other phrases if WtL appears offensive. Some may dislike its philosophical heritage (Schopenhauer 1948). Others may decry its uncritical use in various contexts. A "pure" concept it is not. Perhaps we would be better advised to formulate a new term that is not contaminated

by previous use. We tend to think, however, that development of a more adequate concept (or set of concepts) will follow more naturally from systematic exploration of the starting point, WtL. The WtL concept has at least three advantages: (a) by observing the contexts in which it has already been used we are directed to significant human problems, (b) there is much to be learned from the attitudes and behaviors that group themselves around the WtL concept, and (c) the conceptual and empirical questions one must raise about the concept are fairly evident for all to see. The hasty substitution of a made-up term might well introduce conceptual problems that are more difficult to uncover, while proferring the illusion of greater scientific rigor. For the time being, we opt for an active and critical use of the WtL concept.

(3) The concept calls attention to the integrative functioning of the person. Both the research enterprise and mass-oriented administration techniques tend to accentuate the opposite of the person as integer. Observational and statistical techniques allow us to differentiate the person into a cross-hatch of dimensions each with its own name (even when the person has lost his). Administrative processes sort and resort not people as such, but abstracted statistical ghosts such as Selective Service and Internal Revenue Service numbers. Against this admittedly useful penchant for dividing and conquering individuality, one might suggest the continued support of a few concepts which strongly imply that the person should also be taken seriously as a unit, an integer in his own right.

(4) The WtL concept may form a useful tandem with hope. However one chooses to define it, hope generally implies an intrapsychic state. WtL (and its companion concept, Will-to-Die) direct attention immediately to action. The actions or action-tendencies may be explicit or subtle. But we find ourselves concerned with what the person is *doing* to protect or endanger his life, as contrasted with the tint of optimism-pessimism with which he colors futurity. By retaining both terms we increase our likelihood of discovering the complex relationships that obtain between phenomenologic state (as exemplified by hope), and organismic commitment to action (as exemplified by WtL). Collapsing hope and WtL into a single concept might prove a costly economy.

Our own interest in the WtL concept was aroused during clinical encounters with people who seemed to be waging a campaign for survival against high odds. One writer had the occasion to work intensively with gravely ill aged men and women (R.K.), the other with children and adults stricken by a variety of conditions (genetic and acquired) with grim prognoses (B.K.S.). At first we wondered if we were deviant in perceiving some patients as having a strong will-to-live, but soon found that this was a recognized, familiar perception among health personnel of various types. Absence of WtL was also something that one saw (or thought that he saw) on some occasions. We would find ourselves speaking variously of a patient who had "lost" his WtL or had developed an orientation toward the hastening of his own death. It appeared that the classification of a patient as a "Willer," "Unwiller," or "Anti-Willer" had some importance in the minds of staff. What and how much would be done for the patient seemed to be at least in part a function of his classification. (The perception and classification was not always as conscious and explicit as this discussion may have implied; but conversation usually could bring out the implicit judgments that had been formed without their owner's "official" certification.) Unsurprisingly, in the continuing circuit of service-oriented work, few hospital staff took time out to check their fleeting impressions of patients' WtL status with other factors, including survival itself. Especially interesting cases would be remembered, but nothing systematic or self-correcting would be learned.

Our first study of WtL was prefaced with the suggestion that "*Will* may be regarded as the organization of personality toward a specific direction of action—the 'unity of personality' that puts specific factors to work in service of a central (temporary or enduring) orientation. The *will* concept does not imply unlimited capability of action, but simply the stance of the organism toward or against its total milieu, or some perceived force within the milieu." It has long been recognized in this concept that some things happen *willy-nilly*, i.e., regardless of our strongest desires and efforts. To speak of a will-to-live, then, does not prejudge the questions of efficacy and processes; we merely enter the central state of the organism as a potential variable in its own survival (Kastenbaum 1965).

The purpose of this study was to learn whether or not the WtL classification, as employed by physicians, "behaved" systematically. Do general patterns seem to emerge, or is idiosyncratic, random, unreliable usage the order of the day? More specifically, we hoped to learn something of the accuracy with which physicians could predict the longevity of elderly patients when WtL was included as an explicit variable, the nature of the cues employed in making the ratings, and whatever else might be gleaned from these data regarding the physician-patient relationship when survival is at issue.

The data-gathering procedure will be described here because it illustrates one possible approach to operationalizing the broad concept and, in fact, choosing among several ways in which the concept itself might be formulated. The limitations of this procedure should be fairly evident. It was an attempt to assess WtL at a level that would make sense to the practicing physician, permitting him to use his routine judgmental processes, rather than requiring him to adopt a very special attitude for purposes of the study. Although the physician was invited—urged—to contribute detailed information concerning the bases of his judgment, he was required only to answer a set of conclusion-type questions. This seemed sufficient for an exploratory study, although hardly adequate for fine-grained follow-up research.

The WtL Rating Scale is reproduced in Table 19-1. It will be noticed that the first section actually is not concerned with WtL at all. The focus is upon prediction of remaining longevity from medical status alone. This information

Table 19-1
Rating Scale

I. Prediction from Medical Status

A. Based upon medical status exclusively, this patient's remaining life-span is most likely to be (write in 1 and 2 for the most likely and second most likely time periods):

Less than 1 month _____ Less than 3 months _____ Less than 6 months _____
Less than 1 year _____ Less than 2 years _____ Less than 3 years _____
Less than 4 years _____ Less than 5 years _____ Five years or more _____

B. Concerning my estimate of this patient's longevity from medical status, I am
_____ rather confident _____ fairly confident _____ not very confident
_____ just guessing

C. For this patient, death is likely to come
_____ rather suddenly _____ rather gradually _____ no opinion

---

II. Prediction from "Will-To-Live"

A. If this patient's "will-to-live" should operate as a factor in his longevity, it is more likely to:
_____ extend or _____ shorten his life expectancy

B. The prospect that "will-to-live" will have any effect upon this patient's life expectancy is:
_____ very likely _____ possible but not likely _____ quite unlikely

C. Does this patient have an exceptionally strong "will-to-live"?
_____ Yes _____ No

D. Does this patient have a "will-to-die"?
_____ Yes _____ No

E. What psychological factors or events, if any, might affect this patient's longevity?

PHYSICIAN'S COMMENTS:

was considered important in its own right. However, we also wished to establish a clear distinction between medical status and WtL judgments. By providing the opportunity for physicians to provide medical status judgments first, we reasoned it should be easier for them subsequently to concentrate upon WtL. At this point, then, our attempt to operationalize WtL did not assume any particular relationship between medical status and the individual's (perceived) orientation toward his own survival; this would be a question that could be explored empirically.

Each of the questions in the WtL section was presented to the physician as being theoretically independent from the others. A patient might, for example, be considered to have an exceptionally strong WtL (Question C), yet this orientation may be deemed quite unlikely to have any actual effect upon his life expectancy (Question B). Similarly, a physician might judge in a particular case that a patient who he sees as having an exceptionally strong WtL may also manifest a WtD (Question D). Another patient might be regarded as having neither an exceptionally strong WtL nor a WtD. Obviously, our aim was to avoid the premature "jelling" of the WtL concept. Relationships between the directionalities (live/die), and between will and effectiveness were posed as questions requiring empirical answers. The option was even left open for negative or paradoxical conclusions. Perhaps with some patients, for example, it would be judged that a strong WtL might have the effect of shortening life expectancy (Question A). In addition to the open-ended Question E, the physician was asked, in the space provided for his comments, to identify the cues he employed or thought he employed in reaching his conclusion.

The entire medical staff of an all-geriatric hospital voluntarily consented to complete the WtL Rating Scale for new admissions to the institution. In preliminary discussion it was mutually agreed that the WtL concept was both familiar and poorly understood. We were all curious to learn how it would prove to work out when made explicit. The physicians understood that we were not testing their perceptions of WtL against some secret superscientific formulation that had already been established. We were simply trying to learn through them.

Men and women newly admitted to the hospital were seen individually by the physician who would be primarily responsible for their care, at least at the beginning. The patient's status would then be presented to the other physicians at the weekly admission meeting, and the patient himself introduced to the group for a quick "looksee." Ordinarily, new admissions per week ranged between three and six. Each physician would make an independent rating after the patient had been seen by the medical staff (representatives of nursing, social work, and psychology departments were also present, but not asked to complete WtL ratings—which, in retrospect, seems to be a glaring oversight).

Results from the first series of WtL ratings (51 consecutive admissions, Sample I) were supported and strengthened by a second series of 51 admissions (Sample II). The sixty-four women and thirty-eight men ranged in age from 66 to 98, with a mean of 78.2. "Chronic brain syndrome" was the most frequent primary diagnosis, but 27 other categories were also utilized. Within the limits of this exploratory study there was the overall impression that WtL ratings were being made in a rather systematic fashion. There were also indications that physician attitude variables may have systematically influenced the medstatus ratings as well—despite our attempt to keep the two apart. In Sample I *no* patients were predicted for death within the next 12 months, and only 10 percent mortality for that time span was cited in Sample II. Yet the hospital's baseline statistics (with approximately five years of history behind her) indicated that 26 percent of new admissions die within one year. The marked disparity between future projections and past death rate existed only for the near future; agreement became close thereafter. Thus, although physicians knew (not necessarily through statistics but through their own experience) that many patients die soon after admission, when rating individuals they reached quite another conclusion. And patients did continue to die more or less "on schedule" as a cohort. It is difficult to avoid an interpretation of these results that would emphasize the physician's own attitudes and needs in contrast to the (supposedly) "objective" medical facts from which survival status was to be assessed.

A motivational component in the physician's ratings is further suggested by comparison of the "first guess" and "second guess" of longevity (Section 1, Question A). The first or best guess extended further into the future than the second guess in 81 of the 102 instances, a highly significant difference. This finding would go along with the emerging circumstantial case that physicians *wanted* to see their patients live (or not die) and permitted this orientation to influence judgments they thought were being made on a strictly medical basis. (It should be kept in mind that these judgments were made at the point of the elderly person's admission to the hispital; it need not be assumed that either the physician or the patient retained his initial orientation throughout the subsequent period of hospitalization.)

Data from the WtL section strengthened the impression that physicians emphasized every potentially favorable (life-extending) indice they could discover. For example, patients seen as strong "Willers" were regarded as more likely actually to influence their longevity than those classified as "Anti-Willers" or "Shorteners." Confidence in their own ratings was higher for patients with a positive as compared with a negative will orientation, and many more patients were classified as strong "Willers" than as "Anti-Willers." The lack of comparable data from other populations was one of the limitations that hampered generalization from this study at the time it was first reported, and this remains substantially true today as well.

Three alternative lines of explanation were sketched. These remain of interest not only with respect to hospitalized geriatric patients but for the larger issue of the relationship between a vulnerable person and the significant people in his environment:

". . . Might it be that physicians *must* regard aged patients in a sanguine way in order to involve themselves in the daily care of persons whose life-span is rather limited? If this is the case, one might hypothesize the specific need to deny the possibility of death within the near future, as perception of same might lead to a handicapping negative affect on the physician's part.

"However, it might be that there is a genuine 'spark of life' that a sensitive observer can discern in many persons whose superficial appearance would indicate otherwise because of advanced age and multiple ailments. Were this the case, then further investigation might disclose the processes by which WtL operates 'beneath the surface.'

"Still again, the crucial point might be found in the interaction between the physician's tendency to regard his elderly patient in a favorable light, and the patient's response to this orientation. WtL might turn out to be a variable strongly conditioned by interpersonal relationships, with the tacit understanding between physician (and other persons in the environment) and the patient constituting the key to extended or foreshortened longevity" (Kastenbaum 1965).

To these considerations might be added the possibility that a temporary dyadic identity or common cause is established on an emotional level between the physician and his patient. By seeing the patient as potentially "keep-aliveable," the physician may also be indirectly bolstering his own thoughts of death-avoidance. This notion will strike some readers as irresponsibly wild, although perhaps not those familiar with research on physicians' death attitudes (Feifel 1965). We do not mean to push this specific hypothesis very far. But it illustrates the possibility that—in general—we may have *personal* reasons for viewing others as life or death striving.

It is interesting to wonder about what might happen after the hypothetical common cause has been established. There is a point at which one can convince himself that it is possible to preserve life (the patient's and my own) by adroit and diligent management. All available positive indicators are upgathered for this effort. It is plausible to conjecture that the common cause might well result in the patient's survival of one or more potentially lethal hazards. But somewhere along the line the pushed-to-one-side negative indicators may demand the physician's full attention. He becomes aware (as he has known but not quite "registered" for a while) that his efforts are doomed to failure. It is at this juncture that common cause or dyadic identity may be dissolved—and so swiftly that it may be hard to believe in retrospect that it ever existed. The physician must now act to save his own skin. "I cannot loan or invest in you my own longevity strivings any further. It is too dangerous. You are on your own now." The physician (or other helping person) withdraws first in an emotional sense that will be virtually imperceptible to those who have not learned to read people, but which will soon have its concrete behavioral effects. Behavioral indexes of reduced interest in a vulnerable person have been described by a number of observers in recent years. (Duff and Hollingshead 1968; Glaser and Strauss 1966). These include not only clearly psychosocial actions (e.g., visiting vs. nonvisiting), but also life-guarding behaviors (e.g., prompt and accurate provision of required medication).

The study cited above continued with replications and variations beyond the data that have been summarized here. There have been hints that patients seen as oriented toward their own death (WtD) did in fact tend to die sooner than one would have predicted on medical status alone. Thus far it has not been possible to control statistically for complicating, potentially contaminating factors and arrive at a clear evaluation of this seeming trend. It is probable that a new research program will be required to do this satisfactorily. There have also been indications that WtL could be affected strongly by cues received from the environment, as in some of the material developed during the psychological autopsy series (Weisman and Kastenbaum 1968).

WtL research with people who are not physically ill is also in its early stages.

In an attempt to reduce WtL to operational definition, Richard M. Heavenrich used a brief, objective self-rating scale. The strength of motivation to live was assessed by five questions drawn from a battery of death-related questionnaires developed at the Center for Psychological Studies of Dying, Death, and Lethal Behavior. With his sample of 154 college undergraduates, Heavenrich found several relationships between WtL scores and other variables. Perhaps the most important relationships were those between WtL, future optimism, and objective lethality. The objective lethality (OL) variable was defined (on its high extreme) as being represented by a person "who thinks about the possibility of committing suicide and who considers suicide as a behavior within his present or potential repertoire (Heavenrich 1970).

Those whose responses were scored as indicative of strong WtL tended to be low in OL and high in future optimism. In fact, these three variables formed the most significant cluster in a large correlation table, supporting one of Heavenrich's basic hypothesis in his masters thesis research. Although this study comprised only a first approach to a complex program of proposed research, Heavenrich found sufficient evidence to support his belief that "Strength in these areas (WtL and future optimism) is the single most important buffer against vulnerability to isolating experiences and lethal outcomes."

As Heavenrich notes, his approach has much in common with the theory of suicide proposed by Maurice Farber, and may be said to lend some empirical support to that position. Farber's main contention is that suicide is a function of hope. The greater the threat that confronts one, the more competence he needs to cope with it; conversely, the less competent the person feels, the more vulnerable he becomes to such threats. He suggests that "It may well be that the best short-term predictor of suicide is an estimate of the individual's hope" (Farber 1968). Heavenrich takes the combination of strong WtL and high future optimism as a fair approximation to Farber's view of hope. Again, there seems to be something important going on among hope, WtL and vulnerability.

Neither Heavenrich nor the present writers offer the self-report WtL scale as an adequate representation of the larger concept. However, it appears to be a window for acquiring a dependable view, at one level, of the individual's orientation toward his own survival. It is encouraging to learn that responses to this scale, whatever else they might mean, do behave in a proper fashion in terms of their seeking association with variables for which they "ought" to have affinity. It is also useful to see the WtL concept applied to potential self-destructive behavior as well as to illness.

Up to this point we have been emphasizing the individual's internal state (as exemplified by hope) and his organismic commitment to action (as exemplified by WtL). Now an effort must be made to place the individual within his environmental context with special reference to vulnerability and survival.

Survival

This term seems pertinent only when it is in question. There is little point in speaking of survival unless there is a prospect of nonsurvival or extinction.

Typically, then, we find ourselves interested in survival under one or both of the following conditions: (1) a specific threat to life, (2) a system of time coordinates. Did our former colleague survive the typhoon that ravaged a large area in Pakistan? Before the typhoon it had not occurred to us to wonder about her survival status. How many of our gradeschool classmates are still alive? There has now been considerable movement along the time dimension. A casualty rate must be expected, even though we cannot single out one dominant threat to survival during the interim.

Despite the specificity of the stimuli which bring the survival question into focus, it may be useful to consider survival as a constant question for both theoretical and applied purposes. The constancy is that survival is always a question; the specific terms seem to be forever in flux. We have a probability of nonsurvival at every moment of our lives. Survival always implies an interaction between an individual (or a number of individuals) and the environment. Usually emphasis is upon survival of the individual in his environment. But the survival of the environment itself is also problematic. We may ask questions such as: Will the individual out-live the environment, or vice-versa? Do the factors which favor survival of the one also favor survival of the other, or is it necessary to choose between individual-protecting and environment-protecting actions? Is the individual disposed to place equal or higher priority on survival of the environment as compared to his own survival?

There will be opportunity later to return to some of these distinctions and questions when we attempt to draw together the concepts of survival, hope, and the caring environment.

"Hard Core Unemployed": A Case History

Let us start to bring together a few of the strands which have already been presented in solo fashion. The continued survival of some people is in special jeopardy because of their particular conjunction of demographic and personal characteristics. For a specific example, here is a black man of limited educational background and occupational skills who lives in one of our famous inner cities. The probabilities of his survival over a given period of time seem smaller than that of a white man in similar straits, or of a black man with more culturally-valued achievements behind him, or of any man dwelling in a less violent environment, etc. Without knowing anything about him as a specific person, we would be inclined to classify him as vulnerable.

It remains now to bring in the terms of hope and the caring environment. A sample of black men who fit the above description became available for research interviews. The context was their participation in an industrial program intended to make successful job placements for hard core unemployed males. The circumstances were something less than ideal for a thorough exploration of the phenomenologic-ecologic relationship, but it did prove possible to learn something of their orientations toward futurity and longevity. The men responded to several of the questions which were also included subsequently in the Heavenrich study. They spoke of their past experiences, future expectations, and likely longevity (including probable mode of death).

As a group, these men viewed their past lives as having been on the "rough" and unsatisfactory side. But within the group there was an important differentiation with respect to future outlook—and this differentiation was itself related to a point of environmental contact. Divide the hard cores into those who express optimism for the future and who also anticipate a relatively long life ahead, and those who hold a more pessimistic and foreshortened perspective. Now divide the group crosswise into those who remained on the new job, and those who departed (for any combination of reasons). Teahan and Kastenbaum report that the men high on future optimism and subjective life expectancy were also those who would hold on to their jobs. (Teahan, in press.)

On the phenomenologic side, it is interesting to note that similar interpretations of *past* experiences ("rough") did not necessarily lead to similar projections into the future. It is also worth remarking that the foreshortened perspective of those leaving their job seemed to have much in common with the outlook that people expect to find in geriatric patients.

What can be said of the "caringness" of the environment in this instance? For brevity and focus, suppose that we concentrate upon the new environment represented by the opportunity for employment in this industrial demonstration program. It seems reasonable to propose:

(1) The larger environment (federal, state, and city officialdom) explicitly committed itself to a caring orientation for a specific group of citizens.
(2) The paper-and-planning version of this caring environment did translate itself into concrete form: job opportunities in a local industry.
(3) The caring was not directed to the problem of longevity or survivorship as such; there is no indication that this was ever recognized as a factor, or as a desirable outcome variable. The caring was at a more general level (and perhaps heavily freighted with political motivation that had not very much to do with the fate of the participants as individuals).
(4) From the viewpoint of the potential employees, the new environment was not especially meaningful as such. It did represent an opportunity to become solvent, perhaps a basis for bolstering self-respect and sense of competence. But there was little reason for supposing that the hard core corps would have developed any positive sentiment for the industrial environment before their actual entry. Survival, or enhancement of the caring environment would not have much representation within the individual's phenomenologic field (i.e., he might have hopes for himself and his family, but not for the new environment per se).
(5) Although the caring environment was new in two ways, it was old in another. The industrial situation was new in its official revision into a caring environment, and it was new to the hard cores. But the environment had already existed for many years in its "pre-caring" form. It could not be altered completely by a new demonstration project. Especially relevant is the

fact that the "old" employees would comprise a significant aspect of the effective environment for the new employees. The old-timers presumably had an investment in maintaining the existing environment against the "invaders." Survival of the pre-existing environment might be seen by the old-timers as a positive goal that would be jeopardized by survival of the newcomers. While there may have been no serious question about the maintenance of the industrial environment as such, there may well have been concern about its threatened transformation into a different kind of environment. Caring for strangers of bad repute might be equivalent to caring less about those who had been responsible for successful functioning of the environment all along.

(6) The survival of the newcomers was mentioned above in a somewhat ambiguous sense. Did we intend to say that there was opposition to the newcomers becoming permanent employees? If so, this would seem to have no relevance to survival in the life-or-death sense. It would pertain only to nonsurvival as a resident of a specialized environment, rather than nonsurvival in the total human environment. But the ambiguity is worth preserving. Incidents occurred (and others seemed on brink) which suggested the existence of murderous rage within the caring environment. Some of the hard cores themselves had difficulty in controlling assaultive impulses apparently aroused by the new challenges and demands of the situation. For their part, some of the old-timers may not have distinguished firmly between the wish for the newcomers to be turned away and the wish for them to vanish from the face of the earth. Anxiety and anger do not encourage the development of fine cognitive discriminations.

(7) It is likely, we think, that at least some of the newcomers felt themselves to be the target of negative attitudes verging on lethal intensity. This feeling of being on the spot—in an environment earmarked for its caringness—might well have been an outcome of private expectations and prejudgments in addition to negative cues from the environment. Teahan and Kastenbaum report that among those who left the new employment opportunity within a few months there seemed to be an unusually large number who expected to die fairly soon and by violent means. There is no firm basis for supposing that these expectations were created by the new environment, although they may have been exacerbated.

What might eventuate, then, as an outcome of the encounter between a vulnerable individual (black man with problematic work history) and his new caring environment, when the latter is also an old and noncaring environment? We would suggest a high probability of heightened expectation of sudden, violent death—and perhaps despair over this hurtful opportunity, and a plunge into a lifestyle that will in fact decrease the vulnerable man's probabilities for survival.

Vulnerability: Three Hypotheses

How vulnerable is *what* person to *which* environment? Refined theories of the relationship between the individual and his environment may be premature. But enough observations have been made to encourage the formulation of a few hypotheses. We have selected three hypotheses that might prove heuristic. Each of them bear upon the relative vulnerability of different individuals to hazards in their proximal and distal environments.

These hypotheses will first be offered in their general form, i.e., specifying basic characteristics of the individual's relationship to his environment. It will then be possible to focus upon implications for vulnerability.

(1) *The developmental hypothesis*: Dependence upon the proximal environment is greatest at both extremes of the life cycle, infancy and advanced age. From infancy onward the individual gradually differentiates himself from the world. Simultaneously he becomes more liberated from his immediate environment and more involved in sociophysical systems that are remote in time, in space, or both (Werner 1957).

(2) *The docility hypothesis*: "The greater the degree of competence of the organism, the less will be the proportion of variance in behavior due to environmental factors. Conversely, limitations in health, cognitive skills, ego strength, status, social role performance, or degree of cultural evolution will tend to heighten the docility of the person in the face of environmental constraints and influences." This hypothesis has been offered by M. Powell Lawton and his associates (Lawton 1970). We would modify this formulation for the present purposes: Decrements in the individual's competence increase his dependency upon the proximal environment (a matter of emphasis that we believe is in keeping with Lawton's intent). And we would omit status and degree of cultural evolution, as these factors seem to be rather unlike the others cited in his hypothesis and better served in a separate statement as below.

(3) *The social echelon hypothesis*: The lower the individual's echelon of socioeconomic status, the greater his immersion in the proximal environment. He is more dependent upon, and his behavior is more predictable from, the close-in environment than is the case for a person similar in age and ability but occupying a higher social echelon.

The same person may be deeply embedded in his proximal environment for any or all of the reasons mentioned. An impoverished aged woman with poor health and limited mobility, for example, would be a far from fictitious instance. It is probable that these sources of dependence upon the proximal environment interact dynamically, rather than additively. Advanced age increases one's probability of serious financial concern (Brotmann 1968). Age and impecunity may conspire to reduce future optimism, social interaction, and level of health maintenance. The resulting phenomenological constriction, social isolation, and failing health can then serve to accelerate deteriorative changes with age, increase the discrepancy between funds available and those required, etc. This example is just one of many that could be given.

Although there are directional similarities in such instances, the three hypotheses each retain their individual character. When an aging person shows decreased coping ability he might be regarded from the standpoint of both the developmental and the docility hypotheses (or even from the social echelon hypothesis, considering the low status often ascribed to the elderly in our society) (Slater 1964). However, aging individuals differ widely in the amount and type of impairment manifested, and there are many sources of impaired functioning apart from aging. Furthermore, even the nonaged and nonimpaired within a low social echelon may find themselves in straits somewhat similar to the aged or impaired in higher echelons.

Now let us move on to vulnerability. To say that a person is highly dependent on his proximal environment is to imply that he would be quite vulnerable to deficiencies or stresses within that sector. This implication is acceptable, but it is only part of the story that may eventually be told. The infant is obviously at the mercy of his mother in particular, and his immediate environment in general. He would not long survive without constant and adequate care. Somewhat less obviously, the very aged person is also at the mercy of his proximal environment. Lawton predicts from his docility hypothesis that geographical distance would have its most powerful limiting effects upon those who are most impaired (Lawton 1970). For a resource (food, health care, a place for peace and quiet) to exist just a little beyond the elder's effective operational range may be functionally equivalent to its nonexistence. The person who does not venture out of his proximal environment because he does not feel welcome anywhere else could perhaps be regarded as no less deprived and vulnerable.

There is something in common among the factors already mentioned. The developmental, docility, and social echelon hypotheses imply that those who fall into these categories are especially vulnerable to failures in the sustaining power of their proximal environments. The environment fails if it no longer "cares," or it no longer offers the essential support regardless of its disposition toward the individual.

Another element can be added here. As his continued survival becomes more problematic, one may either heighten, diminish, or reverse his WtL. This orientation will be perceived (or misperceived) by the environment and may influence what comes next. Caringness might be reinstated by a strong display of WtL, i.e., the individual "earns" his continued survival. It is also possible that a clear manifestation of WtD could have the same effect. We are thinking, for example, of self-destructive behavior that calls attention to the individual's needs in a manner too obvious to be neglected. Yet people with a strong WtL have been known to perish in an environment that could have kept them alive, and behavior of high lethal intent has also been ignored.

At this point in our lack of detailed and organized knowledge of behavioral ecology it would be unwise to suggest that there is any dependable relationship between WtL and the environmental conditions which both precede and follow this orientation. But it is timely to propose that WtL be introduced as a relevant variable at every opportunity. The men studied by Teahan and Kastenbaum, for example, were vulnerable as a group in terms of both the social echelon (black and impoverished) and docility (deficient in occupational and other adaptive skills) models. Yet there were appreciable individual differences in future optimism and subjective life expectancy—variables that are relevant to WtL. Moreover, these phenomenologic differences were predictive of significant behavioral outcomes (hold on to new job vs. leaving/quitting). Vulnerability, WtL, and the life-protecting/endangering characteristics of the environment are closely intertwined but not related to each other in a simple one-to-one manner.

Spreading the net a little further, we begin to see that a person may be caught in more ways than one, and that even those apparently free from overdependency have their own special problems. In their well-known work on suicide and murder, Henry and Short (1954) have reported material which suggests that the favored people in our society may be especially vulnerable on some counts. A plummetting stock market may upset the affluent person more immediately and drastically than the man who has not been worrying about investing the money he never had. Although by no means firmly established as a sociopsychological fact, it is at least a compelling hypothesis that suicides and other self-destructive behaviors may be related closely to high level economic fluctuations in those who are in a position to see themselves affected. Ordinarily, this would not be the very young or very old person, the markedly impaired, or the dweller in the socioeconomic basement. Various forms of so-called psychosomatic disorder have also been attributed, either wholly or in part, to stresses that are most likely to confront those who are "making it" or endeavoring to do so.

The formulation of vulnerabilities can be enlarged as follows: Those on the low end of the developmental-docility-social echelon axis are particularly vulnerable to problems generated within the proximal environment; those on the high end of this axis are particularly vulnerable to problems generated within the distal environment. The aged, impoverished, and ailing woman is jeopardized by the lack of nutritious food on the table. The healthy middle-aged executive is jeopardized by his own anxiety and despondence related to the numbers that are tapping over the ticker tape. Proximal deprivation the one, distal stress the other—in both cases, a threat to continued survival exists.

Add one more factor—the double vulnerability of the person who is embedded in the proximal environment. It was appropriate to emphasize, as above, the urgent plight he faces should his proximal environment reject or fail to nurture him. This kind of threat is likely to be concrete and identifiable: the empty cupboard, the undiagnosed and untreated malady, the assailant springing out from the alley. But the same person may also be in considerable jeopardy from the distant environment. This threat is not as easily perceived—indeed, the invisibility or amorphousness of the distal environment to this person may itself constitute the primary threat. When he finds himself forced to interact with the distal environment on its terms he may blunder out of anxiety or inexperience. When the distal environment intrudes upon his own "turf" he may similarly behave in a manner that increases rather than diminishes his vulnerability. He does not really know (care for) the outer world and it does not really know (or care for) him an an individual. The ill or impoverished person fails to obtain the benefits and opportunities which are rightfully his. Blunders and misunderstandings get him into further trouble with the authorities. Thus he finds his life disjointed and threatened by the end effects of policies that began far away in the distal environment (e.g., the ghetto adolescent headed for Vietnam, the old man dislocated in an urban renewal project, headed . . . where?).

Learned Hopelessness

Absence of WtL has emerged as a salient consideration. People who appear to be equally vulnerable to their environment may prove to differ in WtL. Why? Survival of people regarded as terminally ill and precipitous death of those thought to be in no unusual danger have been attributed to variations in WtL (LeShan and Gassman 1958; Weisman and Kastenbaum 1968; Kubler-Ross, 1969). Why? Occasional or systematic actions of the environment may result in heightened, diminished, or reversed WtL. Why?

One interesting line of possible explanation derives from experimental studies of animal behavior. We will focus upon the recent contributions of Martin Seligman and his colleagues (Seligman and Groves 1970; Maier et al. 1969). Their published findings at this time are based largely upon dogs, but comparable results have now been obtained with other species. The striking feature of Seligman's research is that it produces creatures who fail to escape from painful stimuli (electric shock) when, in fact, escape is objectively possible. Even the triple inducement of an open door, a coaxing researcher, and a slice of Hebrew National Salami fails to induce the dog to leave his paining environment.

Unlike most observations of paradoxical or hard-to-explain human behavior, those of Seligman and his colleagues are linked to a clear picture of the antecedent conditions. They are in the position to make at least a highly informed guess because the observers themselves were responsible for creating this peculiar behavior. "Learned helplessness" is the term employed by Seligman. Since we will be adding a few speculations and applying the paradigm to human behavior in complex situations, we do not wish to distort Seligman's concept. We will speak instead of learned *hope*lessness, a term compatible with the original but giving us more room for maneuvering.

Apparently, what the animals learn is that their behavior has no effect upon avoiding the undesired. At any rate, it has no power to rid them of the shock. They learn this through prior exposure to inescapable shock. It is necessary to emphasize that exposure to shock itself does not produce this helpless/hopeless orientation.

Furthermore, the giving up orientation becomes entrenched. In new situations and at later times the animal still behaves as though there were no point in attempting to gain relief. "The expectation that responding will produce relief provides the incentive for responding; learning that responding is ineffective undermines this incentive and produces failure to escape." (Seligman and Groves 1970, p. 191.) Shock may or may not end, but this outcome will have nothing to do with one's own efforts. And one has not learned any successful association between a particular behavior and its outcome. The animals do not learn how to control the environment. It might be said they fail to develop faith or confidence in their own competence (cf. the docility hypothesis above). The Seligman group itself suggests "that learning that shock is uncontrollable produces a motivational depletion not unlike clinical depression in humans (which) . . . contributes to the failure to escape shock . . . (furthermore) both failure to escape and the greater stress produced by inescapable shock have a common cause: learning that responding and trauma are independent" (p. 192).

It would be absurd to weld this interpretation to human behavior, but plausible to consider the implications. Some human behavior does have the look of learned hopelessness. Why does he not try harder to recover? To escape this punishing and threatening environment? To change the environment? WtL may develop from a life history of some success with environmental control. Not every effort and perhaps not even most efforts would have to have met with success. But there would have been enough success to have created a phenomenologic background of confidence; the precedent would be there.

Perhaps it would be worthwhile to distinguish three types of success.

(1) "I got my way." We learn that our own actions can fulfill positive goals. Future optimism is likely to be stimulated by such experiences. One of the many implications here is that a greater multiplicity of future goals and prospects unfolds within one's mind, and a greater multiplicity of goal-attaining techniques develop from subsequent behaviors. Therefore, the loss of one particular goal or the blockage of any particular goal-seeking maneuver may be less likely to induce hopelessness/helplessness. "I can focus on another goal; I can try another method."

(2) "I escaped in one piece." This type of success more closely parallels the Seligman experiments. The person has managed to extricate himself from jeopardy. The general outcome should be a sense of resiliency. "Having come through a few tough scrapes, I know that you don't have to give up when things look bad." The well-known animal experiments of Curt Richter suggest that even a single successful escape experience may insulate the organism against sudden death when things "look bad" (1959).

(3) "When I do something, something usually happens." Actions have not necessarily led to the effects one desired. One blunders or miscalculates; the goal slips away, the predicament worsens. But the environment was responsive. One has validated his power to contact and impress the

environment. It is possible to develop and maintain a "will" from such experiences, we think. The effectiveness of the will is another story.

Although these three types of success seem difficult to avoid completely, one may nevertheless find himself, at critical times, in a situation where none of these resources are available. The person who is low man in all three vulnerability models (developmental, docility, and social echelon) comes up against an establishment that acts upon him without truly acknowledging his existence. The very first point of contact may instantly convey the message: "You have no power." We may be talking about an employment, educational or health-services establishment, for example. Objectively, there could be many opportunities for the individual to achieve his own goals or to obtain a relevant response from the environmental system. But one quick encounter may be enough to freeze him into the learned hopelessness position. Indeed, he has never really succeeded when coping with The Establishment, why should he expect to succeed this time?

The Establishment itself does not have a fair chance. The vulnerable one scans what The Establishment puts forth in a highly biased style, looking for confirmations of what he already suspects. This process is probably less certain and rapid in those who occupy a less vulnerable position at the beginning. But sooner or later some environmental cue may be interpreted as confirmation of one's self-suspected inability to impose his will on the world. The dynamics of learned hopelessness may undergo the clinical picture of "willessness."

Both long term and situational environmental influences contribute to the fragile WtL. Recent critics of our educational and correctional systems seem to be making some points in common, points relevant to WtL. The schools are said to discourage initiative, spontaneity, and a sense of one's being able to act creatively upon the environment. Detention centers and prisons are said to keep men removed from the possibility of competent action until their motivation and skills have deteriorated. Both instances, if the criticisms are well-founded, exemplify long-term influences that would make it difficult to develop and maintain a viable WtL. To these would be added situational influences such as the unresponsiveness of hospital routine to the needs of a particular person, the welfare agency maze that faces a desperate family, etc. (We are stressing here the general case; the exceptions should not be overlooked.)

There is an obvious implication for those who are in contact with vulnerable people, or with any person who is at a vulnerable point in his life. We might be well advised to improve sensitivity to the metacommunication of our own actions. What are we conveying that might be read as a confirmation of the individual's feared powerlessness? Sudden giving up of WtL leaves the would-be helping person with a puzzlingly and annoyingly inert object. The response can easily exacerbate the problem—strengthening the learned hopelessness and actually increasing the probability of foreshortened survival.

Consideration of the learned hopelessness model might alert us to warning signals. Negativistic or seemingly self-defeating behavior can provoke or alienate the helping person. We interpret the same behavior differently, however, if it is viewed as a possible last-ditch maneuver before succumbing to a powerless, futureless orientation. The vulnerable person may have already given up any hope of attaining positive goals. He doesn't expect to get his way. Next, he may relinquish the prospect of successful avoidance of negative goals. His fate (death or other threatening outcome) seems inescapable. What he has left is the sense of still being able to act upon his environment. The response, whatever form it takes, confirms his continued existence and potency, even if it does not offer much comfort otherwise. Actually, continued give-and-take might enable him to return eventually to a higher level of willing (toward goal-fulfillment or away from pain-disaster).

When a person is clinging to this minimal level of will-support, what is the worst response the environment might offer? Avoidance, withdrawal, nonresponsiveness in general would probably comprise the most jeopardizing action. It should be noted that the caring environment may be essentially nonresponsive even when it is providing services. The services are provided at the discretion and convenience of the environment. Little that is said or done by the recipient affects the system. At least, this is the reasoning that would seem to follow from the learned hopelessness model. It might be more will-bolstering and life-protecting for the environment to deny or withhold services directly because "You got us angry at you," or "You did the wrong thing," as compared with placing the vulnerable person into the role of a one-hundred percent recipient of routinized or arbitrary action.

Additionally, we could speculate that a clear manifestation of opposition from the environment might lead to different alterations in WtL status. The nonresponse environmental syndrome seems calculated to wither the individual's ability to maintain any motivational stance at all. WtL would falter, dissipate. Opposition seems more likely to challenge and thus stimulate WtL, or precipitate transformation into WtD—still an orientation, but now with a new direction.

Although we have not taken space to spell out many of the implications or to detail further research and action possibilities, it should be evident that the learned hopelessness model lends itself to application in situations where human life is in jeopardy. Because it has roots in an experimental paradigm, this model also carries the promise of being amenable to controlled investigation. Nothing that has been proposed in this (or preceding) sections is necessarily beyond the scope of psychosocial research. We also wish to note that emphasis upon the learned hopelessness model is meant to illustrate the type of explanatory frameworks that can be found or developed. Other approaches certainly should be explored as well.

Where Have We Been? Where Are We Going?

We started out with the recognition that all the variables which influence survival do not march up and announce themselves to us, neatly prelabeled and enrolled on a finite and stable list. Specialized models of predictions can limit attention to a small, tightly-defined set of variables. These models often have valuable applications—not the least of which is their willingness to organize our perceptions, thoughts, and habits for us. But we were concerned about the premature closure of models for predicting survival. Somehow we should be able to include more. The "more" should include events that transpire too fast or too slow to fit into existing systems of analysis, events that are too subjective, too hard to observe reliably, too multileveled to encompass easily within a simple framework, too anything.

It was our intention to show something of the complexity and relevance of factors which deserve more systematic attention. This required brief visits to a variety of content areas (although too few to be more than suggestive). It also required concentration upon a few selected concepts. We have tried to describe and define these concepts by setting them to work upon a sampling of phenomena whose relevancy were simultaneously hoping to convey. Thus it is that our journey has involved circular as well as forward motion. The reader might prefer an alternative set of concepts to encompass the same material, or he might prefer to apply the concepts to other specific phenomena. We are less invested in the particular connections set forth than in the generation of systematic research—and action—efforts.

Future developments could well make use of resources that were not incorporated into the present paper. Special mention should be made of the ecological contributions offered over the years by Roger Barker and his colleagues (1968), and the psychoanalytic insights of Otto Rank (1945). There are many people we can learn from. It is clear enough that our fund of empirical knowledge in this area should be increased by sophisticated research efforts. But there is a corresponding need for theoretical integration.

Predicting longevity is one thing—enhancing and protecting life is something else. There would be sufficient justification for predictive efforts even without the intent to protect life. So far as the present writers are concerned, however, the prime motivation is to reduce the waste of human lives. It is hardly disputable that people have been known to squander their hours or years. But death withdraws the option of change, or developing a more rewarding quality of life. Specialists in the study of aging or death sometimes are perceived as narrowly morbid folk. This is as good a time as any to say that this view is superficial. Infirmity, poverty, inequality, depression and loss are among the trials faced by many elders. These problems limit the range of action and opportunity, threaten authentic existence as a person as well as physical survival. Death places the ultimate limitation on our prospects for continued development. It is not lack of concern for the quality of life that arouses interest in life protection and extension, nor is it an infatuation with the subject matter. Those processes which cripple life or snatch it away prematurely must be identified if we are to have at least the option for a life of quality.

This brings us to one final concern. The psychosocial case in favor of prolonging human life is not without opposition. The opposition is both historical and contemporary. There are individuals who prefer death to life;

there are social trends which imply that life-shortening or life-denying actions are preferable (Gruman 1966; Kastenbaum, in press). Thus, the same research efforts that improve our ability to predict and perhaps safeguard or extend longevity could also be put to other use. The task for the future includes monitoring—critically—our own sentiments and actions. The predictor variables and the life/death differentials are within us as well as "out there."

References

Barker, R.: *Ecological Psychology*. Stanford: Stanford University Press, 1968.
Brotmann, H.: *Who Are The Aged: A Demographic View*. (Occasional Papers in Gerontology, No. 1) Ann Arbor, Michigan: Institute of Gerontology, 1968.
Duff, R. and Hollingshead, A.: *Sickness and Society*. New York: Harper and Row, 1968.
Farber, M.: *Theory of Suicide*. New York: Funk and Wagnalls, 1968.
Feifel, H.: The function of attitudes toward death. In Symposium of group for Advancement of Psychiatry: *Death and Dying: Attitudes of Patient and Doctor*, pp. 633-641, 1965.
Gruman, G.: *A History of Ideas about the Prolongation of Life*. Philadelphia: American Philosophical Society, 1966.
Glaser, B. and Strauss, A.: *Awareness of Dying*. Chicago: Aldine, 1966.
Heavenrich, R.: *Lethality As A Function of Experienced Isolation, Motivation to Live and Social Resources: An Exploratory Study in Suicidology*. Wayne State University, Detroit: Masters Thesis, 1970.
Henry, A. and Short, J., Jr.: *Suicide and Homicide*. Glencoe, Ill.: The Free Press, 1954.
Kastenbaum, R.: The structure and function of time perspective. *J. Psychol. Research*, (India) 1963.
Kastenbaum, R.: The realm of death: an emerging area in psychological research. *J. Human Relations*, 13:538-552, 1965.
Kastenbaum, R.: While the old man dies. In Kutscher, A. (ed.), *Psychosocial Care of the Terminally Ill Patient*. New York: Columbia University Press, in press.
Kubler-Ross, E.: *On Death and Dying*. London: Collier-Macmillan, 1969.
Lawton, M.: Ecology and Aging. In Pastalan, L. and Carson, D. (eds.), *Spatial Behavior of Older People*. Ann Arbor, Michigan: Institute of Gerontology, pp. 40-67, 1970.
LeShan, L. and Gassman, M.: Some observations on psychotherapy with patients suffering from neoplastic disease. *Amer. J. Psychotherapy*, 12:723-734, 1958.
Rank, O.: *Will Therapy and Truth and Reality*. New York: A.A. Knopf, 1945.
Ritchter, C.: The phenomenon of unexplained sudden death in animals and man. In Feifel, H. (ed.), *The Meaning of Death*. New York: McGraw-Hill, pp. 302-316, 1959.

Schopenhauer, A.: *The World as Will and Idea*. Haldane, T. and Kemp, J. (trans.), London: Routledge and Kegan Paul (1883) 1948.

Seligman, M. and Groves, D.: Nontransient learned helplessness. *Psycho. Sci.*, 19:191-192, 1970.

Seligman, M.; Maier, S. and Solomon, R.: Pavlovian fear conditioning and learned helplessness. In Campbell, B. and Church, R. (eds.), *Punishment and Aversive Behavior*. New York: Appleton-Century-Crofts, pp. 299-342, 1969.

Slater, P.: Cross-cultural views of the aged. In Kastenbaum, R. (ed.), *New Thoughts on Old Age*. New York: Springer, 1964.

Teahan, J. and Kastenbaum, R.: Future optimism and subjective life expectancy in "Hard-Core Unemployed" men. *Omega*, in press.

Weisman, A. and Kastenbaum, R.: The psychological autopsy: a study of the terminal phase of life. *Community Mental Journal*. Monograph No. 4. New York: Behavioral Publications, 1968.

Werner, H. *Comparative Psychology of Mental Development*. New York: International Universities Press, 1957.

20 Added Years: Social Issues and Consequences

RICHARD A. KALISH

Introductory Framework

Despite the possible dangers of scientific developments, the prospect of leashing scientists until the long-range significance of their work is completely understood is both impractical and inappropriate. However, it is possible to involve scientists in discussion of the future implications of their research, so that responsibility not be delegated to the allegedly amoral and objective *science*, which is a concept rather than an entity and thus obviously incapable of either defense or retaliation. As we learn more about the variables contributing to human survival and as we find ways to extend life expectancy, we need to give consideration to the social meaning of our actions and to participate in making certain that, by the time the fruits of our research are borne, the community is ready for coping with the outputs.

If this polemic sounds platitudinous, it is only because it has been written before—not because it has been heeded before. The natural scientist who talks about slowing *aging* frequently evinces little concern about the *aged*; the behavioral scientist who studies behavior change seems to ignore the behaver; the social scientist who attempts to affect individual attitudes may pay little attention to the individual.

Life has, of course, already been extended by many years since the turn of the century, but by far the greatest part of the increased life span comes from reduced infant mortality and from reduced impact of childhood diseases. Relatively little extension has been obtained from improving the health of the elderly. Evidence is also prevalent that even the elimination of heart disease, stroke, and cancer would not increase life by more than a handful of years, ten or a dozen at the most. Therefore, it appears logical that, if more years of alertness and vitality are to be added to the life expectancy of middle-aged people, it must be done through affecting those processes which appear to cause the decremental correlates of aging.

In April, 1970, the Center for the Study of Democratic Institutions, based at Santa Barbara, held a five-day conference under the leadership of Dr. Alex Comfort, titled *Project Life Span*. The premise of this conference was that by

Richard A. Kalish is Associate Professor, School of Public Health University of California, Los Angeles, and Department of Psychiatry, University of California, San Francisco.

1990 biologists will have discovered how to slow down the aging process in such a way as to provide an extra decade of healthy and alert life for each person. This chapter is based in large part on the stimulation and conversation of those five days, and readers are encouraged to pursue this discussion themselves by reading the Center's forthcoming report, edited by Harvey Wheeler (in press).

The plan for the remainder of this chapter is to outline some of the issues involved with the increased life span, as proposed above. The first half of the paper will briefly discuss several issues that evolve directly from the biological changes to be produced; the second half will touch on some of the possible social implications inherent in an extra decade of life. My purpose is breadth rather than depth, uncovering issues rather than probing issues. This chapter may provide a social Rorschach into which the reader may project his own angers and anxieties and hopes and speculations regarding the reviving of the spirit of Ponce de Leon.

Biological Parameters

Issue: How can the world, already overcrowded, handle yet another source of population increase? This most obvious of all questions cannot be answered without knowledge concerning some of the other issues to be cited below. One possible response would be to cease all research of cancer and heart disease, while turning full attention to aging research. The former often extends senility, leaving the old to die of something else, probably equally degrading and discomforting; the latter would (depending upon the response to the next issue) add to good years without prolonging the duration of the exit.

If the notion of eliminating cancer and heart research is too macabre even to contemplate, let me suggest an alternative. I will take as axiomatic the thought that the purpose of cancer research is to provide a large number of people with a life that is both longer and healthier and to reduce the amount of suffering they will have to undergo. Implicit is the notion that persons who are thus saved from death by cancer will eventually die a less grotesque (if the word is fair) death. If half the money for cancer research were put into aging research and the other half were to be used to develop medication that would reduce the suffering of cancer patients without reducing their alertness, it would be of equivalent value to cancer patients and of much greater value to all others. Aging research would provide extra years of life; the new medication would reduce substantially the pain and discomfort of death from cancer; hence the person would live longer and die more comfortably, which is exactly what cancer research proposes, but the results of the aging research would also benefit other people.

I recognize that I will be accused of opposing cancer research, although this is not the case. Indeed, much valuable information regarding aging accrues from such research, as well as precious understanding of cancer. I only wish to emphasize that there are alternative priorities. I would also suggest that many people may become less than sanguine when they realize that other forms of dying may inflict kinds of deterioration that might be perceived as worse than cancer.

Issue: To what degree will increased human survival merely extend the terminal months and years and to what degree will the extension be in years of vigor and health? The respected biogerontologist, Harry Sobel, once remarked that the present research trend will enable men to "live for 300 years, 50 years of virility and 250 years of senility." Psychologist Oscar Kaplan has already warned the geriatric-caretaking community of the coming need for facilities for persons whose organic brain changes will require virtually total care. Will the new biomedical advances merely verify the Sobel and Kaplan pronouncements, or will they add the kind of years of life that can be enjoyed? Will the processes to be used to extend life of the organism also extend, comparably, the life of all organs, including the brain?

Issue: To what degree will sensory and motor capacities and good general health be extended? Losses in the sensory and motor capacities and in general health increase geometrically with age. As Leroy Duncan has pointed out, cumulative effects of exposure to sun or to noise would be accentuated in importance if the life expectancy is increased, eventuating in dermatological damage or hearing loss (Wheeler, in press). Since more people would be living into their eighties and nineties, we could see more of the debilitating effects of such long-term environmental influences. However, these are not beyond remedying, Duncan emphasizes, either through direct interventions or prosthetic devices.

Alvin Goldfarb adds another dimension to this concern by posing the psychosocial counterpoint to Duncan: will the effects of psychological insults be cumulative? Goldfarb is not persuaded that adding to the middle years, as has been suggested, will necessarily have a beneficial effect, since the stresses and anxieties of middle age seem to be as great as those of most other age groups (Wheeler, in press).

Issue: How will the added years be distributed across the age range? Previously I asked whether life would be extended primarily in the late years, but the matter becomes infinitely more complex. For example, life extension could conceivably occur by prolonging infancy, the preschool years, or the first decade of life, a prospect which parents might view with mixed feelings. Or the years immediately following puberty might be extended, a circumstance which would probably advance the cause of antiscientism manyfold. Those more optimistic claim that the additional years will be added only during the optimum period, when the gradient of youthfulness and vigor crosses the gradient of wisdom and experience. If what takes place is a slowing-down of the decremental qualities of aging, the added years would be distributed roughly from the mid-twenties onward. The nature of this distribution of years will inevitably shape many institutions, e.g., the family, education, work, and leisure, for the foreseeable future.

Issue: Will all aspects of the aging process be retarded or will age-related decrements follow a different pattern than at present? Although the 250 years of senility proposed by Sobel, not completely facetiously, is undoubtedly an extreme version, it is logical to hope that the brain and the other body organs will fail at roughly the same time. Otherwise we risk the possibility of, on the one hand, the lengthy senility mentioned by Sobel or, on the other hand, an alert brain existing for an indefinite period in a useless organism. The latter offers some possibility of remedy or prosthetics, but our history of helping the aged and the disabled is not a healthy prognosis for the wide distribution of such facilities.

Issue: What will be the nature of the process that extends life? If we can increase productive life by taking a harmless, inexpensive pill, few people would reject the service. Evidence is already substantial, however, to indicate that certain regimens would find less than 100 percent acceptance. People appear unable to alter such life habits as eating, smoking, and exercising, in spite of good evidence that making certain changes would, in all probability, increase healthy years. Few people undertake the suggested annual medical check-up, with finances being only one reason for reluctance, and physicians have many patients who appear unable to follow even the simplest of treatment programs.

If extended life comes at the cost of major dietary changes, elimination of certain enjoyable habits, regular visits to medical centers to undergo unpleasant treatment, or such home programs as self-innoculations, many people will not avail themselves of the resources.

Issue: What is the duration of the increase? For the previously cited Santa Barbara conference, an arbitrary period of ten added years was selected along with a target date, felt reasonably by many conferees, of 1990. Dr. Alex Comfort and others, however, emphasized that once even a small breakthrough was made in slowing the process of aging, it would bring up the possibility of subsequent discoveries. Thus, the 20-year-old of 1990 who saw his life expectancy extended by a decade might well anticipate that future research would add additional decades. Inevitably the prospect of eternal life would begin to glow upon the horizon. Although most of this article is addressed to the possibility of a normal life span of 100 to 120 years at the outside, the notion of living four or five centuries or more involves many more issues and much more innovative thinking. It is no longer strictly in the realm of science fiction to contemplate a time when one would need to request permission to die.

Issue: At what age will this process be effective? Assume for the moment that it is 1990 and that the announcement of a successful treatment program has been made public: human life expectancy jumps for a 20-year-old from 55 more years to 65 more years. You, however, are now 60 years old: how much longer than your previously allotted time will your new life charts predict?

Issue: Who will have access to increased longevity? Who will control its source? Caused in part by inequitable distribution of medical services, not every human conception has an equivalent chance to live out its present maximum life span. If the increased life span is available at low cost to everyone, the present inequities will relatively not be changed; if the cost is high, then the wealthy will inevitably have greater access to this opportunity. Prehoda discusses the actuarial aspects of this consideration (Wheeler, in press).

Perhaps even more important is the possibility that governments might retain control of the life extending commodity or service, using it to reward selectively those who fulfill its needs. Thus we might find extra years doled out to high producers, docile workers, political loyalists, professional athletes, or whatever categories happen to be in favor with the controllers at the time.

Not all the issues presented above are of vital importance; not all are equally simple to explain. I have attempted to provide a brief discussion of some of the concerns which the nonacademic community will undoubtedly consider as they decide whether to reward the biogerontologist or to reject him. But the previous comments represent only one type of concern: those directly related to the biological aspects of change. Perhaps even more important are the ways in which the many societies of the world might be affected. What is the significance of life extension for family structure, for the educational system, for delivery of health care services, for employment and recreation, for the economy, and so on and on.

Psychosocial Implications

The remainder of this paper must become a bit speculative, delving sporadically into the domain of fantasy and science fiction. How then might an increased life expectancy affect the family structure? Building upon what I have discussed elsewhere I would suggest an upsurge in the already increasing divorce rate of those in their fifties and sixties, as well as a comparable increase in marriage and remarriage rates of those in their sixties and seventies. In the fifties, the cementing influence of dependent children has dissolved; retirement and an increase in time together is imminent; sexuality has diminished; the bases for the original marriage may not have retained their substance over the three intervening decades. With a weaker base in human interrelationships to hold the marriage together, and with greater acceptance of divorce from the general community, the dissolution of marriage becomes increasingly possible. At the time that life is extended, another potentially important reason for maintaining a minimally adequate marriage disappears: if, by the time children become independent and retirement is approaching, the aches and pains of aging begin, the terminal illnesses of age peers become known, and one's own future years are statistically known to be ten or twelve, entering new relationships may loom as menacing. If, however, health, vitality, and sexuality are present, if friends remain similarly healthy, and if a quarter of a century of future life appears likely, new relationships become more enticing, and the obstructions to severing a longstanding relationship become less acute. Therefore, divorce would probably become more common in this age group.

For the same basic reasons, marriage in these now middle-age years will also become more common. Sociologist Andrea Tyree has expressed the belief that the need for secure and dependable companionship will not diminish and that remarriage, or at least a comparable relationship, will follow the increase in late middle-years (*Los Angeles Times*, 1970).

Another change in family structure, less speculative than the above, is that four-generation families will be common and five-generation families will be far from unique. What, if any, role does a great-great-grandmother have with her forty-five year grandson and her three year old great-great-granddaughter? Is 80 years and five generations too much to be spanned? Evidence is undoubtedly available, but little has been done to look now at a relationship which will become more common.

The impact of increased life span upon work and retirement may be considerable. Already we are concerned about people required to retire, who may have the physical and personal resources and the motivation to work for another ten, fifteen, or twenty years. More familiar is the retired person who, although not really liking his former work, feels personally diminished by the combined loss of identifiable role, of time structure, of social relationships, and of income. If retirement age remains the same or, as is likely, is lowered by two or three years, a new retiree will be able to bet upon twenty-five to thirty-five good years ahead, a time period which almost matches the number of years that he has worked previously. Unless adequate income and services are available, people may have to anticipate one-third of their lifetimes being spent in financially marginal, socially frustrating circumstances.

The well-known biologist, Bernard Strehler, labels this concern as "Myth Number Four: Postponement of senescence will impose great economic burdens on society" (Wheeler, in press). He subsequently avoids closing the trap he has sprung by explaining that this is a myth *if* previous productivity is high enough to cover all age groups. I heartily agree with Dr. Strehler, but I do not share his optimism that income redistribution is likely to occur in time to make pleasant retirement years for more than a portion of these persons. Our past record in this area has not been good. The other possibility that he discusses, continuation of active work for an additional time period, also has merit, but overlooks some of the difficulties inherent in postponing promotions, maintaining employees with outmoded skills and the problem of motivating workers who are just plain bored with their work.

However, if we do supply adequate income, so that retirees with discretionary income and discretionary time became more numerous, I strongly suspect that the capitalistic system will come to the rescue by offering needed services. Fields involving recreation and travel will boom, with retirees undoubtedly on both the giving and receiving ends of goods and services.

Another option is education for second careers. People with outmoded skills may turn to another job field in which their present experience, interests, and skills permit success. Since a 55-year-old could anticipate an additional quarter century of healthy, alert life, the probable pay-off for training to enter a new kind of job would be ample. The trend toward second careers for those in their fifties and early sixties, like the trend for this age group to participate in second marriages, is very likely to accelerate.

Assuming the knowledge explosion continues and that certain kinds of experience and wisdom are valued, continuing education or re-education become prime considerations. Adult education, the stepchild of the educational system, may emerge as the most important link in the chain of higher education. Such continuation programs will update skills and awareness for some older students, will offer others the opportunity to enter new job fields, and will provide still others with the intellectual stimulation and personal growth that makes life worthwhile.

Continuing education may have an additional purpose. With additional decades separating family patriarchs and new arrivals as well as upper echelon management and lower levels, teachers and students, continuing education will be increasingly needed to enable the older person to be aware of the changing values and demands of younger persons. The rigidities of age that emanate from fear of illness and death, pain suffered from loss, and anxiety over impending role change, all these may be diminished; however, the rigidities imposed by having been socialized in an era when the world was different, when technology and social values were based on considerations that no longer exist, this source of rigidity will remain. Not only will it remain, but it will impede progress on a variety of fronts. Hopefully, continuing education will perform an important task in this regard.

Before leaving the topic of work, I wish to touch on an important economic matter, imposed by increased longevity: pension programs. I suspect that a sudden and unexpected increase in life span would bankrupt every retirement fund in the country and would seriously threaten the present structure of the Social Security system. A recent article titled "Warning, These People Can Be Dangerous," makes this same point (*Forbes Magazine*, 1970).

For a final thought, I would wonder whether the role of the traditional religions and of man's relationship with his God might not also be reconsidered. The very definition of being a mortal implies that one is vulnerable to death. If death can be postponed by ten years, then the next 10 or 100 or 1000 may not be too far off to contemplate. If death ceases to be relevant; will man continue to adhere to religious doctrine that posits after-life as a core tenet? If life is for 1000 years, of what cogency is after-life? And if man can postpone death and—as I assume he eventually will do also—create life, then perhaps man becomes his own god and the Judeo-Christian God ceases to exist. The important point is that the 1000 year extension is not required for this to occur. It may occur with merely the possibility that such a breakthrough is potentially in the foreseeable future.

In the previous pages, I have attempted to probe the parameters of (a) the biological boundaries of the projected increase in life expectancy and (b) the social implications of setting the operation into motion. I have undertaken the relatively easy task of asking the questions; much more difficult is the job of giving satisfactory answers. The basic question is similar to the war-time one, "If we win the war, what will we do with the peace?" It is imperative that we now contemplate what we will do with longer life, if we succeed in attaining it.

References

Forbes Magazine: "Warning, these people can be dangerous." October 1, 1970.
Los Angeles Times: page 1, May 10, 1970.
Wheeler, H. (ed.): Report on *Project Life Span*; Conference held at the Center for the Study of Democratic Institutions, Santa Barbara, California, April, 1970 (in press).

Part V
Summary and the Future

21 Summary and the Future

ERDMAN PALMORE

This book has presented many recent findings on different physiological, psychological, and social predictors of longevity, based on research with several types of groups ranging from normal community residents of middle and older ages to the institutionalized aged. It is important in such a book to summarize the diverse findings and to attempt some integration and interpretation of their significance on a broader scale.

Summary Propositions

We will begin by summarizing the main findings with twenty-one propositions about the prediction of life span. These propositions are usually stated on a somewhat higher level of generality than were the specific findings presented in the previous chapters. For this reason they should be regarded primarily as hypotheses suggested by the findings which should be tested further on the other groups and perhaps by other methods to evaluate how generally they apply and under what conditions they should be modified.

A. Physiological Predictors

1. Maximum possible life span is determined by genetic inheritance. (Chapter 3.)
2. Hereditary factors (genetic and nongenetic) influence longevity. However, the importance of hereditary factors relative to environmental factors is unknown, because persons with similar heredity tend to have similar environments. (Chapters 1 and 2.)
3. Women tend to live longer than men, but this may be entirely due to differences in the environment, roles, and life-style of men and women. (Chapter 1.)
4. Physicians' ratings of impairment and disability are powerful predictors of mortality among patients in hospitals even after accounting for age and other factors. (Chapter 4.)
5. Sudden death from atherosclerosis and heart disease is much less frequent among middle-aged persons who are physically active, maintain moderate weight, and avoid cigarette smoking. (Chapter 5.)

283

6. Physical activity, weight control, and avoiding cigarettes also contribute to less illness and greater longevity among normal aged. (Chapters 6 and 10.)
7. Among the institutionalized aged, the strongest predictors of mortality are incontinence, physical disability, and chronic brain syndrome. (Chapter 7.)
8. Among the psychiatrically disturbed aged, physicians' rating of functional capacity is the strongest predictor of survival. (Chapter 12.)
9. Among the normal aged, physical health is one of the strongest predictors of longevity. (Chapters 2, 11, 17 and 18.)
10. Brain impairment with relatively early onset among the aged predicts shorter longevity, but brain impairment with late onset does not. (Chapter 8.)

B. Psychological Predictors

11. A marked decline in cognitive functioning among the aged predicts a high mortality rate within one to five years. (Chapters 9, 11, 13, and 15.)
12. Among the normal aged, higher intelligence or mental status predicts greater longevity even when other factors are controlled. (Chapters 10, 11, 15, and 18.)
13. Among the psychiatrically disturbed aged, cognitive functioning is the second strongest predictor of survival. (Chapter 12.)
14. Among those aged undergoing stress (such as awaiting entrance into homes for the aged), cognitive functioning is one of the strongest predictors of survival. (Chapter 13.)
15. Among preindustrial men (such as the Navajo and the Druze), an active-productive personality predicts better health and longevity. (Chapter 14.)

C. Social Predictors

16. Higher social class and occupation predicts greater longevity, but this may be primarily due to factors other than the direct effects of class and occupational life-style. (Chapters 1, 2, 17, and 18.)
17. Among hospital patients (such as those with heart attacks), behavioral adjustment is a significant predictor of survival even after severity of illness is controlled. (Chapter 16.)
18. Among the normal aged, higher financial status, more social activity, and more life satisfaction are significant predictors of survival or number of years remaining. (Chapters 10, 11, 17, and 18.)
19. Among the normal aged, work satisfaction and happiness rating are the two best predictors of age-standardized longevity, with work satisfaction (or active and organized behavior) being most important for men and happiness being most important for women. (Chapters 10 and 18.)
20. Hope and will-to-live may be predictors of survival, especially among hospital patients. (Chapter 19.)

21. By 1990 life span will have increased by at least ten years, which will create many psychosocial problems as well as opportunities. (Chapter 20.)

Summary Comments

It may be worthwhile to speculate on the broader implications of these propositions. These comments should be understood as my own impressions and guesses based on research and reading of literature. Others may well come to different conclusions.

As for the relative influence of genetic factors, although it will probably be conclusively demonstrated some day that maximum possible life span is determined by genetic inheritance, at the present time it seems that the many intervening environmental factors such as nutrition, disease, stress, psychological attitudes, social roles, and life-styles probably outweigh the genetic factors in accounting for longevity, especially among the aged. But it may also be true that as we learn to control chronic and acute diseases and as we learn to eliminate the psychological and social stresses which produce excess mortality, the genetic factor may tend to grow in importance.

Although no studies at present have been able to separate out the effects of the hereditary factors from environmental factors, it would seem theoretically possible to do this either by deliberately manipulating the environment of persons with similar or identical heredity (as in the case of identical twins), or in the future by directly manipulating the genetic factor through operations on the chromosomes themselves. Whether this sort of experimentation would be desirable and socially acceptable or not is an open question, but it would seem to be at least a theoretical possibility which may grow in importance as our knowledge advances.

As for the question of why women tend to live longer than men, perhaps an answer will begin to emerge as the environment, role, and life-styles of men and women become more similar. This assumes that the present trends toward more equality between the sexes and less discrimination against women in various fields will produce less sexual differentiation in our society. For example, if it is true that the higher mortality of men is mainly due to their greater cigarette smoking, the recent increases in cigarette smoking among women should make their mortality rate increase to approximate that of men. If the increasing equality between men and women does *not* result in increasing similarity of longevity, this would indicate that hereditary differences are the main explanation of the differences in longevity between men and women.

There seems to be a remarkable agreement from several studies that physical activity, weight control, and avoiding cigarettes are strongly related to greater longevity. The hopeful thing about these three variables is that they can all be manipulated at almost any point in life, although there are, of course, in actuality many reasons why people do not manipulate them in the theoretically desired direction. There is also the nagging possibility that the associations between these three variables and longevity are entirely or partly due to their association with some other unknown variables such as personality type, intelligence, or even genetic predisposition.

Looking over these findings one gets the impression that physiological predictors are especially important among the very old, the institutionalized, or the otherwise physically impaired. As a corollary, psychological and social predictors seem to be better predictors of longevity among more normal populations and among the "younger aged." There are two interpretations of this impression: psychological and social impairment may be simply early concommitants or warning signs of later decline in health which leads to death; or it may be that psychological and social impairments reveal stress and maladaptation which directly cause a decline in health and early death. We are a long way from having sufficient evidence to distinguish between these alternative interpretations.

As for psychological predictors, the evidence indicates that among both the normal aged and the institutionalized aged, higher intelligence or cognitive functioning has a long-term association with greater longevity. Furthermore, it appears that a marked decline in cognitive functioning predicts an abrupt decline in longevity and a high mortality rate within a few months or a year. The model would appear to be that persons who start with lower cognitive functioning or whose cognitive functioning has begun a gradual decline may expect to have a somewhat shorter longevity over a period of several years, but that those with a sharp decline in cognitive functioning usually die within a short period.

As for social predictors, at present it is as difficult to untangle the direct effects of social from nonsocial factors as it is to untangle genetic from nongenetic factors. However, it does appear clear that regardless of the interpretation, such social measures as behavioral adjustment, financial status, social activity, work satisfaction, and organization of behavior are highly predictive of longevity. Indeed, among the normal aged, the social predictors often come out with the highest correlations even when other factors are controlled in a multivariate analysis. This strongly suggests that there are important direct and indirect effects of social factors on longevity which are independent of the other factors.

As a final summary statement, it seems clear that there are many variables, hereditary, physiological, psychological, and social, which significantly predict longevity. Furthermore, no one variable by itself can be an adequate or complete explanation of longevity. Present and future research will deal with the complex problem of specifying which predictors are most closely related to longevity under which circumstances and why.

Future Research

It is relatively easy to describe the ideal type of research needed to improve our knowledge about longevity; it is another to design feasible and practical research within limited budgets and time spans. We will suggest several types of research, beginning with the most ideal but also most expensive and time-consuming and moving on down to the less expensive and more practical types.

The ideal research on longevity would appear to be a classical experiment combined with a long-term series of follow-ups until all the participating subjects had died. In such an experiment one would take two large groups of persons, matched as carefully as possible on all variables which might affect longevity (the poorer the matching, the larger the numbers required), and then deliberately introduce an experimental variable in one of the groups while keeping the other group as a control. Thus, one might pay (or otherwise motivate) one group to give up smoking, or to control weight, or to increase exercise, or to increase their education, or to avoid retirement, or become more active socially. Then one would restudy these subjects at intervals and keep track of them until all members of both groups had died. Such an experiment would obviously be very expensive and require many years before completion. The length of time could be reduced by studying mortality rates at ten-year intervals from the beginning of the experiment as a means of estimating ultimate longevity. Or a method such as computing a Longevity Index (see Chapter 18) at some period ten or twenty years after the beginning of the experiment could also estimate ultimate longevity. Some such experiments with limited numbers and quite limited time spans have been attempted; there have also been some proposals for large-scale experiments with various drugs and chemicals, but at the present time we are unaware of any substantial progress along these lines.[1]

A somewhat less rigorous type of research is the "natural experiment." In this type of study, one deliberately seeks out two different groups with different characteristics whose effects on longevity are to be studied. Thus, one might select out a group of people who were "naturally" more physically active, or who did not smoke, or who were highly satisfied with their work, and match them as far as possible against their opposites so that there would be a "natural" control group. Then one follows both groups over a period of years as above and determines mortality rates, or until all have died in order to determine ultimate longevity. Several such studies as these have in fact been carried out, for example, in studying the effects of cigarette smoking. The main weakness with such types of research is that one can never be sure of complete matching on all the relevant factors or on the presence of some unknown selection factor which might affect the result. Thus, the objection to the smoking research is that nonsmokers may live longer than smokers because of some unknown personality or genetic factors which just happen to be characteristic of nonsmokers.

An even less rigorous research method is to select a random sample of some population and study all possible variables for a long duration, preferably until all the subjects have died. One then performs a multivariate analysis on all the factors measured to see which ones are most associated with longevity and which

---

[1]Richard A. Passwater recently reported plans for such a large-scale long-term experiment for testing a group of nutrient and chemical substances. "Plan large-scale human tests of chemicals to retard aging," *Geriatric Focus*, March, 1971, p. 5.

remain important when other factors are statistically controlled. Several such studies are reported in this book. Again, the difficulty with such research is that it involves a host of assumptions about the statistical nature of the variables and their interrelations which may be more or less unfounded. Also there are many problems of measurement error, interpretation of covariance, and uncertainty concerning the best ways of attempting statistical control of variables. At best, such studies only suggest hypotheses for further testing with more ideal methods. There is also the usual longitudinal problem of following the subjects long enough to get an accurate measure or estimate of ultimate longevity.

A solution to the long time-span required by longitudinal studies is that of a retrospective study in which records or recall are used for data at some earlier point of time. Although such studies solve the time-span problem, all the other problems are compounded by the insufficiency and inaccuracy of available records and recall. However, some approximate solutions to these problems have been attempted in the past and better solutions may be achieved in the future. Because they can be done at one time, such studies are the least expensive and most feasible of those previously described.

All these various types of research have their own unique advantages and disadvantages, and presumably all types will continue to be used. Hopefully, there will be a shift from the less rigorous but less expensive types to the more rigorous though more expensive and time-consuming types.

Regardless of which types of research are used, we venture to predict that the number of longevity studies will increase at a logarithmic or exponential rate. There are several reasons for such an optimistic prediction. Scientific research in general is increasing at logarithmic rates. This is due to the well-known "snowball effect" in which as more is learned, more interest develops, a broader knowledge base develops for research, more research support becomes available. Furthermore, as records improve and as more scientific measures are made of factors which may be ultimately related to longevity, more retrospective and follow-up studies become feasible in the future. Finally, as infectious and childhood diseases are reduced, interest and research will shift toward controlling the chronic diseases, which are more closely related to longevity in the middle and later years. Thus, this general shift in emphasis in medical science should also contribute to more and better research related to longevity.

As stated in the first chapter, since it appears probable that the factors associated with longevity are usually associated with such generally desirable qualities as life satisfaction, productivity, and adequate functioning, the expanding longevity research of the future should not only increase the *quantity*, but should also improve the *quality*, of human life-span.

About the Editors

Erdman Palmore received his B.A. at Duke University, his M.A. at the University of Chicago, and his Ph.D. at Columbia University in 1959. He has taught sociology at Finch College in New York City, Yale University, University of Maryland, and Duke University. From 1963 to 1967 he was a Research Sociologist at the Social Security Administration, working on their surveys of the aged and disabled. Since then he has been Associate Professor of Medical Sociology in the Department of Psychiatry, Associate Professor in the Department of Sociology, and Coordinator for the longitudinal studies of aging at the Duke Center for the Study of Aging and Human Development. He is a Fellow in the Gerontological Society, the American Sociological Association, the Southern Sociological Society, and the American Association for the Advancement of Science. His publications include NORMAL AGING published by Duke University Press, and over 30 articles in professional journals or books.

Frances C. Jeffers received her B.A. at the University of Missouri and her M.A. at Columbia University. She has taught nursing at the University of Alabama and at Duke University. Since 1954 she has been Research Associate in the Department of Psychiatry, Executive Secretary and Editor of the Duke Center for the Study of Aging and Human Development. She is a Fellow in the Gerontological Society and a member of the National Association of Social Workers, the Academy of Certified Social Workers, and the American Association of University Women. She has published 16 articles on gerontology in professional journals or books.

Index